T0348643

Management of Infections in Solid Organ Transplant Recipients

Editor

SHERIF BENIAMEEN MOSSAD

INFECTIOUS DISEASE CLINICS OF NORTH AMERICA

www.id.theclinics.com

Consulting Editor
HELEN W. BOUCHER

September 2018 • Volume 32 • Number 3

ELSEVIER

1600 John F. Kennedy Boulevard • Suite 1800 • Philadelphia, Pennsylvania, 19103-2899.
http://www.theclinics.com

INFECTIOUS DISEASE CLINICS OF NORTH AMERICA Volume 32, Number 3
September 2018 ISSN 0891–5520, ISBN-13: 978-0-323-64167-8

Editor: Kerry Holland
Developmental Editor: Donald Mumford

© **2018 Elsevier Inc. All rights reserved.**

This periodical and the individual contributions contained in it are protected under copyright by Elsevier, and the following terms and conditions apply to their use:

Photocopying

Single photocopies of single articles may be made for personal use as allowed by national copyright laws. Permission of the Publisher and payment of a fee is required for all other photocopying, including multiple or systematic copying, copying for advertising or promotional purposes, resale, and all forms of document delivery. Special rates are available for educational institutions that wish to make photocopies for non-profit educational classroom use. For information on how to seek permission visit www.elsevier.com/permissions or call: (+44) 1865 843830 (UK)/(+1) 215 239 3804 (USA).

Derivative Works

Subscribers may reproduce tables of contents or prepare lists of articles including abstracts for internal circulation within their institutions. Permission of the Publisher is required for resale or distribution outside the institution. Permission of the Publisher is required for all other derivative works, including compilations and translations (please consult www.elsevier.com/permissions).

Electronic Storage or Usage

Permission of the Publisher is required to store or use electronically any material contained in this periodical, including any article or part of an article (please consult www.elsevier.com/permissions). Except as outlined above, no part of this publication may be reproduced, stored in a retrieval system or transmitted in any form or by any means, electronic, mechanical, photocopying, recording or otherwise, without prior written permission of the Publisher.

Notice

No responsibility is assumed by the Publisher for any injury and/or damage to persons or property as a matter of products liability, negligence or otherwise, or from any use or operation of any methods, products, instructions or ideas contained in the material herein. Because of rapid advances in the medical sciences, in particular, independent verification of diagnoses and drug dosages should be made.

Although all advertising material is expected to conform to ethical (medical) standards, inclusion in this publication does not constitute a guarantee or endorsement of the quality or value of such product or of the claims made of it by its manufacturer.

Infectious Disease Clinics of North America (ISSN 0891–5520) is published in March, June, September, and December by Elsevier Inc., 360 Park Avenue South, New York, NY 10010-1710. Periodicals postage paid at New York, NY and additional mailing offices. Subscription prices are $319.00 per year for US individuals, $629.00 per year for US institutions, $100.00 per year for US students, $379.00 per year for Canadian individuals, $785.00 per year for Canadian institutions, $428.00 per year for international individuals, $785.00 per year for international institutions, and $200.00 per year for Canadian and international students. To receive student rate, orders must be accompanied by name of affiliated institution, date of term, and the *signature* of program/residency coordinator on institution letterhead. Orders will be billed at individual rate until proof of status is received. Foreign air speed delivery is included in all *Clinics* subscription prices. All prices are subject to change without notice. **POSTMASTER:** Send address changes to *Infectious Disease Clinics of North America,* Elsevier Health Sciences Division, Subcription Customer Service, 3251 Riverport Lane, Maryland Heights, MO 63043. **Customer Service: 1-800-654-2452 (US). From outside of the US and Canada, call 1-314-447-8871. Fax: 1-314-447-8029. E-mail: JournalsCustomerService-usa@elsevier.com (print support) or JournalsOnlineSupport-usa@elsevier.com (online support).**

Infectious Disease Clinics of North America is also published in Spanish by Editorial Inter-Médica, Junin 917, 1er A 1113, Buenos Aires, Argentina.

Reprints. For copies of 100 or more, of articles in this publication, please contact the Commercial Reprints Department, Elsevier Inc., 360 Park Avenue South, New York, New York 10010-1710. Tel. 212-633-3874, Fax: 212-633-3820, E-mail: reprints@elsevier.com.

Infectious Disease Clinics of North America is covered in *MEDLINE/PubMed (Index Medicus), Current Contents/ Clinical Medicine, Science Citation Alert, SCISEARCH,* and *Research Alert.*

Contributors

CONSULTING EDITOR

HELEN W. BOUCHER, MD, FIDSA, FACP
Director, Infectious Diseases Fellowship Program, Division of Geographic Medicine
and Infectious Diseases, Tufts Medical Center, Associate Professor of Medicine, Tufts
University School of Medicine, Boston, Massachusetts, USA

EDITOR

SHERIF BENIAMEEN MOSSAD, MD, FACP, FIDSA, FAST
Staff Physician, Department of Infectious Diseases, Respiratory Institute, Cleveland Clinic,
Section of Transplant Infectious Diseases and Transplant Center, Professor of Medicine,
Cleveland Clinic Lerner College of Medicine of Case Western Reserve University,
Cleveland, Ohio, USA

AUTHORS

LUTHER A. BARTELT, MD
Assistant Professor, Division of Infectious Diseases, University of North Carolina at Chapel
Hill, Chapel Hill, North Carolina, USA

MICHELE BARTOLETTI, MD, PhD
Infectious Diseases Unit, Department of Medical and Surgical Sciences,
Sant'Orsola-Malpighi Hospital, University of Bologna, Bologna, Italy

BARBRA M. BLAIR, MD
Director, Medical Education for Transplant Infectious Diseases/Immunocompromised
Host Program, Department of Medicine, Division of Infectious Diseases, Beth Israel
Deaconess Medical Center, Instructor of Medicine, Harvard Medical School, Boston,
Massachusetts, USA

ELIZABETH BUGANZA-TORIO, MD
Division of Gastroenterology, University of Alberta, Edmonton, Alberta, Canada

CHRISTIAN DONATO-SANTANA, MD
Division of Infectious Diseases and Immunology, University of Massachusetts Medical
School, Worcester, Massachusetts, USA

KAREN ELIZABETH DOUCETTE, MD, MSc
Division of Infectious Diseases, University of Alberta, Edmonton, Alberta, Canada

NISSREEN ELFADAWY, MS, MD, FASN, FAST
Nephrology Fellow, Department of Nephrology and Hypertension, University Hospitals,
Cleveland Medical Center, Cleveland, Ohio, USA

DAVID J. EPSTEIN, MD
Division of Infectious Diseases and Geographic Medicine, Clinical Assistant Professor, Department of Medicine, Stanford University, Stanford, California, USA

STACI A. FISCHER, MD, FACP, FIDSA
Associate Professor of Medicine, The Warren Alpert Medical School of Brown University, Providence, Rhode Island, USA; Employer, Accreditation Council for Graduate Medical Education, Chicago, Illinois, USA

RACHEL J. FRIEDMAN-MORACO, MD
Assistant Professor of Medicine, Division of Infectious Diseases, Emory University School of Medicine, Atlanta, Georgia, USA

MADDALENA GIANNELLA, MD, PhD
Infectious Diseases Unit, Department of Medical and Surgical Sciences, Sant'Orsola-Malpighi Hospital, University of Bologna, Bologna, Italy

JONATHAN HAND, MD
Department of Infectious Diseases, The University of Queensland School of Medicine, Ochsner Clinical School, Ochsner Medical Center, New Orleans, Louisiana, USA

JUSTIN HAYES, MD
The University of Alabama at Birmingham, Birmingham, Alabama, USA

CHRISTINE E. KOVAL, MD
Section Head, Transplant Infectious Disease, Infectious Disease, Transplant Center, Assistant Professor of Medicine, Cleveland Clinic Lerner College of Medicine of Case Western Reserve University, Cleveland, Ohio, USA

ANNE M. LACHIEWICZ, MD, MPH
Assistant Professor, Division of Infectious Diseases, University of North Carolina at Chapel Hill, Chapel Hill, North Carolina, USA

TRACY L. LEMONOVICH, MD
Assistant Professor, Department of Medicine, Division of Infectious Diseases and HIV Medicine, University Hospitals, Cleveland Medical Center, Case Western Reserve University School of Medicine, Cleveland, Ohio, USA

MARICAR F. MALINIS, MD, FACP, FIDSA, FAST
Assistant Professor of Medicine and Surgery (Transplant), Section of Infectious Diseases, Yale School of Medicine, New Haven, Connecticut, USA

JEREMY S. NEL, MD
Fellow, Division of Infectious Diseases, University of North Carolina at Chapel Hill, Chapel Hill, North Carolina, USA; Faculty of Health Sciences, University of the Witwatersrand, Johannesburg, South Africa

ANOMA NELLORE, MD
The University of Alabama at Birmingham, Birmingham, Alabama, USA

STEPHANIE M. POUCH, MD, MS
Assistant Professor of Medicine, Division of Infectious Diseases, Emory University School of Medicine, Atlanta, Georgia, USA

NAGARAJU SARABU, MD
Assistant Professor, Department of Nephrology and Hypertension, University Hospitals, Cleveland Medical Center, Cleveland, Ohio, USA

ARUNA K. SUBRAMANIAN, MD
Chief, Immunocompromised Host Infectious Diseases, Division of Infectious Diseases and Geographic Medicine, Clinical Associate Professor, Department of Medicine, Stanford University, Stanford, California, USA

ALAN J. TAEGE, MD
Assistant Professor of Medicine, Department of Infectious Disease, Cleveland Clinic, Cleveland, Ohio, USA

SARAH TAIMUR, MD
Assistant Professor of Medicine, Division of Infectious Diseases, Icahn School of Medicine at Mount Sinai, New York, New York, USA

SARA TEDESCHI, MD
Infectious Diseases Unit, Department of Medical and Surgical Sciences, Sant'Orsola-Malpighi Hospital, University of Bologna, Bologna, Italy

NICOLE M. THEODOROPOULOS, MD, MS, FAST
Assistant Professor, Division of Infectious Diseases and Immunology, University of Massachusetts Medical School, Worcester, Massachusetts, USA

DAVID VAN DUIN, MD, PhD
Associate Professor, Division of Infectious Diseases, University of North Carolina at Chapel Hill, Chapel Hill, North Carolina, USA

PIERLUIGI VIALE, MD
Infectious Diseases Unit, Department of Medical and Surgical Sciences, Sant'Orsola-Malpighi Hospital, University of Bologna, Bologna, Italy

MASAAKI YAMADA, MD
Transplant Nephrology Fellow, Division of Nephrology, University of Cincinnati College of Medicine, Cincinnati, Ohio, USA

Contents

Infection is an inevitable complication of solid organ transplant. Unrecognized infection may be transmitted from a donor and result in disseminated disease in the immunosuppressed host. Recent outbreaks of deceased donor–derived infections resulting in high rates of mortality and severe morbidity have emphasized the need to be cautious in using donors with possible meningoencephalitis. Screening of organ donors for potential transmissible infections is paramount to improving transplant outcomes.

Living safely after organ transplant starts before transplant and continues after transplant. To minimize a solid organ transplant (SOT) recipient's risk for infection and risk for injury, it is important to plan for numerous potential exposures after transplant. These include potential exposure to others with viral or bacterial illness, potential exposure to food and water sources, participation in recreational activities, resuming sexual activity, living with pets, and opportunities for travel, especially internationally. Addressing these risks head-on ensures that SOT recipients and their providers can plan accordingly and anticipate measures that will assist with maintaining such health.

This article discusses the recommended vaccines used before and after solid organ transplant period, including data regarding vaccine safety and efficacy and travel-related vaccines. Vaccination is an important part of the preparation for solid organ transplant, because vaccine-preventable diseases contribute to the morbidity and mortality of these patients. A pretransplant protocol should be encouraged in every transplant center. The main goal of vaccination is to provide seroprotection before transplant, because iatrogenically immunosuppressed patients posttransplant have a lower seroresponse to vaccines.

Complications of antimicrobial therapy, such as multidrug-resistant organisms and *Clostridium difficile*, commonly affect solid-organ transplant recipients and have been associated with graft loss and mortality. Although opportunities are abundant, antimicrobial stewardship practices guiding appropriate therapy have been infrequently reported in transplant patients. A patient-centered, multidisciplinary structure, using established antimicrobial optimization principles, is needed to create nuanced approaches to protect patients and antimicrobials and improve outcomes.

The current era is ruled by an alarming evolution of antimicrobial resistance. Solid organ transplant recipients are prone to develop infections caused by multidrug-resistant pathogens. The current challenges in this setting include screening of donors and recipients and prevention/treatment of donor-derived and posttransplant infections. The epidemiology of these infections varies between centers, type of transplanted organ, and pathogen. Treatment options are limited. Efforts to reduce carbapenem antibiotic pressure and infection control measures are necessary to reverse the spread of multidrug-resistant pathogens. Novel drugs for gram-negative multidrug-resistant bacilli may contribute to reduce carbapenemase diffusion and reduce the rate of treatment failure.

Despite advances in prevention and treatment, cytomegalovirus (CMV) infection and disease remain an expected problem in solid organ transplant recipients. Because of the effect of immunosuppressing medications, CMV primary, secondary, and reactivated infection requires antiviral medications to prevent serious direct and indirect effects of the virus. Side effects and drug resistance, however, often limit the capacity of traditional antiviral therapies. This article updates the clinician on current and promising approaches to the management and control of CMV in the solid organ transplant recipient.

BK virus (BKV) can cause graft dysfunction or failure in kidney transplant recipients and hemorrhagic cystitis in allogeneic hematopoietic stem cell transplant patients. BKV-associated nephropathy (BKVAN) emerged as a common complication in the late 1990s, probably due to the introduction of potent immunosuppressive agents. BKVAN occurred in up to 5% of kidney transplant recipients, with graft failure in up to 70%. Since universal implementation of effective screening and treatment strategies, BKV is no longer a common cause of graft failure; reported graft loss is only 0% to 5%. This article briefly describes BK virology, epidemiology, diagnosis, and management.

Human immunodeficiency virus (HIV) has become a chronic disease with a near-normal life span resulting in increased risk of organ failure. HIV organ transplant is a proven and accepted intervention in appropriately selected cases. HIV-positive organ transplant into HIV-positive recipients is in its nascent stages. Hepatitis C virus, high rates of organ rejection, and immune dysregulation are significant remaining barriers to overcome. This article provides an overview of the transplant needs in the HIV population focusing on kidney and liver transplants.

With potent nucleos(t)ide analogue (NA) therapy, hepatitis B virus (HBV) is now an uncommon indication for liver transplant (LT) in North America. NA therapy, with or without hepatitis B immunoglobulin, results in low recurrence rates and excellent outcomes after LT. Direct-acting antiviral therapy for hepatitis C virus (HCV) results in cure in most patients, either before or after transplant. There are now descriptions of good clinical outcomes of transplant from HBV- and HCV-infected donors, as treatments are so effective and well tolerated. Hepatitis E virus in transplant requires a high suspicion to diagnose, and optimal therapy remains incompletely defined.

Invasive candidiasis remains the most common invasive fungal infection following solid organ transplant (SOT), but risk factors are evolving. Current challenges include infection due to drug-resistant nonalbicans and emerging novel species such as Candida auris. Preventive antifungal use in SOT needs to be reexamined in light of these current challenges. Cryptococcosis is the second most common invasive fungal infection following SOT. Cryptococcus gattii is an emerging pathogen that can have reduced in vitro susceptibility to antifungal agents. Cryptococcus-associated IRIS in SOT is a clinical entity that warrants heightened awareness for timely recognition and management.

The endemic mycoses are a group of thermally dimorphic fungal pathogens occupying a specific geographic range. In North America, the chief endemic mycoses are histoplasmosis, coccidioidomycosis, and blastomycosis. Endemic fungi can cause serious infections in solid organ transplant recipients from primary infection, reactivation of latent disease, or donor-derived infection.

Mold infections carry a substantial clinical and economic burden in solid organ transplant (SOT) recipients with a high overall mortality of near 30%. The most important pathogens include Aspergillus, the Zygomycetes, Fusarium, Scedosporium/Pseudallescheria, and the dematiaceous (dark) molds. Risk factors for the infections vary by transplant type but include degree of immune suppression and loss of skin or mucosal integrity. Correct diagnosis usually requires histopathology and/or culture. Management often requires a multidisciplinary team approach with combined antifungal and surgical therapies. This article reviews the epidemiology, risk factors, microbiology, diagnostics, and treatment approach to mold infections in SOT recipients.

Solid organ transplant recipients are at an increased risk of tuberculosis, and transplant candidates should be screened early in their evaluation with a detailed history, tuberculin skin test or tuberculosis interferon-gamma release assay, and chest radiograph. For latent tuberculosis treatment, isoniazid and rifamycin-based regimens have advantages and disadvantages; treatment decisions should be customized. Tuberculosis after solid organ transplant generally occurs after months or years; early infections should raise the possibility of donor-derived infections. Tuberculosis diagnosis and treatment in solid organ transplant recipients may be complicated by protean manifestations, drug interactions, and adverse drug reactions.

Mycobacteria other than tuberculosis are important pathogens to consider in solid organ transplant recipients. Delay in recognition and treatment may incur significant morbidity and mortality. Management of mycobacteria other than tuberculosis requires a knowledge of treatment specific for each species and drug-drug interactions between antimicrobial and immunosuppressive drugs. Therapy in solid organ transplant can be prolonged and may require a reduction in immunosuppression to improve outcomes.

Clostridium difficile infection is a significant cause of morbidity and mortality in solid organ transplant recipients. Risk factors in this population include frequent hospitalizations, receipt of immunosuppressive agents, and intestinal dysbiosis triggered by several factors, including exposure to broad-spectrum antimicrobials. The incidence and potential for significant adverse outcomes among solid organ transplant recipients with *C difficile* infection highlight the evolving need for strategic *C difficile* infection risk factor modification and novel approaches to disease management in this patient population. This article focuses on current concepts related to the prevention and treatment of *C difficile* infection in solid organ transplant recipients.

Justin Hayes and Anoma Nellore

Strongyloides stercoralis is a threadworm parasite with the unique capacity to complete its entire life cycle in a human host. Although asymptomatic in normal hosts, *S stercoralis* infection in solid organ transplant recipients is often severe, disseminated, and fatal. Risk factors for disease acquisition include travel to endemic regions. Antihelminth therapy should be instituted before transplant for optimal clinical outcomes. Herein the authors review the epidemiology, biology, immune response, and diagnostic and screening strategies, as well as treatment modalities for *S stercoralis* in the solid organ transplant population.

INFECTIOUS DISEASE CLINICS
OF NORTH AMERICA

THE CLINICS ARE AVAILABLE ONLINE!
Access your subscription at:
www.theclinics.com

Preface

Management of Infections in Solid Organ Transplant Recipients

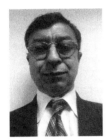

Sherif Beniameen Mossad, MD, FACP, FIDSA, FAST
Editor

It has been 5 years since the last update on infections in solid organ transplant (SOT) recipients was published in *Infectious Disease Clinics of North America* in 2013. There has been a 20% increase in the number of organ transplants over the last 5 years,[1] largely driven by increase in the number of deceased donors, with more than 33,000 transplants performed annually in the United States. Our nation is facing an unprecedented opioid epidemic, which is currently accounting in several parts of the country for a quarter of organ donors who die of overdose. These donors are considered at increased risk for transmitting blood-borne pathogens, including hepatitis B virus (HBV), hepatitis C virus (HCV), and human immunodeficiency virus (HIV). However, data have accumulated, documenting the long-term survival benefit of accepting such organs. One recent article[2] showed that only a third of kidney transplant candidates who were offered and declined an increased risk donor (IRD) later received non-IRD kidney transplants. The irony is that the kidney donor risk profile index (which predicts the likelihood of graft failure) of these non-IRD kidneys was more than double that of the IRD kidneys that had been declined. Although the mortality risk in the first 30 days following acceptance of IRD kidneys was higher compared with non-IRD kidneys, mortality risk was 33% lower 1 to 6 months, and 48% lower beyond 6 months after decision, respectively.

The transplant community has benefited greatly from the infectious diseases practice guidelines first published by the American Society of Transplantation Infectious Diseases Community of Practice in 2004 and then updated in 2009 and 2013.[3] Authors of the current issue of *Infectious Disease Clinics of North America* have set out to provide the transplant community with an update in several pertinent topics in this field.

While the need for organs is ever increasing, more than 115,000 people are currently on the waiting list, identifying donors that are safe from the infectious diseases perspective remains of paramount importance. On average, 2 to 3 organs are procured

Infect Dis Clin N Am 32 (2018) xiii–xvii
https://doi.org/10.1016/j.idc.2018.06.001
0891-5520/18/© 2018 Published by Elsevier Inc.

from each donor; range is 1 to 8 organs. It thus befits to start the current issue with an update of this topic. In addition, several other articles in this issue address specific aspects of this topic, such organs from donors colonized or infected with multidrug-resistant bacterial infections, and organs from HCV- or HIV-infected donors. Certain infections, such cytomegalovirus (CMV), are "expected" to be transmitted from donors to recipients; thus specific guidelines for surveillance and prevention have been published. Most organ donor–derived infections present within the first 6 weeks after transplantation. However, certain infections, particularly latent infections with long incubation periods that are not readily recognized to be transmitted, may cause disseminated disease in the immunosuppressed organ recipient. Donors with possible meningoencephalitis are particularly associated with dire consequences.

Immunizations are considered the "seatbelts" of health care. While the majority of immunizations are provided by primary care providers who are currently caring for a large number of patients awaiting SOT, many of these patients are immunocompromised due to their end-organ disease and its consequences, or due to immunosuppressive medications attempting to support organ function while awaiting transplant. It is important to vaccinate transplant candidates as early as possible during transplant evaluation. Barring the holy grail of tolerance, SOT recipients are expected to remain on immunosuppressive medications for life to prevent organ rejection. While inactivated vaccinations are safe before or after transplantation, live-attenuated vaccines usually cannot be safely administered to patients receiving immunosuppressive medications. Thus, updating immunizations before transplantation may represent the only opportunity to administer live-attenuated vaccines. As importantly, certain vaccines may allow SOT recipients to accept organs they may not have otherwise, as in the case of the hepatitis B core antibody positive donor organs. To improve vaccine-induced immunogenicity posttransplant, most centers start vaccinating SOT recipients 3 to 6 months after transplant.

We live in a microbial world, mostly in symbiosis. While this may be true for the majority of the population, immunosuppressed individuals, particularly SOT recipients, view microbes surrounding them as their primary enemy, and rightly so. It's true that after transplantation they should return, as much as possible, to their normal activities, and not "live in a bubble." However, patients, their families, and health care providers (HCP) hold many beliefs about safe living that may or may not be true. The transplant community needs sound advice on a variety of issues ranging from leisurely activities, food and water safety, safe sex, animal contact, and travel. Precious lives extended by SOT should be protected by education before and after transplantation, providing the knowledge and measures to mitigate exposures to various infections in the community.

Almost all health care systems currently have an antimicrobial stewardship program (ASP) in place. Judicious use of antibiotics is "expected" of all HCP, but implementing programs to oversee such practice is actually in its infancy. The Infectious Diseases Society of America and the Society of Healthcare Epidemiology of America published its first edition of such guidelines in 2016.[4] Perhaps no more important than in SOT recipients, should ASP be implemented, given the rising rates of antimicrobial resistance in this patient population. Such ASP should be specifically customized to the SOT population, accounting for the multidisciplinary nature of the care for these patients, and the particularly important aspect of integrating the microbiology laboratory in this process, also known as "diagnostic" stewardship.

Infections due to multidrug-resistant organisms (MDRO) disproportionately affect SOT recipients and are associated with a 3-fold increase in mortality. In endemic areas, the incidence of infections due to carbapenem-resistant enterobacteriaceae

(CRE) is 5%; most of which occur within 2 to 4 weeks of transplantation. Several new antibacterial agents have been developed to treat these infections, including ceftolozane-tazobactam, ceftazidime-avibactam, and meropenem-vaborbactam. Studies have shown a mortality advantage in using these agents, compared to older agents, such as polymyxin in treating infections due to CRE. It is important to use these agents judiciously, since resistance can develop. Outcomes of SOT in patients colonized with MDRO vary with the organ transplanted and type of organism. For example, pretransplant colonization of lung transplant candidates with MDR *Pseudomonas aeruginosa* strains does not affect short- or long-term survival following transplantation.

Morbidity and mortality associated with invasive fungal infections (IFI) in SOT recipients remain high. Candida infections remain the most common cause of IFI in these patients. Invasive mold infections (IMI) are associated with mortalities ranging from 20% to 60%, because they are difficult to diagnose; commonly requiring invasive procedures, and difficult to treat, possibly with combination antifungal medications. IMI most commonly affect the lungs, except for dematiaceous (pigmented) molds and paecilomyces, which most commonly cause localized skin infections. Endemic mycoses are rare in SOT recipients, but are also difficult to diagnose, with progressive disseminated disease as the most common form of presentation, and therapy typically recommended for 12 months or more. In the last 5 years, no new classes of antifungal agents have come on the market, but new members of antifungal classes have been developed, such as isavuconazole. Better formulated antifungal agents, such the extended-release posaconazole, are now available. Combinations of antifungal agents have been studied in transplant recipients, with some success. While antifungal prophylaxis in SOT recipients has been relatively successful, it is clear that "one size does not fit all." As expected, breakthrough fungal infections with both commonly and rarely encountered fungi continue to occur. In addition, newly described fungi, such as *Candida auris*, have been encountered in SOT recipients.

CMV is arguably the most important pathogen in SOT recipients. High CMV seroprevalence, unique viral biology, and "sicker" transplant recipients contribute to this fact. Adoption of the World Health Organization CMV standard based on international units per milliliter, rather than copies per milliliter, has allowed labs to standardize quantitative polymerase chain reaction results. One important caveat is that tissue-invasive CMV disease, particularly gastrointestinal disease, can occur in the absence of CMV viremia, particularly in CMV seropositive recipients. Prophylactic ganciclovir and valganciclovir have been very successful in preventing CMV-related events, but late infections after completing prophylaxis course and the emergence of ganciclovir resistance have been formidable problems facing the transplant community. Letermovir, the only new agent active against CMV that has been approved in the United States in the last 5 years, has a different mechanism of action than previously approved classes; it inhibits CMV deoxyribonuclease terminase complex, thus inhibiting viral packaging. It is currently approved only for prevention of CMV reactivation in CMV seropositive allogeneic hematopoietic stem cell transplant recipients, but studies in SOT recipients are underway. Newer diagnostic tests assessing the cell-medicated immune response to CMV are currently available and may soon be integrated in risk stratification for duration of primary or secondary prophylaxis.

Although BK polyomavirus is the most common opportunistic viral infection occurring in kidney and pancreas transplant recipients, there is currently no specific antiviral treatment for BK viremia and the associated nephropathy. Reduction of immunosuppression remains the mainstay of management. Systematic surveillance is currently standard of care, and early recognition is crucial for graft survival.

Infection prevention interventions have been successful in reducing several hospital-acquired infections, with the exception of *Clostridium difficile*–associated diarrhea (CDAD). Rates of CDAD have actually doubled in the last decade. Heavy use of antimicrobial agents in SOT recipients puts them at a particularly high risk for recurrent CDAD. The highest incidence is in lung transplant recipients. A 2-fold increased risk of graft loss has been observed, even with mild clinical presentation of CDAD. Diagnostic stewardship has become a cornerstone of preventing *C difficile* infection. Treatment in SOT recipients is similar to that in immunocompetent patients. Fecal microbiota transplantation has been safely used in SOT recipients, but randomized trials in this population are lacking. Fidaxomicin was approved in 2011, and a study is currently underway comparing its use to standard of care in SOT recipients. Bezlotoxumab, a human monoclonal antibody binding *C difficile* toxins A and B, decreases the rate of recurrent CDAD, but studies in SOT recipients are lacking.

Nucleoside or nucleotide analogues with or without hepatitis B immunoglobulin have resulted in excellent outcomes in all SOT recipients with HBV infection. All SOT candidates should receive the 40 μm/mL preparation 3-dose series of HBV vaccine. Donors who are positive for anti-HB core antibody can be safely used for recipients who are immune to HBV (anti-HB surface antibody >10 IU/mL), or with appropriate prophylaxis of the nonimmune recipients. Limited data exist regarding the use of HBsAg-positive donors. We are in the "golden age" for management of HCV infection. Directly acting antivirals, particularly with pangenotypic combinations, have significantly improved the outcomes in SOT candidates and recipients. Timing of whether to treat HCV infection before or after SOT remains controversial. There is growing interest in transplanting HCV viremic organs in HCV-negative recipients. Hepatitis E virus (HEV) infection is much less prevalent than HBV and HCV infections, but it becomes chronic in 60% of cases and results in cirrhosis in 10%. HEV antibodies may be absent in 20% of patients; thus, diagnosis relies on the detection of HEV ribonucleic acid in serum or stool. Most transplant recipients with HEV infection respond well to ribavirin.

Tuberculosis (TB) is not endemic in the United States, but screening of SOT candidates is recommended, as well as epidemiological assessment of SOT donors for TB. Treatment of active TB is much more complicated than treatment of latent tuberculosis infection (LTBI) in SOT candidates and recipients, given the myriad of drug interactions with immunosuppressive medications, and overlapping side effects. Isoniazid for 9 months is the preferred therapy for LTBI. Risk of TB following SOT is at least 4 times that of the general population, and about twice as common as the risk in patients with end-organ disease. Most cases of TB following SOT are due to reactivation of LTBI due to iatrogenic immunosuppression and occur months to years following SOT. Thus, diagnosis of TB in the early period following SOT should raise suspicion for a donor-derived infection. In general, treatment of active TB following SOT should follow the same guidelines as for the general population.

Mycobacteria other than tuberculosis (MOTT) are ubiquitous in the environment. Lung transplant candidates are particularly at higher risk for colonization and infection with MOTT, which may pose significant risks, particularly in the early period after transplantation. Explanting the infected lungs at the time of transplantation significantly reduces the burden of infection, but anastomotic sites remain at risk. Different MOTT organisms require specific combination of antimicrobials; many have significant drug interactions with immunosuppressive medications. Several antimicrobials have been added to the list of agents active against MOTT, including clofazimine, bedaquiline, tedizolid, tigecycline, and inhaled amikacin.

Strongyloidiasis remains endemic in the southern United States. Reactivation after SOT is rare, but should be eliminated by pretransplant surveillance and targeted treatment. Ideal screening method is yet to be determined, but treatment with ivermectin appears to be well tolerated in SOT candidates and recipients.

Life expectancy of patients infected with HIV is currently similar to the general population, thanks to effective antiretroviral agents. Progress of SOT in these patients has been slow. Efforts should be made to refer HIV-infected patients for assessment for SOT, before they become too ill for transplant. New hope came with the HIV Organ Policy Equity "HOPE" act, which was implemented in 2015. This will allow for standardized research into transplanting organs from HIV-positive donors into HIV-positive recipients.

I thank the authors of the 16 articles in this issue of *Infectious Diseases Clinics of North America*. I especially thank Dr Helen Boucher, who invited me as editor for this exciting issue.

Sherif Beniameen Mossad, MD, FACP, FIDSA, FAST
Department of Infectious Diseases
Respiratory Institute
Cleveland Clinic
Section of Transplant Infectious
Diseases and Transplant Center
Lerner College of Medicine of
Case Western Reserve University
9500 Euclid Avenue G21, Room 131
Cleveland, OH 44195, USA

E-mail address:
mossads@ccf.org

REFERENCES

1. Increasing the number of transplants in the United States. 2016 in review. Available at: https://unos.org/about/annual-report/2016-annual-report/. Accessed December 27, 2017.
2. Bowring MG, Holscher CM, Zhou S, et al. Turn down for what? Patient outcomes associated with declining increased infectious risk kidneys. Am J Transplant 2018;18(3):617–24.
3. Special Issue: The American Society of Transplantation Infectious Diseases Guidelines, 3rd edition. Am J Transplant 2013;13(s4):1–371.
4. Barlam TF, Cosgrove SE, Abbo LM, et al. Implementing an Antibiotic Stewardship Program: guidelines by the Infectious Diseases Society of America and the Society for Healthcare Epidemiology of America. Clin Infect Dis 2016;62(10):e51–77.

Is This Organ Donor Safe?
Donor-Derived Infections in Solid Organ Transplantation

Staci A. Fischer, MD[a,b,*]

KEYWORDS

- Transplant infections • Donor-transmitted infections • Donor-derived infections
- Organ donor screening • Lymphocytic choriomeningitis virus

KEY POINTS

- Organ donor–derived infections are uncommon but may cause significant morbidity and mortality in transplant recipients.
- Diagnosis of infection in deceased donors may be challenging due to reliance on next of kin to provide critical medical and social history, the short time available for evaluation and testing, and the lack of rapid, sensitive assays for uncommon organisms.
- Growing experience with the use of donors at increased risk for infection with human immunodeficiency virus, hepatitis B virus, and hepatitis C virus suggests that these donors may be used with caution and informed consent of the recipients.
- Donors with unrecognized meningoencephalitis may transmit multiple infections including viruses, for which limited therapies exist.
- Careful screening of donors is paramount to improving the safety of organ transplantation.

In 2017, more than 10,000 deceased donors provided organs for more than 28,000 patients in the United States.[1] Although advances in critical care and immunosuppressive therapy have facilitated the use of more deceased donors and improved the outcomes of many transplant procedures, infection remains a common and significant complication of solid organ transplantation (SOT).[2] Causes of post-transplant infection include health care–associated infection during hospitalizations, community-acquired infection, and reactivation of latent infection in the recipient. Transmission of infection from donor to recipient, although less common than the other etiologies, ranges from the routine to the devastating. Although donor-derived infections, such as cytomegalovirus (CMV), are well-studied, anticipated, and able to be prevented in most

Disclosure Statement: The author has nothing to disclose.
[a] The Warren Alpert Medical School of Brown University, 222 Richmond Street, Providence, RI 02903, USA; [b] Accreditation Council for Graduate Medical Education, 401 North Michigan Avenue, Suite 2000, Chicago, IL 60611, USA
* 470 North Lane, Bristol, RI 02809.
E-mail address: sfischer@acgme.org

Infect Dis Clin N Am 32 (2018) 495–506
https://doi.org/10.1016/j.idc.2018.04.001
0891-5520/18/© 2018 Elsevier Inc. All rights reserved.

id.theclinics.com

cases, the number and variety of pathogens transmitted with transplantation continue to grow (**Box 1**).[3–31]

RISK OF INFECTION IN ORGAN DONORS

Most organs transplanted in the United States are from deceased donors, who often require intensive medical care prior to becoming candidates for donation, with mechanical ventilation, indwelling vascular and urinary catheters, and administration of broad-spectrum antimicrobials. As a result of intensive care, donors may become colonized or infected with resistant bacterial pathogens as well as fungi, including *Candida* and *Aspergillus*. In many cases, donors with documented bacterial infections on effective antimicrobial therapy may be used when the recipients are also treated; caution should be used with multidrug resistant organisms and infections of the allograft itself. Donors may also harbor latent infections (eg, *Histoplasma*, *Coccidioides immitis*, *Mycobacterium tuberculosis*, and strongyloidiasis), based on their epidemiologic exposures. When transplanted into a recipient on immunosuppressive therapy, these latent infections may reactivate, causing disseminated disease. Because 1 donor may provide organs to as many as 8 recipients, who may be scattered across multiple transplant centers, states, and regions, prompt recognition of donor-derived infections and communication between transplant centers and organ procurement organizations (OPOs) is critical to improving outcomes of these often devastating infections.

WHEN TO SUSPECT DONOR-DERIVED INFECTION

In most cases, infections transmitted from an organ donor present early post-transplant, often in the first 6 weeks. Some pathogens with long incubation periods or latent infection, however, may take months to even years to present in the immunocompromised transplant recipient. Most outbreaks of infection have been identified when more than one recipient of an organ from a common deceased donor develops similar symptoms and signs.[8–12] Because recipients are often hospitalized in different transplant centers and may be under the care of different teams within the same institution, recognition of a pattern of clinical findings may be difficult. If a recipient develops fever, leukocytosis, leukopenia, or other potential signs of infection early post-transplant, and donor-derived infection is considered a possibility, the responsible OPO should be contacted to discuss the findings and determine whether other recipients of organs from the same donor are experiencing similar illnesses. State public health departments and the Centers for Disease Control and Prevention (CDC) can also be of assistance in investigating the cause of an outbreak of infection.

SCREENING ORGAN DONORS FOR INFECTION

Screening potential donors for infection remains crucial to improving the safety of organ transplantation. The United Network for Organ Sharing is contracted by the Department of Health and Human Services to serve as the Organ Procurement and Transplantation Network (OPTN), responsible for policy development and oversight of SOT in the United States. The policies of the OPTN and the experience of the transplant infectious disease community have resulted in recommendations for routine screening of potential donors for several pathogens (**Box 2**).[32–35] Screening for antibodies to HTLV types I and II had been routine for many years, but with the prevalence

Box 1
Pathogens reported to be transmitted via solid organ transplantation

Bacteria

Acinetobacter species

Bartonella species

Brucella species

Ehrlichia species

Enterobacter species

Enterococcus species

Escherichia coli

Klebsiella species

Legionella pneumophila

Listeria monocytogenes

Mycoplasma hominis

Nocardia species

Pseudomonas aeruginosa

Salmonella species

Serratia species

Staphylococcus aureus

Streptococcus species

Treponema pallidum

Veillonella species

Yersinia enterocolitica

Fungi

Aspergillus species

Blastomyces dermatiditis

Candida species

Coccidioides immitis

Cryptococcus neoformans

Histoplasma capsulatum

Prototheca

Scedosporium apiospermum

Zygomyces

Microsporidia

Encephalitozoon cuniculi

Mycobacteria

Mycobacterium tuberculosis

Nontuberculous *Mycobacteria*

Parasites/protozoa/prions/amebae

Babesia species

Balamuthia mandrillaris

Creutzfeld-Jakob disease

Naegleria fowleri

Plasmodium species

Schistosoma species

Strongyloides stercoralis

Toxoplasma gondii

Trypanosoma cruzi

Viruses

Adenovirus

BK virus

CMV

Epstein-Barr virus

HBV

HCV

Hepatitis D virus

Hepatitis E virus

Human herpesvirus 6

Human herpesvirus 7

Human herpesvirus 8

HIV

Human T-lymphotropic virus

Influenza virus

Lymphocytic choriomeningitis virus

Parainfluenza virus

Parvovirus B19

Rabies virus

Varicella-zoster virus

West Nile virus

Data from Refs.[3–31]

of infection in the United States and few donor-transmitted events, serologic screening for this viral pathogen is no longer indicated.[36]

All potential donors should be screened for blood-borne pathogens, such as HIV, hepatitis B, and hepatitis C; those living in endemic areas should also be tested for hepatitis E, an increasingly recognized pathogen in transplant recipients. Serology for CMV and Epstein-Barr virus should be performed to predict the risk of transmission and guide post-transplantation monitoring and CMV prophylaxis. Donors with specific epidemiologic risk factors for infection with endemic fungi, *Strongyloides*, *Trypanosoma cruzi*, *Cryptococcus*, West Nile virus, and other pathogens should be screened for infection with these organisms; in some cases, prophylactic therapy may be

---

Box 2
General screening for potential organ donors

Required by OPTN policy
    Serology for HIV, hepatitis B, and hepatitis C (repeat within 28 days of donation in living donors)
    CMV IgG
    Epstein-Barr virus IgG
    HIV-1/2 antibody or HIV antigen/antibody assay
    Hepatitis B surface antigen and core antibody; consider NAT
    Hepatitis C NAT
    Syphilis screening
    Toxoplasma IgG
    Blood, urine, and sputum cultures

Recommended additional screening:
    Tuberculosis screening (purified protein derivative or interferon-γ release assay)
    Testing based on prior history of living in an endemic area
        Strongyloides antibody
        Trypanosoma cruzi antibody
        Histoplasma antibody
        Blastomyces antibody
        Coccidioides immitis antibody
        Hepatitis E antibody
    Testing based on epidemiologic exposures
        Brucella antibody
        Cryptococcus antigen
        West Nile virus antibody

Organ-specific testing: urine culture for kidney donors, bronchoalveolar lavage fluid/sputum culture for lung donors

Data from Refs.[32–35]

---

indicated.[18,31–35] The risk of infection is related to the tissue tropism of specific pathogens (eg, *Toxoplasma* and *Trypanosoma* in heart transplants and BK virus in kidney transplants) as well as viability of the organisms.

Because screening for many infections is based on serology, the sensitivity and specificity of the assays used must be considered in choosing a donor screening methodology. Results of these tests may also be affected by dilution from transfusion of multiple blood products and crystalloid into deceased donor candidates.

The key to assessing the risk of infection from a particular donor is obtaining an accurate history of exposures. OPOs are responsible for reviewing available medical records and interviewing family members to ascertain this information. Questionnaires used to guide next of kin discussions are not standardized across the United States but generally address medical and social factors to help assess organ quality and the risk of infection. The information gathered is dependent on the accurate knowledge of those questioned with the prospective donor's circumstances. In evaluating potential living donors, transplant centers have time to assess medical, social, and exposure histories and treat any identified infections prior to donation to prevent transmission.

SELECTED PATHOGENS THAT CAN BE DONOR TRANSMITTED

Balamuthia mandrillaris

Two outbreaks of donor-transmitted *Balamuthia mandrillaris* have recently been described.[20,21] This free-living ameba, known to cause granulomatous amebic encephalitis, is found in soil in multiple areas of the world, including the United States, where infection seems more common in patients of Hispanic ethnicity. Infection is believed to result from inhalation or inoculation into broken skin, with spread to the brain and spinal cord. In both transplant-related clusters, the organ donor presented with headache and focal brain lesions on CT or MRI; 1 donor had a several month history of neurologic symptoms. One donor had fever; the other was afebrile but demonstrated lymphocytic pleocytosis on cerebrospinal fluid (CSF) testing. In both cases, some recipients developed neurologic symptoms (eg, headache, blurred vision, and ataxia), whereas others were asymptomatic; fever was variably present. CSF revealed lymphocytic pleocytosis and MRI demonstrated multiple ring-enhancing lesions in some of the recipients. Histopathologic testing of brain tissue from symptomatic recipients at the CDC revealed evidence of *Balamuthia* infection, for which therapy was initiated with combinations of flucytosine, pentamidine, sulfadiazine, fluconazole, azithromycin, and miltefosine, with variable outcomes, including infection clearance, significant neurologic sequelae, and death.[21]

Coccidioides immitis

Coccidioides immitis is an endemic fungus in the southwestern United States, Mexico, and parts of Central and South America, which can be transmitted with transplantation. Deceased or living donors who have visited or lived in an endemic area may have viable organisms that reactivate in the setting of immunosuppression in the recipient, regardless of whether they or their families recall previous infection, which is usually asymptomatic. Guidelines for treatment of exposed recipients recommend fluconazole, 400 mg daily for 3 months to 12 months, for nonlung recipients and lifelong therapy for lung transplant recipients when the donor has evidence of pulmonary coccidioidomycosis.[34] Screening of potential donors from endemic areas has been recommended to guide informed consent and treatment of the recipients.

Lymphocytic Choriomeningitis Virus

Multiple outbreaks of donor-derived infection with lymphocytic choriomeningitis virus (LCMV) and related arenaviruses have been described in recent years.[8–10] Because infection is most commonly asymptomatic, recognition of donor infection is difficult. Some donors may present with aseptic meningitis; the timeframe for deciding whether to use a deceased donor generally precludes CSF testing (eg, by culture, polymerase chain reaction [PCR], and/or enzyme immunoassay), which is available through the CDC and some state health departments. Exposure to wild or pet mice or hamsters, which may harbor lifelong asymptomatic infection, may be an important clue to the possibility of LCMV infection, for which no screening tests are routinely available. Decreasing immunosuppressive therapy and administration of ribavirin may be of use in treating infected recipients, in whom the mortality rate has been high.[8,10]

Strongyloides stercoralis

Strongyloides stercoralis is endemic in tropical and subtropical areas, including the southern United States. Infection may be asymptomatic, with reactivation causing disseminated disease (termed, *hyperinfection syndrome*) in immunocompromised hosts. Most donor-derived infection cases present within the first 6 months after transplantation, with variable symptoms; fever and eosinophilia, hallmarks of infection in immunocompetent hosts, are often absent.[18,19] Screening donors who have traveled to or lived in endemic areas with serology may be useful in preventing infection, by treating the living donor prior to procurement and/or treating the recipients with ivermectin and/or albendazole.[19]

Trypanosoma cruzi

Chagas disease, caused by *Trypanosoma cruzi*, is endemic throughout much of Mexico, Central America, and South America. Several outbreaks of donor-derived infection have occurred in the United States.[17] The risk of transmission is highest in heart and intestine recipients, due to chronic infection of myocardial and enteric tissues, although recipients of liver and kidney transplants have also developed infection. Donors from endemic areas should be screened for infection with serologic testing, and caution used when considering heart or intestinal transplantation. Monitoring noncardiac recipients with PCR and serology may be of assistance in diagnosing donor-derived infection. Treatment with nifurtimox and/or benznidazole may be challenging in the United States, where these agents are not readily available.

USE OF DONORS AT RISK OF HEPATITIS B VIRUS, HEPATITIS C VIRUS, OR HUMAN IMMUNODEFICIENCY VIRUS INFECTION

Transplantation of organs from donors at risk for HIV, hepatitis B virus (HBV), and hepatitis C virus (HCV) poses inherent risk of transmission of infection to recipients. With increasingly effective therapies now available against these pathogens, centers are gaining experience with transplantation of organs from donors with treated (nonviremic) infection in selected recipients.[37–40]

All potential organ donors, regardless of risk, should undergo testing for HIV (anti-HIV 1/2 or HIV antigen/antibody), HBV (hepatitis B surface antigen and core antibody), and HCV (anti-HCV antibody and HCV-RNA by nucleic acid testing [NAT]), with results available prior to procurement. For potential living donors, testing should be repeated within 28 days of donation.

Although NAT has improved the sensitivity of testing potential organ donors for infection with these viruses, those with recent infection in the window period of current diagnostic testing may transmit infection. The US Public Health Service has developed guidelines for the testing and use of organs from donors at higher than average risk of infection with hepatitis B, hepatitis C, and HIV, which are termed, *increased risk donors* (*IRDs*) (**Box 3**).[41] It has been estimated that approximately 30% of donors in the United States and Canada meet these criteria.[42,43] As the opioid epidemic spreads in the US, more donors meet these criteria.

Those potential organ donors meeting criteria for increased risk should undergo more sensitive testing (eg, HIV NAT) prior to procurement, although results may not be available prior to transplantation from deceased donors. Living IRDs should undergo repeat testing using NAT within 28 days of surgery. Informed consent of recipients accepting organs from IRDs is critical, as is rigorous post-transplant NAT testing. Use of IRDs has been successful in many centers, proving an important resource in the current organ shortage. A recent registry review demonstrated a significant long-term survival benefit for recipients who accepted IRD kidneys, in which only 31% of those who declined an IRD offer had undergone transplant with a non-IRD donor after 5 years.[44]

MENINGOENCEPHALITIS

In recent years, outbreaks of donor-derived infections, such as rabies, West Nile virus, LCMV, and *Balamuthia*, have emphasized the difficulty in diagnosing encephalitis in potential deceased organ donors and the risk of transmission of infection if undetected (**Box 4**).[45,46] Donors with bacterial meningitis may be used if antimicrobial therapy is administered to the donor and all recipients. Undiagnosed meningoencephalitis of viral etiology may pose the greatest risk of donor-derived infection, due to high rates

Box 3
The US Public health service–defined increased risk donors

Men who have had sex with a man (MSM) in the past 12 months

Nonmedical injection drug use in the past 12 months

Having sex in exchange for money or drugs in the past 12 months

Having sex with a person known or suspected to have HIV, HBV, or HCV infection in the past 12 months

Women who have had sex with a man with a history of MSM behavior in the past 12 months

Having sex with a person who had sex in exchange for money or drugs in the past 12 months

Having sex with a person who injected drugs by intravenous, intramuscular, or subcutaneous routes for nonmedical purposes in the past 12 months

A child less than or equal to 18 months of age born to a mother known to be infected with or at increased risk for HIV, HBV, or HCV infection

A child who has been breastfed in the past 12 months whose mother is known to be infected with or at increased risk for HIV infection

In lockup, jail, prison, or a juvenile correctional facility for more than 72 consecutive hours in the past 12 months

Newly diagnosed with, or previously treated for, syphilis, gonorrhea, *Chlamydia*, or genital ulcers in the past 12 months

On hemodialysis in the past 12 months (HCV only)

When a deceased potential organ donor's medical/behavioral history cannot be obtained or risk factors cannot be determined, the donor should be considered at increased risk for HIV, HBV, and HCV infection because the donor's risk for infection is unknown.

When a deceased potential organ donor's blood specimen is hemodiluted, the donor should be considered at increased risk for HIV, HBV, and HCV infection because the donor's risk for infection is unknown.

From U.S. Department of Health & Human Services Organ Procurement and Transplantation Network. Understanding the risk of transmission of HIV, hepatitis B, and hepatitis C from PHS increased risk donors. Available at: https://optn.transplant.hrsa.gov/resources/guidance/understanding-hiv-hbv-hcv-risks-from-increased-risk-donors/. Accessed January 27, 2018.

Box 4
Central nervous system pathogens transmitted through solid organ transplantation

Aspergillus Species

Balamuthia mandrillaris

Coccidioides immitis

Cryptococcus neoformans

Herpes simplex virus

LCMV and related arenaviruses

Mycobacterium tuberculosis

Rabies virus

West Nile virus

of transmissibility, morbidity, and mortality and the lack of effective antiviral therapies. Recognition of infection may be limited by the myriad etiologies for fever and altered mental status in potential deceased organ donors as well as the limited diagnostic testing available for some of these pathogens (**Box 5**). Guidelines have been developed to assist OPOs in recognizing the potential donor with meningoencephalitis.[46]

When evaluating a potential donor with a presumed cerebrovascular accident (CVA) or stroke, OPOs and transplant centers should consider the following questions:

- Do the donor's age and comorbidities (eg, previous stroke, hypertension, and diabetes mellitus) support a diagnosis of CVA? Meningoencephalitis should be considered in younger donors and those without underlying comorbidities, in whom CVA is less likely.
- Were fever, altered mental status, and/or seizures noted on presentation? If there is not a clear explanation for these symptoms and signs, meningoencephalitis should be considered.
- Is there unexplained CSF pleocytosis, hypoglycorrhachia, or elevated protein (eg, no identified bacterial pathogen prior to initiation of antibacterial therapy)?
- Is there unexplained hydrocephalus, which could be a sign of infection?
- Is the donor immunosuppressed, so that the risk of infection is higher and atypical presentations possible?
- Does the donor have a history of potential environmental exposures to pathogens causing meningoencephalitis (eg, bats, rodents, and mosquitoes) or of living in areas endemic for or in the midst of epidemic spread of CNS pathogens (eg, West Nile virus and *Coccidioides*)?
- Was the donor homeless? This could result in exposure to rodents and their excreta.

In several investigations of transplant-related outbreaks of LCMV and rabies, risk factors for infection were not identified during pretransplant evaluation of the donors.[8,10,12] Caution should be used when the next of kin of a potential deceased donor is unfamiliar with the donor's recent history and exposures so that risk may not be accurately assessed.

INVESTIGATING AND REPORTING DONOR-DERIVED INFECTIONS

Prevention, identification, and treatment of potential donor-derived infections is a fundamental role of the transplant infectious disease specialist. The OPTN/UNOS, which regulates SOT in the United States, has an Ad Hoc Disease Transmission Advisory Committee (DTAC) that investigates possible transmission of infection and diseases (eg, malignancy) from donors to recipients and publishes its findings.[4–6,47]

Box 5
Challenges in recognizing central nervous system infections in potential deceased donors

Suspecting infection
   May be clinically silent
   May be difficult to differentiate from stroke or drug overdose

Diagnosing infection
   Limited time prior to procurement
   Specialized testing (eg, PCR) not available in a timely manner

Lack of effective treatments for many pathogens

When suspicious of donor-transmitted infection, notification of the responsible OPO and DTAC may help facilitate recognition of similar symptoms in other recipients and testing for possible donor-derived infections in the hope of improving outcomes of these uncommon events.

REFERENCES

1. U.S. Department of Health & Human Services Organ Procurement and Transplantation Network. Transplants by donor type. Available at: https://optn.transplant.hrsa.gov/data/view-data-reports/national-data/#. Accessed January 27, 2018.
2. Kotloff RM, Blosser S, Fulda GJ, et al. Management of the potential organ donor in the ICU: Society of Critical Care Medicine/American College of Chest Physicians/Association of Organ Procurement Organizations consensus statement. Crit Care Med 2015;43:1291–325.
3. Morris MI, Fischer SA, Ison MG. Infections transmitted by transplantation. Infect Dis Clin North Am 2010;24:497–514.
4. Ison MG, Grossi P, AST Infectious Diseases Community of Practice. Donor-derived infections in solid organ transplantation. Am J Transplant 2013;13:22–30.
5. Ison MG, Nalesnik MA. An update on donor-derived disease transmission in organ transplantation. Am J Transplant 2011;11:1123–30.
6. Ison MG, Hager J, Blumberg E, et al. Donor-derived disease transmission events in the United Stated: data reviewed by the OPTN/UNOS Disease Transmission Advisory Committee. Am J Transplant 2009;9:1929–35.
7. U.S. Department of Health & Human Services Organ Procurement and Transplantation Network. Pathogens of special interest. Available at: https://optn.transplant.hrsa.gov/media/1911/special_pathogens_list.pdf. Accessed January 27, 2018.
8. Fischer SA, Graham MB, Kuehnert MJ, et al. Transmission of lymphocytic choriomeningitis virus by organ transplantation. N Engl J Med 2006;354:2235–49.
9. Palacios G, Druce J, Du L, et al. A new arenavirus in a cluster of fatal transplant-associated diseases. N Engl J Med 2008;358:991–8.
10. Mathur G, Yadav K, Ford B, et al. High clinical suspicion of donor-derived disease leads to timely recognition and early intervention to treat solid organ transplant-transmitted lymphocytic choriomeningitis virus. Transpl Infect Dis 2017;19: e12707–15.
11. Iwamoto M, Jernigan DB, Guasch A, et al. Transmission of West Nile virus from an organ donor to four transplant recipients. N Engl J Med 2003;348:2196–203.
12. Srinivasan A, Burton EC, Kuehnert MJ, et al. Transmission of rabies virus from an organ donor to four transplant recipients. N Engl J Med 2005;352:1103–11.
13. Meije Y, Piersimoni C, Torre-Cisneros J, et al. Mycobacterial infections in solid organ transplant recipients. Clin Microbiol Infect 2014;20:89–101.
14. Kay A, Barry PM, Annambhotla P, et al. Solid organ transplant-transmitted tuberculosis linked to a community outbreak – California, 2015. Am J Transplant 2017; 17:2733–6.
15. Kusne S, Taranto S, Covington S, et al. Coccidioidomycosis transmission through organ transplantation: a report of the OPTN *Ad Hoc* disease transmission advisory committee. Am J Transplant 2016;16:3562–7.
16. Serody JS, Mill MR, Detterbeck FC, et al. Blastomycosis in transplant recipients: report of a case and review. Clin Infect Dis 1993;16:54–8.
17. Huprikar S, Bosserman E, Patel G, et al. Donor-derived *Trypanosoma cruzi* infection in solid organ recipients in the United States, 2001-2011. Am J Transplant 2013;13:2418–25.

18. Roxby AC, Gottlieb GS, Limaye AP. Strongyloidiasis in transplant patients. Clin Infect Dis 2009;49:1411–23.
19. Le M, Ravin K, Hasan A, et al. Single donor-derived strongyloidiasis in three solid organ transplant recipients: case series and review of the literature. Am J Transplant 2014;14:1199–206.
20. Centers for Disease Control and Prevention. *Balamuthia mandrillaris* transmitted through organ transplantation – Mississippi, 2009. Am J Transplant 2011;11: 173–6.
21. Farnon EC, Kokko KE, Budge PJ, et al. Transmission of *Balamuthia mandrillaris* by organ transplantation. Clin Infect Dis 2016;63:878–88.
22. Fischer SA. Emerging and rare viral infections in transplantation. In: Ljungman P, Snydman D, Boeckh M, editors. Transplant infections. 4th edition. Switzerland: Springer; 2016. p. 911–24.
23. Mirazo S, Ramos N, Mainardi V, et al. Transmission, diagnosis, and management of hepatitis E: an update. Hepat Med 2014;6:45–59.
24. Behrendt P, Steinmann E, Manns MP, et al. The impact of hepatitis E in the liver transplant setting. J Hepatol 2014;61:1418–29.
25. Kamar N, Garrouste C, Haagsma EB, et al. Factors associated with chronic hepatitis in patients with hepatitis E virus infection who have received solid organ transplants. Gastroenterology 2011;140:1481–9.
26. Schlosser B, Stein A, Neuhaus R, et al. Liver transplant from a donor with occult HEV infection induced chronic hepatitis and cirrhosis in the recipient. J Hepatol 2012;56:500–2.
27. Hocevar SN, Paddock CD, Spak CW, et al. Microsporidiosis acquired through solid organ transplantation: a public health investigation. Ann Intern Med 2014; 160:213–20.
28. Lion T. Adenovirus infections in immunocompetent and immunocompromised patients. Clin Microbiol Rev 2014;27:441–62.
29. Smibert OC, Wilson HL, Sohail A, et al. Donor-derived *Mycoplasma hominis* and an apparent cluster of *M. hominis* cases in solid organ transplant recipients. Clin Infect Dis 2017;65:1504–8.
30. Vora NM, Basavaraju SV, Feldman KA, et al. Racoon rabies virus variant transmission through solid organ transplantation. JAMA 2013;310:398–407.
31. Kauffman CA, Freifeld AG, Andes DR, et al. Endemic fungal infections in solid organ and hematopoietic cell transplant recipients enrolled in the Transplant-Associated Infection Surveillance Network (TRANSNET). Transpl Infect Dis 2014;16:213–24.
32. Len O, Garzoni C, Lumbreras C, et al. Recommendations for screening of donor and recipient prior to solid organ transplantation and to minimize transmission of donor-derived infections. Clin Microbiol Infect 2014;20:10–8.
33. Fischer SA, Lu K, American Society of Transplantation Infectious Diseases Community of Practice. Screening of donor and recipient in solid organ transplantation. Am J Transplant 2013;13:9–21.
34. Singh N, Huprikar S, Burdette SD, et al. Donor-derived fungal infections in organ transplant recipients: guidelines of the American Society of Transplantation, Infectious Diseases Community of Practice. Am J Transplant 2012;12:2414–28.
35. Levi ME, Kumar D, Green M, et al. Considerations for screening live kidney donors for endemic infections: a viewpoint on the UNOS policy. Am J Transplant 2014;14:1003–11.
36. US Department of Health & Human Services Organ Procurement and Transplantation Network. Guidance for HTLV-1/2 screening and confirmation in potential

donors and reporting potential HTLV-1 infection. Available at: https://optn.transplant.hrsa.gov/resources/guidance/guidance-for-htlv-1-screening-and-confirmation-in-potential-donors-and-reporting-potential-htlv-1-infection/. Accessed January 27, 2018.

37. Huprikar S, Danziger-Isakov L, Ahn J, et al. Solid organ transplantation from hepatitis B virus-positive donors: consensus guidelines for recipient management. Am J Transplant 2015;15:1162–72.

38. Levitsky J, Formica RN, Bloom RD, et al. The American Society of Transplantation consensus conference on the use of hepatitis C viremic donors in solid organ transplantation. Am J Transplant 2017;17:2790–802.

39. Muller E, Barday Z, Mendelson M, et al. HIV-positive-to-HIV-positive kidney transplantation – results at 3 to 5 years. N Engl J Med 2015;372:613–20.

40. Wright AJ, Rose C, Toews M, et al. An exception to the rule or a rule for the exception? The potential of using HIV-positive donors in Canada. Transplantation 2017; 101:671–4.

41. U.S. Department of Health & Human Services Organ Procurement and TransplantationNetwork. Understanding the risk of transmission of HIV, hepatitis B,and hepatitis C from PHS increased risk donors. Available at: https://optn.transplant.hrsa.gov/resources/guidance/understanding-hiv-hbv-hcv-risks-fromincreased-risk-donors/. Accessed January 27, 2018.

42. L'Huillier AG, Humar A, Payne C, et al. Organ utilization from increased infectious risk donors: an observational study. Transpl Infect Dis 2017;19:e12785–92.

43. Irwin L, Kotton CN, Elias N, et al. Utilization of increased risk for transmission of infectious disease donor organs in solid organ transplantation: retrospective analysis of disease transmission and safety. Transpl Infect Dis 2017;19:e12791–7.

44. Bowring MG, Holscher CM, Zhou S, et al. Turn down for what? Patient outcomes associated with declining increased infectious risk donors. Am J Transplant 2017;1–8. https://doi.org/10.1111/ajt.14577.

45. Basavaraju SV, Kuehnert MJ, Zaki SR, et al. Encephalitis caused by pathogens transmitted through organ transplants, United States, 2002-2013. Emerg Infect Dis 2014;20:1443–51.

46. U.S. Department of Health & Human Services Organ Procurement and Transplantation Network. Guidance for recognizing central nervous system infections in potential deceased organ donors. Available at: https://optn.transplant.hrsa.gov/resources/guidance/guidance-for-recognizing-central-nervous-system-infections-in-potential-deceased-organ-donors/. Accessed January 27, 2018.

47. U.S. Department of Health & Human Services Organ Procurement and Transplantation Network. Disease Transmission Advisory Committee. Available at: https://optn.transplant.hrsa.gov/members/committees/disease-transmission-advisory-committee/. Accessed January 27, 2018.

Safe Living Following Solid Organ Transplantation

Barbra M. Blair, MD

KEYWORDS

- Solid organ transplantation • Vaccination • Food safety • Travel advice
- Infection prevention

KEY POINTS

- Infections after transplant can have significant impact on a patient's as well as their organ's survival. Several strategies can be used to minimize risk of acquisition of such infections.
- Vaccination against viral and bacterial illnesses, carefully timed preferably pretransplant, as well as safe living strategies posttransplant can afford protection against infections.
- Careful assessment pretransplant combined with a strategy of ongoing patient education pretransplant and posttransplant can assist patients with maintaining their health.

INTRODUCTION

Living safely after organ transplantation requires an integrated care continuum that starts before transplant and ideally even before the development of end organ disease. In order to minimize a solid organ transplant (SOT) recipient's risk for infection and risk for injury, it is important to anticipate the risks after transplantation inherent in living. These risks include potential exposure to others with viral or bacterial illness, to food and water sources, participation in recreational activities, resuming sexual activity, living with pets, and opportunities for travel, especially internationally. It is invaluable to orient potential SOT recipients to these risks, because often leading up to transplant they may likely experience debilitation and significant handicaps due to chronic illness. After SOT, once they overcome the preceding debilitation and surgical effects, they, despite chronic immunosuppression, can go on to live healthy, fruitful lives, which they may not have been able to fully conceive of while debilitated. Thus, in anticipation of SOT, potential transplant recipients should update their vaccinations. Potential recipients need to be made aware of food and water safety important after transplant so they may plan accordingly. In addition, potential recipients

Disclosure Statement: None.
Division of Infectious Diseases, Beth Israel Deaconess Medical Center, 110 Francis Street, Suite GB, Boston, MA 02215, USA
E-mail address: bblair@bidmc.harvard.edu

Infect Dis Clin N Am 32 (2018) 507–515
https://doi.org/10.1016/j.idc.2018.04.014
0891-5520/18/© 2018 Elsevier Inc. All rights reserved.

id.theclinics.com

should be educated as to the risks of pet ownership and animal exposure, again to plan accordingly. Finally, realistic expectations should be set with regard to travel and participation in recreational activities especially within the first year after transplant, the period during which they are at increased risk of infection.[1] The American Society for Transplantation Infectious Diseases Community of Practice has previously set forth informal guidance on strategies for living safely after SOT.[2] The investigators astutely note that, unlike Centers for Disease Control and Prevention (CDC) guidelines set forth in other populations such as hematologic stem cell transplant recipients[3] and those infected with human immunodeficiency virus,[4] no such evidence-based guidance exists for the SOT population. That said, the data available for these groups and other immunocompromised populations can be extrapolated to provide guidance, understanding that this guidance may require tailoring based on an individual patient's situation.[2]

STRATEGIES TO PREVENT INFECTION
Vaccination

Posttransplant infections can have a major effect on a patient's as well as their allograft's survival; thus strategies aimed at preventing infections are likely to have significant impact.[5] One such strategy is vaccination (please see Dr Christian Donato-Santana and Nicole M. Theodoropoulos' article, "Immunization of Solid Organ Transplant Candidates & Recipients: A 2018 Update," in this issue for more details). Although inactivated vaccinations have been demonstrated safe after SOT, so too are these vaccines safe in end-stage liver disease (ESLD) and end-stage renal disease (ESRD), and antibody titer response after vaccination is higher pretransplant.[6–12] Viral infections, such as measles virus and varicella zoster virus that can be prevented by live-attenuated vaccine, can have significant morbidity and mortality after SOT.[13] Varicella disease in the immunocompromised host can lead to severe complications.[14,15] Measles outbreaks unfortunately continue to occur in the present day, and measles in an immunocompromised host can cause pneumonitis and encephalitis and has been associated with high mortality.[16]

Live-attenuated vaccines are not recommended posttransplant; thus, identifying those susceptible hosts pretransplant and vaccinating them are paramount in avoiding devastating consequences of infection in an SOT recipient. Most transplant centers have procedures in place to identify these susceptible patients via pretransplant serologies, and every effort is made to ensure vaccination occurs before transplant with intervals as prescribed by the Advisory Committee of Immunization Practices (ACIP). Two other vaccine-preventable diseases that are more common than measles require attention: influenza and Streptococcus pneumoniae. Because invasive pneumococcal disease can have substantial morbidity and mortality in SOT recipients and in those with chronic lung, heart, renal, and liver disease, the ACIP recommends vaccination with PCV13 followed by PPSV23. Furthermore, there are few contraindications to influenza vaccine in these populations, especially given the severe pulmonary and extrapulmonary complications associated with infection.[5] Live-attenuated influenza vaccine should be avoided posttransplant both in the SOT recipient and, if at all possible, in their household contacts.[17]

In general, in anticipation for SOT, vaccination should occur as soon as possible to afford protection to those with chronic heart, lung, renal, and liver disease but also because live-attenuated vaccinations should not be administered after transplant. Realistically, however, this is not always possible because in those with critical illness, there may not be time to complete vaccination series before transplant. However, transplantation should not be postponed solely for this purpose. Although the optimal timing of vaccination after transplantation is not known, most centers initiate vaccination 3 to 6 months after transplantation.[17] Despite theoretic concerns, no evidence of a link to vaccination and acute episodes of rejection has been found.[14,18,19] Thus, influenza vaccine should be administered yearly as long as at least 3 to 6 months after SOT and not given previously that season. Ideally, any encounter with a potential SOT recipient should prompt a review of vaccine status and update as indicated[5] (**Table 1**).

Everyday Strategies for Disease Prevention

In SOT, most infections occur during the first 6 months after transplant unless there are extenuating circumstances, such as organ rejection and need for augmentation of immunosuppression. After 6 months, most infections seen in the SOT recipient are similar to those seen in the general adult population.[1] Because most pathogens are either acquired via direct contact via hands, ingestion, or inhalation, frequent hand washing and avoidance of those with respiratory or gastrointestinal illnesses are essential ways to minimize acquisition of infectious pathogens.[2] Close contacts of transplant recipients should be encouraged to receive updated vaccines as per the ACIP guidelines and their personal health care providers. There is little risk from family members/close contacts who receive live-attenuated vaccines to transplant

Table 1
Vaccine recommendations

Vaccine	Schedule	Comments
Influenza	Annually	Pretransplant & posttransplant
Hepatitis B	3 doses	Consider 40-μg dose in ESLD & ESRD
Hepatitis A	2–3 dose series depending on vaccine	Recommended in ESLD & high-risk travel
Tdap	Single dose ≤2 y after last Td	Td booster every 10 y thereafter
Pneumococcal		
Prevnar (PCV13)	Once regardless of age	If given after PSV23, then wait ≥1 y
Pneumovax (PPSV23)	≥8 wk after PCV13	If administered before age 65, then booster after 5 y
Varicella	2 dose series if nonimmune	Pretransplant only
MMR	1–2 doses depending on previous vaccination	Pretransplant only
Shingles (Varicella-Zoster)		
Zostavax	Once in adults >50 y	Pretransplant only; may be obsolete with advent of Shingrix
Shingrix	To be determined	Approved by FDA 10/20/17 & voted on by ACIP 10/27/17; official recommendations in immunocompromised hosts pending
HPV	3 doses through age 26	Catch up if not previously vaccinated as child
Meningococcal (MenACWY)	1–2 doses	Only for certain populations per ACIP guidelines & no immunogenicity studies post transplant

Data from Refs.[5,17,20,21]

recipients. The only exceptions are smallpox and oral polio vaccines, which are very rarely indicated.[17] In addition, even with rotavirus vaccine, SOT recipients could refrain from diaper changing and/or use meticulous hand washing rather than not have their close contact vaccinated.[22] Similarly, review of safe sexual practices with SOT recipients can reduce risk for acquisition of several pathogens, including hepatitis B and C, human immunodeficiency virus, herpes simplex virus, *Neisseria gonorrhoeae*, *Chlamydia trachomatis*, syphilis, and other fecally transmitted organisms. Unless the patient is in a long-term monogamous relationship, condom usage should be advised. Furthermore, SOT recipients should be counseled on avoidance of oral exposure to feces and hand hygiene after sexual intercourse.[2,3] **Table 2** lists other approaches and habits to use to avoid contact with environmental objects/individuals to decrease an SOT recipient's chance of exposure to infectious pathogens.

Food and Water Safety

According to the CDC, 48 million persons get sick; 128,000 are hospitalized, and 3000 die from food-borne infection and illness in the United States each year. The most often impacted are those with weakened immune systems,[23] which is why education and guidance should be directed at potential SOT recipients and reiterated frequently after transplantation. Waterborne infections arise from drinking contaminated drinking water or inadvertent ingestion of water during recreational activities, such as boating, enjoying water parks, or swimming.[2] Access to safe drinking water within the United States is as simple as using water from the tap delivered from and US Environmental Protection Agency–regulated public water system.[24] That said, many people in the United States who receive their water from private ground water wells are thus responsible for ensuring their water is free from contaminants.[24] The most common causes of water-associated disease outbreaks due to private water sources per the CDC as of 2010 are as follows[24]:

- Hepatitis A
- Giardia

Table 2
Avoidance strategies against environmental and opportunistic pathogens

Employ hand washing after:	Avoid:
Eating or preparing food	Close contact with persons with respiratory viruses
Changing diapers	Prolonged contact with crowded areas
Touching plants or dirt	Tobacco and marijuana smoking
Using the restroom	Visiting areas with increased risk of exposure to tuberculosis (prisons, homeless shelters, certain health care facilities)
Touching animals, particularly at zoos or fairs	
Touching items in contact with animal or human bodily fluids	Construction areas/areas of excavation
Collecting or deposing of garbage	Areas with possible exposure to fungal spores: caves, barns, bird cages/coops, soil aerosols via mulching
Going outdoors or to a public place	Self-piercing, tattooing, or needle sharing

Data from Avery RK, Michaels MG, the AST Infectious Diseases Community of Practice. Strategies for safe living after solid organ transplantation. Am J Transplant 2013;13:304–10; and Guidelines for preventing infectious complications among hematopoietic cell transplant recipients: a global perspective. Biol Blood Marrow Transplant 2009;15(10):1143–238; and *Adapted from* https://www.fda.gov/downloads/Food/FoodborneIllnessContaminants/UCM312793.pdf.

- Campylobacter
- Shigella
- *Escherichia coli*
- Cryptosporidium
- Salmonella
- *Yersinia enterocolitica*

Thus, private water sources such as these should be avoided by SOT recipients.[2] In addition, SOT recipients should avoid swimming in recreational facilities that are likely to be contaminated with human or animal waste, and if swimming, avoid swallowing such water.[2]

After transplant, many patients may experience a renewed appetite that was suppressed due to previous chronic illness such as ESLD or ESRD. Food safety is paramount to retaining an SOT recipient's health with attention paid to handling, preparing, and consuming foods.[25] Raw fish and meats should be handled on separate surfaces from other food items.[3] Separate cutting boards should be used for each food item or thoroughly washed with soapy warm water between uses for separate foods.[3] Any person preparing raw foods as an SOT recipient or for an SOT recipient should practice meticulous hand hygiene after handling raw foods.[3] Raw vegetables should be washed thoroughly before ingestion. Even fruits with skins should be washed before cutting or peeling to avoid internal contamination from the surface.[25] Canned foods should have the lids washed before opening to avoid contaminating the inner contents.[25] All cooked foods should be heated to US Department of Agriculture–recommended safe minimum internal temperatures, including reheating previously cooked foods, such as hams and deli meats.[25] These practices are simple ways to decrease risk of the many infections outlined in **Table 3**, which can have more fulminant presentations and/or be more difficult to treat and eradicate in SOT recipients. Unfortunately, many of these illnesses present similarly; thus, knowledge of potential risk behaviors can inform the SOT recipient on what to avoid, and if ill, can be highlighted to the care team as a possible source of infection/symptoms.

Pet Safety and Animal Contact

Studies have demonstrated the health benefits of animal-human bonding, especially in the immunocompromised, who may feel isolated as a result of their underlying illnesses.[28] Physicians should advise SOT recipients of the potential risks inherent in pet ownership and animal contact, although in most circumstances, such ownership/contact is not absolutely contraindicated.[3] The SOT recipient should not feed or pet stray animals. In general, pets such as lizards, snakes, turtles, baby chicks/ducklings, and exotic pets should be avoided because of risk of *Salmonella* and *Campylobacter* infections.[28–30] Specific guidance for the care of pets should include the following: feeding pets only high-quality commercial food, not raw meat or raw eggs; allowing pets to drink only from potable water sources; leashing and confining dogs to prevent coprophagy (eating feces); avoiding juvenile cats or dogs because they are more prone to enteric infections.[28] In addition, although routine veterinary care for pets is important, SOT recipients can be at risk for pet vaccines–related illness, and thus, caution must be advised. The "kennel cough" vaccine, which is a mixture of *Bordetella bronchiseptica* and parainfluenza, can pose infection risk.[28,30] The *Brucella* animal vaccine has been associated with human illness.[30] In addition to the risks potentially prevented by obtaining veterinary care, caution must be advised when providing in home pet hygiene. In general, bird cages and litter boxes should be cleaned daily by someone other than the SOT recipient. Although fish are

Table 3
Major pathogens causing food-borne illness in solid organ transplant

Food-Borne Pathogen	Commonly Associated Source	Most Common Symptoms/ Complications in SOT
Campylobacter	Contaminated water; raw meat/ poultry; unpasteurized milk	Diarrhea (often bloody), fever, nausea; can lead to bacteremia
Cryptosporidium	Contaminated (unwashed) food; contaminated drinking/ recreational water	Crampy, watery diarrhea leading to dehydration; in SOT can be prolonged
Listeria monocytogenes	Unpasteurized milk/cheeses; improperly reheated deli meats/ hot dogs; store-bought meat salads	Abdominal pain; diarrhea; fevers; chills; headache; can lead to bacteremia and meningitis
E coli	Undercooked meat; contaminated water; unpasteurized juices	Diarrhea; vomiting; certain strains can lead to hemolytic uremic syndrome
Salmonella	Undercooked meat, poultry, eggs; unpasteurized milk/juices; pet turtles	Abdominal pain; fever; diarrhea (may be bloody); can lead to bacteremia
Toxoplasmosis gondii	Raw & undercooked meats (including deer); handling cat feces	Mononucleosis-like symptoms; severe systemic disease in SOT
Vibrio vulnificus	Undercooked & raw seafood	Diarrhea, nausea, vomiting; severe sepsis in SOT
Norovirus	Contaminated food or water; close contact with infected individual	Watery diarrhea (can be prolonged in SOT), nausea, acute onset vomiting

Data from Refs.[25–27]

generally a lower-risk pet, care must be applied to cleaning of fish tanks because mycobacterial disease associated with skin and soft tissue has been linked to such activities.[28–30] Finally, after any animal contact, whether with a personal pet or at a zoo or aquarium, all individuals, but most importantly SOT recipients, should practice careful hand washing.[28–30]

Travel Advice

As per the CDC, immunocompromised travelers compose 1% to 2% of the travelers seen in US travel clinics.[31] These visit statistics are important to note because travel to destinations outside of North America and Europe are associated with increased exposure to enteric and vector-borne pathogens.[32] In a large travel clinic study in Canada from 2001, two-thirds of the travelers surveyed who were SOT recipients were foreign born[32] and historically, being foreign born increases a traveler's likelihood of staying with friends and family.[32] As such, it is unclear if foreign-born SOT recipients frequent travel clinics as several studies have indicated that those traveling to visit friends and family are more likely to contract travel-related illnesses because they are less aware of their susceptibility, less likely to seek pretravel advice, and adopt higher risk behaviors.[33–35] Because of these data, education and recommendation toward seeking pretravel advice should be targeted at all SOT recipients because improved pretravel consultation can potentially prevent devastating infections.[36] The CDC recommends that several key education points be discussed with immunocompromised travelers: developing an illness contingency plan with an identified clinic/hospital; bringing extra medications in case of travel delay; avoiding procuring medications during travel due to risk of counterfeit; use of sun protection; vigilant food and water precautions; and travel with a health kit.[31] In addition to these measures, travel to high-risk destinations should be postponed until at least a year after transplantation.[31] If a potential SOT recipient has the potential to travel to yellow fever–endemic areas after transplant, consideration should be given to vaccination before transplantation.[36] In addition, household contacts of SOT recipients can and should receive live-attenuated travel vaccinations before travel with the precautions as described above in the vaccination section.[32] As for the SOT travelers themselves, other inactivated or non–live vaccines for typhoid, hepatitis A, hepatitis B, and meningococcus should be administered as indicated.[36] In addition, malaria chemoprophylaxis should be prescribed for SOT recipient travelers to endemic areas because they are by virtue of the SOT susceptible to more serious disease.[31] Care does however need to be used when prescribing malaria chemoprophylaxis because potential drug-drug interactions with immunosuppressive medications and dose adjustment for altered renal or hepatic function need to be considered.[31] In addition, strict vector precautions should be advised because diseases like Chagas and leishmaniasis can disseminate in immunocompromised hosts.[36] Furthermore, Dengue infection accounts for about 10% of the systemic febrile illnesses experienced by travelers, suggesting that SOT recipients would be similarly affected.[37] In addition, Chikungunya and Zika viruses have emerged as important travel-associated vector-borne infections recently. Thus, information about the severity in immunocompromised travelers is still being ascertained.[36] Although such extensive travel counseling may be perceived as excessive especially by those who are foreign born, such measures may assist with preventing substantial life-altering illness by promoting travel yet in the safest way possible.

SUMMARY

Receipt of an organ transplant will most likely extend the recipient's life substantially, and, it is hoped, this extension is associated with good health. The benefits of longevity by virtue of organ transplantation need to be closely protected by education before, during, and after transplantation about potential risks and measures to mitigate such exposures. The topics addressed here ensure that an SOT recipient and their providers can plan accordingly and implement measures that will assist with maintaining such health.

REFERENCES

1. Snydman DR. Epidemiology of infections after solid-organ transplantation. Clin Infect Dis 2001;33(Suppl 1):S5–8.
2. Avery RK, Michaels MG, the AST ID COP. Strategies for safe living after solid organ transplantation. Amer J Trans 2013;13:304–10.
3. Guidelines for preventing infectious complications among hematopoietic cell transplant recipients: a global perspective. Biol Blood Marrow Transpl 2009; 15(10):1143–238.
4. Guidelines for prevention and treatment of opportunistic infections in HIV-infected adults and adolescents. AidsInfo.NIH.gov. Available at: https://aidsinfo.nih.gov/guidelines on 12/26/2017. Accessed January 1, 2018.
5. Chow J, Golan Y. Vaccination of solid-organ transplantation candidates. CID 2009;49:1550–6.

6. Keefe EB, Iwarson S, McMahon BJ, et al. Safety and immunogenicity of hepatitis A vaccine in patients with chronic liver disease. Hepatology 1998;27:881–6.

7. Magnani G, Falchetti E, Pollini G, et al. Safety and efficacy of two types of influenza vaccination in heart transplant recipients: a prospective randomized controlled study. J Heart Lung Transplant 2005;24:588–92.

8. Chalasani N, Smallwood G, Halcomb J, et al. Is vaccination against hepatitis B infection indicated in patients waiting for or after orthotopic liver transplantation? Liver Transpl Surg 1998;4:128–32.

9. Rytel MW, Dailey MP, Schiffman G, et al. Pneumococcal vaccine immunization of patients with renal impairment. Proc Soc Exp Bio Med 1986;182:468–73.

10. Linnemann CC Jr, First MR, Schiffman G. Response to pneumococcal vaccine in renal transplant and hemodialysis patients. Arch Intern Med 1981;141:1637–40.

11. Loinaz C, de Juanes JR, Gonzalez EM, et al. Hepatitis B vaccination results in 140 liver transplant recipients. Hepatogastroenterology 1997;44:235–8.

12. McCashland TM, Preheim LC, Gentry MJ. Pneumococcal vaccine response in cirrhosis and liver transplantation. J Infect Dis 2000;181:757–60.

13. Miyairi I, Funaki T, Saitoh A. Immunization practices in solid organ transplant recipients. Vaccine 2016;34:1958–64.

14. Broyer M, Tete MJ, Guest G, et al. Varicella and zoster in children after kidney transplantation: long-term results of vaccination. Pediatrics 1997;99:35–9.

15. McGregor RS, Zitelli BJ, Urbach AH, et al. Varicella in pediatric orthotopic liver transplant recipients. Pediatrics 1989;83(2):256–61.

16. Kaplan LJ, Daum RS, Smaron M, et al. Severe measles in immunocompromised patients. JAMA 1992;267(9):1237–41.

17. Danziger-Isakov L, Kumar D, the American Society of Transplantation Infectious Disease Community of Practice. Vaccination in solid organ transplantation. Am J Transplant 2013;13:311–7.

18. Kimball P, Verbeke S, Flattery M, et al. Influenza vaccination does not promote cellular or humoral activation among heart transplant recipients. Transplantation 2000;69:2449–51.

19. White-Williams C, Brown R, Kirklin J, et al. Improving clinical practice: should we give influenza vaccinations to heart transplant patients? J Heart Lung Transpl 2006;25:320–3.

20. Recommended immunization schedule for adults aged 19 years or older, United States, 2018. CDC.gov. Available at: https://www.cdc.gov/vaccines/schedules/downloads/adult/adult-combined-schedule.pdf. Accessed January 1, 2018.

21. What everyone should know about Zostavax. CDC.gov. 2018. Available at: https://www.cdc.gov/vaccines/vpd/shingles/public/zostavax/index.html. Accessed February 19, 2018.

22. Smith CK, McNeal MM, Meyer NR, et al. Rotavirus shedding in premature infants following first immunization. Vaccine 2011;29:8141–6.

23. People at risk for foodborne illness - transplant recipients. FDA.gov. 2017. Available at: https://www.fda.gov/Food/FoodborneIllnessContaminants/PeopleAtRisk/ucm312570.htm. Accessed January 1, 2018.

24. Drinking water. CDC.gov. 2017. Available at: https://www.cdc.gov/healthywater/drinking/index.htm. Accessed January 14, 2018.

25. Food safety for transplant recipients. FDA.gov. 2011. Available at: https://www.fda.gov/downloads/Food/FoodborneIllnessContaminants/UCM312793.pdf. Accessed January 14, 2018.

26. Avery RK, Lonze BE, Kraus ES, et al. Severe chronic norovirus diarrheal disease in transplant recipients: clinical features of an under- recognized syndrome. Transpl Infect Dis 2017;19:e12674.

27. Foodborne illnesses and germs. CDC.gov. 2017. Available at: https://www.cdc.gov/foodsafety/foodborne-germs.html. Accessed January 14, 2018.

28. Trevejo RT, Barr MC, Robinson RA. Important emerging bacterial zoonotic infections affecting the immunocompromised. Vet Res 2005;36:493–506.

29. Healthy pets healthy people – organ transplant recipients. CDC.gov. 2014. Available at: https://www.cdc.gov/healthypets/specific-groups/organ-transplant-patients.html. Accessed January 15, 2018.

30. Kotton CN. Zoonoses in solid-organ and hematopoietic stem cell transplant recipients. Clin Infect Dis 2007;44:857–66.

31. Traveler's health. Chapter 8 – Advising travelers with specific needs. CDC.gov. 2017. Available at: https://wwwnc.cdc.gov/travel/yellowbook/2018/advising-travelers-with-specific-needs/immunocompromised-travelers. Accessed January 20, 2018.

32. Boggild AK, Sano M, Humar A, et al. Travel patterns and risk behavior in solid organ transplant recipients. J Travel Med 2004;11:37–43.

33. Ryan ET, Wilson ME, Kain KC. Illness after international travel. N Engl J Med 2002;347:505–16.

34. Held TK, Weike T, Mansmann, et al. Malaria prophylaxis: identifying risk groups for non-compliance. Q J Med 1994;87:17–22.

35. Behrens RH, Curtis CF. Malaria in travelers: epidemiology and prevention. BMJ 1993;49:363–81.

36. Patel RP, Liang SY, Koolwal SY, et al. Travel advice for the immunocompromised traveler: prophylaxis, vaccination, and other preventive measures. Ther Clin Risk Manag 2015;11:217–28.

37. Freedman DO, Weld LH, Kozarsky PE, et al. GeoSentinal surveillance network: spectrum of disease and relation to place of exposure among Ill returned travelers. N Engl J Med 2006;354(2):119–30.

Immunization of Solid Organ Transplant Candidates and Recipients: A 2018 Update

Christian Donato-Santana, MD,
Nicole M. Theodoropoulos, MD, MS*

KEYWORDS

- Vaccine • Immunization • Solid organ transplant • Immunosuppressed

KEY POINTS

- Appropriate vaccines should be administered as early in the pretransplant period as possible.
- Data are lacking regarding the safety of live vaccines in the posttransplant period and are currently contraindicated.
- Vaccines should be given before foreign travel, but yellow fever vaccine is currently contraindicated posttransplantation.

INTRODUCTION

Vaccination in transplant candidates is important, but often overlooked. Vaccine-preventable diseases continue to be a considerable cause of morbidity and mortality in solid organ transplant (SOT) candidates and recipients.[1] Vaccinating SOT candidates pretransplant can improve their posttransplant response to vaccines.[2] Certain vaccines may allow SOT recipients to accept organs they may not have otherwise, as in the case of the hepatitis B core antibody positive donor organs. In addition, in the case of influenza vaccine in particular, vaccination may help avoid organ turndown due to SOT candidate illness.

Ideally, SOT candidates should have their vaccines updated as early as possible before transplantation because vaccine immune response is decreased during organ failure and even more so in the setting of immunosuppression after transplant surgery. It is recommended to make sure measles, mumps, rubella, varicella, tetanus-diphtheria-pertussis, pneumococcal, influenza, and hepatitis A and B

Disclosure Statement: The authors have no conflicts of interest to disclose.
Division of Infectious Diseases & Immunology, University of Massachusetts Medical School, 55 Lake Avenue North, S7-715, Worcester, MA 01655, USA
* Corresponding author. Division of Infectious Diseases, University of Massachusetts Memorial Medical Center, 55 Lake Avenue North, S7-715, Worcester, MA 01655.
E-mail address: nicole.theodoropoulos@umassmemorial.org

Infect Dis Clin N Am 32 (2018) 517–533
https://doi.org/10.1016/j.idc.2018.04.002
0891-5520/18/© 2018 Elsevier Inc. All rights reserved.

id.theclinics.com

vaccines are up to date in all appropriate candidates. If a patient has plans for foreign travel after transplant, it should be ensured that travel-related vaccines, especially live vaccines, are given before transplantation.

There is not a clear consensus about when vaccination should resume after transplantation although many centers vaccinate 3 to 6 months after transplantation. Serologic tests can be used to decide if certain vaccines are necessary pretransplant and should be used in certain instances to assess adequate immunologic response more than or equal to 4 weeks after vaccine administration.[3]

MECHANISMS OF IMMUNOSUPPRESION

It is important to understand the mechanism of immunosuppression in SOT recipients because this can help determine the appropriate timing of the vaccines. The immunosuppressive medications used in SOT recipients reduce B-cell and T-cell immune responses, which decrease the vaccine immune response.[4-7] Vaccine response is inversely proportional to the number of immunosuppressive drugs used.[7,8] Also, the specific immunosuppressive drug used may affect the level of immune response to vaccines. Previous studies have found that mycophenolate use was associated with decreased seroresponse in influenza-vaccinated kidney transplant recipients.[1,9,10] Another study evaluated the response to influenza vaccine in the setting of anti–T-cell therapy impact and did not find a significant difference with thymoglobulin versus basiliximab.[1,11]

TIMING

The current recommendation is to complete updating vaccines at least 4 weeks before transplant.[7,12-14] The American Society of Transplantation Third Edition of the Infectious Disease Community of Practice guidelines recommend at least a period of 4 weeks to repeat serologies after vaccine administration to ensure appropriate seroresponse.[3] Because patients are generally under the highest level of immunosuppression in the first 6 months after transplantation, it is recommended to avoid vaccinations in this period because of a likely lack of response. Patients are also recommended to avoid foreign travel in the early posttransplant period. After 6 months, immunosuppression can be reduced in some cases,[15] and therefore, there is improved immunogenicity and response to vaccination.[3,14] However, if T-cell depleting induction immunosuppression is used (ie, alemtuzumab or antithymocyte globulin), SOT recipients will have severely suppressed immune systems for up to 2 years posttransplantation.[16,17]

Several studies have been performed looking for antibody titers after exposure to monoclonal antibody medications. A study looking at vaccine response in patients with immune thrombocytopenia receiving rituximab after the *Haemophilus influenzae* type b (Hib) conjugate vaccine and the pneumococcal polysaccharide vaccine found that 3/14 (21%) in the rituximab group and 4/6 (67%) in the placebo group achieved a 4-fold increase of titers in antipneumococcal antibodies. On the other hand, 4/14 (29%) and 5/6 (83%) achieved a 4-fold increase for anti-Hib antibodies. This finding showed that the antibody responses were impaired for at least 6 months after rituximab administration.[18] A study on autologous hematopoietic cell transplant recipients showed that live vaccines (measles, mumps, and rubella virus [MMR] and Herpes zoster vaccine) were safe and well tolerated 24 months after transplant on patients with bortezomib maintenance therapy.[19] The use of plasma exchange could also affect antibody titers after vaccination. Renal transplant patients who received plasma exchange sessions were found to have a decrease in antimeasles antibody titers from a mean of 3238 mU/l to a mean of 1710 mU/l, but after a median follow-up of 64 days the titers returned to baseline levels.[20]

LIVE, ATTENUATED VIRUS VACCINES

The most common live, attenuated virus vaccines (LAAV) include intranasal influenza (not recommended for use in the 2017–2018 influenza season), varicella zoster, herpes zoster, measles, mumps, rubella, rotavirus, yellow fever, oral polio, and Japanese encephalitis vaccines. The current recommendation is that all live vaccines must be given in the pretransplantation period, at least 4 weeks before transplantation. To facilitate the administration, live-attenuated vaccines can be administered on the same day with inactivated vaccines, and 2 live-attenuated vaccines can be administered on the same day; otherwise, the live vaccines need to be spaced 28 days apart.[3] The infusion of blood products or intravenous immunoglobulin can interfere with the response to LAAV, and therefore, it is recommended to delay vaccines for 3 months after blood products.[14] In addition, tuberculin skin test response may be rendered falsely negative by live vaccines[21] and for that reason is recommended to perform this test before or on the same day of LAAV, but not within 4 weeks of LAAV.[3] Ultimately, it is important to vaccinate as early as possible in the transplant evaluation period.

It is thought that LAAV are unsafe to administer in the setting of immune suppression, and therefore, post-transplant live vaccines are not recommended. There were prospective studies evaluating pediatric SOT recipients who received varicella or MMR vaccines and no adverse events were reported. There was also a retrospective study in Brazil of 19 SOT recipients who received yellow fever vaccine without adverse outcome.[3,22]

A recent study evaluated SOT recipients who received LAAV to look for a correlation between the vaccine and organ rejection. Three cases of organ rejection were found; 1 patient showed chronic rejection at the time of vaccination, 1 patient had a rejection episode of the liver more than 1 year after the varicella vaccine, and 1 patient had acute organ rejection 3 weeks after measles vaccination.[23] The investigators concluded receipt of LAAV did not increase rates of organ rejection in SOT recipients.[23–26]

SOT recipients should use prevention precautions with family members who have received the rotavirus vaccine. This would include avoiding diaper changing in the infant recipient of the vaccine or frequent hand washing after changing diapers in an infant (if unable to avoid diaper changing), and these precautions should be continued for a period of at least 2 weeks after administration of the vaccine.[3,27] The shedding of the virus may occur up to 1 month after the last dose.[28–30] SOT recipients also need to avoid close contact with household contacts who have received the oral polio vaccine (which is no longer available in the Western Hemisphere). The Infectious Diseases Society of America (IDSA) clinical practice guideline recommends against using the live attenuated oral polio vaccine in persons who live with immunocompromised hosts.[14] Rare cases of vaccine-associated paralytic poliomyelitis have been reported. The transmission of the virus after vaccination is by shedding in the stool.[14,31,32] Otherwise, there are no additional precautions recommended if household contacts receive other live vaccines.

MEASLES, MUMPS, AND RUBELLA VIRUS VACCINE

During transplant evaluation, studies should include MMR serologies, especially if the status of vaccination or previous infection is unknown. The MMR is a live, attenuated vaccine and is only recommended to be administered before transplant but have been administered in selected organ transplant recipients on minimal immunosuppression.[3,33]Adult patients could receive a second dose of MMR if there is no seroconversion by 4 weeks. In a recent article, the only reported adverse effect with the mumps immunization in immunosuppressed patients was transient swelling of the parotid glands.[23]

MMR vaccine administration in pediatric patients is recommended before transplant but the infant must be younger than 6 months; a second dose will be needed if the infant did not receive a transplant before 1 year of age.[3,34–38] A study of pediatric recipients of living donor liver transplantation evaluated the safety and effectiveness of MMR vaccination and the patients achieved seroconversion for the live, attenuated strains of measles, mumps, and rubella administered separately and there was no evidence of infection after the immunization.[1,39] At this time, the MMR vaccine is contraindicated after transplantation due to insufficient data about safety and the concern for the development of vaccine-acquired disseminated infection without available effective treatment.[14]

VARICELLA ZOSTER "CHICKEN POX" VACCINE

Transplant patients are at high risk for severe complications from varicella zoster virus (VZV) infection and for that reason pretransplant serologic studies should include VZV immunoglobulin G antibody titers. Seronegative organ transplant candidates should be offered the varicella vaccine more than 4 weeks before transplantation.[14] However, if an otherwise appropriate organ is offered within this 4-week period, it should be accepted, because prophylactic antiviral agents including acyclovir or valganciclovir would be effective in "turning off" this vaccine, thus effectively preventing vaccine-associated disseminated infection. The varicella vaccine is a live, attenuated vaccine and in adults only 1 dose is needed. A second dose could be administered if the patient does not seroconvert 4 weeks after administration.[3,40–43] The varicella vaccine also can be administered in a 2-dose strategy for patients older than or equal to 13 years, separated by 4 weeks between doses; in patients aged between 1 and 12 years old, greater than or equal to 3 months separation is recommended.[14]

In posttransplant patients, a vesicular rash has been reported after varicella vaccine administration in 2 separate pediatric studies.[1,43,44] The Weinberg study noted an 87% VZV seroconversion rate with a single-dose approach, whereas Posfay-Barbe and colleagues observed that 7 of 32 of children required a third dose of varicella vaccine to achieve seroconversion.[1,43,44] Although LAAV are generally contraindicated post-transplantation, the IDSA guidelines make an exception for seronegative pediatric liver and kidney transplant recipients, because they have a high risk of primary varicella infection.[14] A recent article reported 14/339 SOT transplant recipients had a varicella vaccine-related infection and it was of moderate severity, defined as skin manifestations without complications.[23,43,45,46]

HERPES ZOSTER "SHINGLES" VACCINE

Herpes zoster (HZ) is often seen in SOT recipients, putting them at risk for the complications of postherpetic neuralgia, bacterial superinfection, disseminated disease, and death.[1,47] All SOT candidates should receive HZ vaccine more than 4 weeks before transplantation, but, as with varicella vaccine, if an otherwise appropriate organ is offered within this 4-week period, it should be accepted, as patients will be typically given a prophylactic antiviral post-transplant. Despite the increased risk of these complications posttransplant, the currently available HZ vaccine continues to be contraindicated after transplant because there is a theoretical risk of vaccine-derived HZ and a lack of safety and efficacy data in these patients.[14] A new nonlive recombinant subunit HZ vaccine was approved in the United States as of October 2017.[48] There are currently no data in SOT recipients, but theoretically, given that the new vaccine is not live, it may be preferred in this patient population, including in patients who previously received the live, attenuated HZ vaccine. More data are needed before this can be formally recommended.

INFLUENZA VIRUS VACCINE

The standard dose intramuscular vaccine has been studied the most in SOT recipients. Because of the seasonal nature of influenza, patients are often in the first 6 months posttransplant during influenza season and there is a concern that they will have a decreased immune response to the vaccine. A review article in 2013 demonstrated that although administering the influenza vaccine in the first 6 months after transplant results in poor immunologic response, it was still effective in preventing clinical influenza.[49] A multicenter cohort study in 2015 demonstrated (contrary to common belief) that the time from transplantation had no association with response to vaccination.[50] These 2 studies support the importance of the influenza vaccine in transplant patients, even in the early posttransplant period. A multicenter prospective cohort study showed that the influenza vaccine is safe after SOT and reported 1/798 patients developed renal transplant rejection. That patient had an increasing trend in serum creatinine before the vaccine and was diagnosed previously with chronic rejection making the rejection associated to vaccination unlikely.[50] In addition, a randomized trial of 60 kidney transplant recipients compared the safety and immunogenicity of adjuvanted versus nonadjuvanted influenza vaccine and they did not find an increase in human leukocyte antigen alloantibodies in patients who received the adjuvanted vaccine.[51] In the event of a vaccine shortage, intradermal administration of a smaller dose of influenza vaccine is appropriately immunogenic.[52]

In studies evaluating the outcome of a single-dose versus a two-dose booster vaccine, those that received the booster vaccine have higher titers at 10 weeks than those that received a single dose, but there is no difference after 1 year, and no difference in efficacy in preventing clinical influenza.[53] A clinical trial in 2014 by Felldin and colleagues[5] demonstrated an increase in antibody titers after a yearly booster. In pediatric patients, a double-blind study was performed using a high-dose versus standard dose of an inactivated trivalent vaccine and they showed increased immunogenicity with the high-dose vaccine.[54] Revaccination in 3 to 6 months within the influenza season is also a reasonable approach.[3]

Recently a double-blind randomized trial study was published, which compared the high-dose vaccine (Fluzone HD, Sanofi Pasteur, Swiftwater, PA) and the standard dose vaccine (Fluviral, GlaxoSmithKline, Mississauga, ON) in SOT recipients. In the study, the high-dose vaccine had superior immunogenicity for all the virus strains (A/HINI, A/H3N2, and B/Brisbane). The study also evaluated safety and reported no significant differences in local adverse events. This study suggests the possibility of providing the high-dose vaccine in SOT recipients instead of the standard dose.[55]

Live, attenuated influenza vaccines have been studied in patients with HIV and cancer and have been shown to be safe, but studies are lacking in SOT recipients.[3,56,57]

HUMAN PAPILLOMAVIRUS VIRUS VACCINE

There are limited data regarding the human papillomavirus virus (HPV) vaccine in SOT recipients. However, the HPV vaccine series is important to consider because there is an increased risk of anogenital HPV-associated neoplasia in SOT recipients.[1,58,59] If the vaccine is given, it should be administered previous to the transplantation and consists of 3 doses. If it is not possible to complete the schedule before the transplantation, the vaccine schedule could be resumed 3 to 6 months after transplant. One study evaluated the immune response to the HPV vaccine in posttransplant patients and it found that the vaccine is safe, but immunogenicity was suboptimal.[3,60]

PNEUMOCOCCAL VACCINE

SOT recipients have a high rate of morbidity from pneumococcal disease (*Streptococcus pneumoniae* infection), and therefore, the pneumococcal vaccine is recommended by the IDSA clinical practice guideline for vaccination of the immunocompromised host.[1,14,61] Adults and pediatric transplant recipients older than or equal to 6 years should receive 1 dose of the 13-valent protein-conjugate vaccine (PCV-13) followed at least 8 weeks later by the 23-valent polysaccharide vaccine (PPSV-23).[1,62,63]

Children younger than 2 years should receive the PCV-13 vaccine according to the Advisory Committee on Immunization Practices (ACIP) recommendations depending on the age.[64] Children aged 24 to 71 months should receive the PCV-13 depending on the previous doses (**Table 1**). Children older than 5 years should receive the PPSV-23.[3,64]

In adult posttransplant patients, the PCV-13 vaccine produces a similar immune response as the PPSV-23,[3,65] although one randomized study on adult liver transplant recipients showed that there is no additional benefit for the serotypes contained in the PCV-13 by giving the PPSV-23 8 weeks later[3,66]; an immunization strategy known as "prime-boost" is still recommended.

In adult patients who received more than or equal to 1 dose of PPSV-23, PCV-13 should be administered more than or equal to 1 year after the last dose of PPSV-23. In pediatric patients the recommendation is to administer PCV-13 more than or equal to 8 weeks after the last dose of PPSV-23.[1,63] There are some data supporting annual monitoring of pneumococcal titers because they have been reported to decline.[3,61] However, there are currently no specific recommendations to guide interpretation of these titers in SOT candidates or recipients and when to revaccinate.

TETANUS, DIPHTHERIA, PERTUSSIS VACCINES

Diphtheria, tetanus, pertussis (DPaT or Tdap) vaccine is recommended to be administered before SOT because it is safe and immunogenic in patients with end-stage liver disease and end-stage renal disease.[7,67,68] SOT patients should receive a tetanus booster 5 years after last administration.[7,69] Adults should receive one Tdap followed by Td boosters every 10 years.

ROTAVIRUS VACCINE

The rotavirus vaccine has not been studied well in transplant patients and at this moment the vaccine is not listed as a contraindication because there have not been

Table 1
Summary of pneumococcal vaccine recommendations in children aged 24–71 mo

Previous Dose	Schedule[3,59]
Unvaccinated	2 doses of PCV-13
Incomplete schedule of 3 doses	2 doses of PCV-13, first dose ≥8 wk after most recent dose, second dose ≥8 wk later
4 doses of PCV 7 or other age-appropriate schedule	1 dose of PCV-13, ≥8 wk after most recent dose

reports of vaccine-derived rotavirus infection.[1,28] If an infant in a transplant recipient's household receives the vaccine, the transplant recipient should avoid contact with diapers and stool for 4 weeks after each vaccine administration.[14]

HEPATITIS A VIRUS VACCINE

Hepatitis A virus (HAV) vaccine is recommended before liver and intestinal transplantation and is an important vaccine for foreign travelers. SOT patients need 2 doses of the vaccine to have an adequate antibody response.[7,70] The seroconversion after one dose of HAV vaccine in SOT recipients was found to be 41% in liver transplants and 24% in renal transplants recipients. When a second dose of the vaccine is received the data showed that the seroconversion increases to 97% in liver transplant and 72% in renal transplant recipients.[7,8] In some cases, a booster dose can be considered because the antibody response has been shown to wane by 2 years postvaccination in the SOT population.[7,71]

HEPATITIS B VIRUS VACCINE

Hepatitis B virus (HBV) vaccine is recommended before transplantation in all cases, given the potential for HBV transmission from blood and/or organ donors. The efficacy of repeated HBV vaccination ranges from 32% to 36% in SOT recipients compared with 90% to 95% in healthy controls.[7,72–74] Transplant candidates with liver cirrhosis who receive accelerated HBV vaccine regimen have lower vaccine response rates than patients without liver cirrhosis.[1,75,76] The United States Centers for Disease Control and Prevention (CDC) and IDSA recommend that adult immunocompromised patients receive the higher (40 μg) dose of HBV vaccine.[7,14,77] Vaccine titers should be measured at least yearly to ensure ongoing protective immunity (hepatitis B surface antibody >10 unit/mL).[3]

VACCINES FOR SPECIAL SITUATIONS

During intraabdominal transplant surgery, particularly multivisceral transplantation, occasionally there is injury to the spleen requiring splenectomy. Also, some SOT candidates have had splenectomies in the past for other reasons. The current recommendations are to ensure meningococcal, Hib, and pneumococcal vaccines are up to date before (if possible) or after splenectomy. The pretransplantation evaluation should identify patients with asplenia or those planning to undergo splenectomy. Development of atypical hemolytic uremic syndrome or recipients of human leukocyte antigen or ABO incompatible donor organs may also benefit from these vaccinations. The patients under these circumstances should receive meningococcal, Hib, and pneumococcal vaccines. According to the CDC, both the meningococcal conjugate vaccine and the meningococcal serogroup B vaccine should be administered for Neisseria meningitidis protection in asplenic patients.[30] In patients older than or equal to 10 years with persistent complement deficiencies, patients taking eculizumab, or those at increased risk from serogroup B meningococcal disease outbreak, ACIP recommends the meningococcal serogroup B vaccine in addition to the meningococcal conjugate vaccine.[1,30,78] For Hib protection, transplant candidates or recipients with asplenia should receive a 1-time dose of Hib conjugate vaccine.[30]

Patients who are traveling to N. meningitidis endemic areas should receive a meningococcal vaccine. A 2015 study by Wyplosz and colleagues evaluated the immunogenicity of quadrivalent meningococcal vaccine in SOT recipients. The study showed that 2 of 5 patients developed seroprotective titer (hSBA $\geq$4) for the MenC serogroup with the nonconjugate vaccine. With the conjugate vaccine, 6 of 10 patients had protective meningococcal titers, but only 1 developed a booster response (a 4-fold increase in hSBA titers) and only for the MenC serogroup.[79] This study demonstrates a low immune response to the quadrivalent meningococcal vaccine in SOT recipients but because it does provide some seroprotection to patients at risk, the recommendations remain to administer the vaccine when indicated in SOT recipients.

VACCINES FOR TRAVEL OUTSIDE THE UNITED STATES

Transplant recipients can receive travel vaccines but the schedule should be individualized to the area visited and the increased risk of infection for that area.

The *inactivated polio virus vaccine (IPV)* response rates in renal transplant patients were comparable to healthy individuals.[80] If the patient is planning to travel to a polio endemic region, he/she is recommended to have a booster dose of IPV every 10 years.[7,81] The live, attenuated oral polio vaccine should be avoided in post-SOT patients and their household contacts.

Cholera vaccines have been used to reduce diarrhea rates in healthy travelers going to areas of *Vibrio cholerae* outbreaks, but the efficacy data in immunocompromised hosts are limited.[7,82] The live, attenuated form should be avoided in SOT recipients, but the inactivated form may be considered for travel to cholera endemic and outbreak areas.

Patients going to *Japanese encephalitis virus* endemic areas should receive this inactivated vaccine if they will be in high-risk locations or have a prolonged trip to the area. There are limited data for vaccine efficacy in the SOT population. Accelerated regimens or boosting with 2 doses (days 0 and 28) in SOT recipients are recommended with a booster every year for high-risk travelers.[7,13,83–85]

There are case reports of successful *rabies virus* inactivated vaccine preexposure prophylaxis in renal transplant and pediatric SOT recipients.[86–88] The recommendation for preexposure prophylaxis is a 3-dose regimen (days 0, 7, and 28) for high-risk travelers.[89] Postexposure prophylaxis is recommended in transplant recipients who are discovered retrospectively to have unexpectedly received organs from rabies-infected donors with a 5-dose schedule recommended (days 0, 3, 7, 14, and 28)[90] in conjunction with immunoglobulin depending on the category of exposure.[7,89]

In case an SOT patient needs to receive the *typhoid fever vaccine* for *Salmonella typhi* before travel to an endemic country, the inactivated Vi polysaccharide vaccine is preferred to the oral live, attenuated vaccine.[13] The greatest risk area for travelers is South East Asia.[7,91] A single dose of the vaccine confers protection for 2 years and a booster should be given every 2 years to patients at risk.[1,92]

Yellow fever virus vaccine before SOT can have prolonged seropositivity posttransplantation. In one study, protective antibody level was detectable in 52 of 53 patients.[93] A retrospective review published in 2012 of 19 SOT patients who received the live, attenuated yellow fever vaccine posttransplant did not show any significant side effects.[94] Death has been reported after vaccine administration in immunosuppressed individuals in the past due to viscerotropic and neurotropic vaccine–related disease and for that reason it remains contraindicated after SOT.[7,95] SOT recipients will need a physician note to excuse them from the vaccine in order to enter certain countries that require vaccination for entrance.

Table 2
Summary of vaccine recommendations for solid organ transplant candidates or recipients

Vaccine	Inactivated/ Live Attenuated (I/LA)	Candidates	Dose	Timing	Monitor Vaccine Titers	Comments
MMR	LA	Seronegative for ≥1 of the 3 viruses, especially for measles or mumps	1–2 doses	• 4 wk before transplant	Yes	Check for seroresponse >4 wk after vaccine
Varicella	LA	Seronegative for VZV	1–2 doses	• 4 wk before transplant	Yes	Check for seroresponse >4 wk after vaccine
Herpes Zoster	LA	Aged ≥50 y regardless of VZV immunity	1 dose	• 4 wk before transplant	No	New inactivated vaccine approved in October 2017
Influenza	I	All candidates	1 dose	Before Influenza season	No	Consider the high-dose formulation
HPV	I	Ages 9–26 y	3 doses	Before or after transplant	No	
Pneumococcal PPSV-23	I	All candidates if ≤2 doses in the past	Every 5 y	Before or after transplant	No	
Pneumococcal PCV-13	I	All candidates if not yet received	1 lifetime dose (give 1 y after last PPSV-23 dose)	Before or after transplant	No	
DPaT/Tdap	I	All candidates if not previously received	Every 7–10 y	Before or after transplant	No	

(continued on next page)

Table 2
(continued)

Vaccine	Inactivated/ Live Attenuated (I/LA)	Candidates	Dose	Timing	Monitor Vaccine Titers	Comments
Inactivated polio	I	All candidates if not previously received; one booster dose recommended to adults traveling to endemic areas	3 doses to children or unvaccinated adults	Before or after transplant	No	
Cholera (CVD 103-HgR)	LA	Candidates traveling to endemic areas or outbreaks	1 dose	Before transplant only if high-risk travel	No	There are no safety or efficacy data in immunosuppressed patients There are inactivated oral cholera vaccines available directly from the manufacturer
Japanese encephalitis	I	Candidates traveling to endemic areas for >1 mo or <1 mo in areas of increased transmission	2 doses at 0 and 28 d	Before or after transplant	No	
HAV	I	Seronegative for anti-HAV	2 doses at 0 and 6 mo	Before or after transplant	Yes	Recommended for foreign travel or before liver or intestinal transplant
HBV	I	Seronegative for anti-HBs	3 doses at 0, 1 and 6 mo	Before or after transplant	Yes	
Rabies	I	High-risk travelers defined by WHO[a]	3 doses at 0, 7, and 21 or 28 d	Before or after transplant	No	Postexposure 5 doses at 0, 3, 7, 14, and 28, plus rabies immunoglobulin
Typhoid fever	LA or I	Candidates traveling to endemic areas	1 dose	Before or after transplant	No	Use inactivated vaccine only after transplant

Yellow fever	LA	Candidates traveling to endemic areas	1 lifetime dose	Before transplant	No	Posttransplant patients will require medical note to enter certain countries without vaccine because it is contraindicated after transplant
Meningococcal conjugate (MenACWY and MPSV4)	I	Candidates with asplenia, college students, and military personnel	2 doses, 8 wk apart	Before or after transplant	Yes	Every 3 y as needed depending on titers
Serogroup B meningococcal	I	Candidates aged ≥10 y with persistent complement deficiencies, patients taking eculizumab, or those at increased risk from serogroup B meningococcal disease outbreak	MenB-FHbp: 3 doses MenB-4C: 2 doses	Before or after transplant	Yes	Asplenic patients should receive both the meningococcal conjugate and serogroup B vaccines
Hib	I	Candidates with asplenia	1–2 doses separated by 4–8 wk	Before or after transplant	Yes	Measuring titers at least once may be helpful

Abbreviation: WHO, World Health Organization.

[a] Candidates at high risk are those who will be at increased risk of exposure to rabies virus (eg, laboratory workers dealing with the virus, veterinarians, and animal handlers). Other group that is at high risk includes travelers with extensive outdoor exposure in rural high-risk areas where immediate access to appropriate medical care may be limited.[84]

SUMMARY

A vaccination protocol pretransplantation is the best way to provide all the needed vaccines to an SOT candidate or recipient (**Table 2**). The recommendation is to complete all necessary vaccines before transplantation, ideally at least 4 weeks before transplantation, because after transplantation the immunosuppressive therapy will decrease the vaccine immune response. Live, attenuated vaccines remain contraindicated after transplantation, but inactivated vaccines can be given after transplant safely. The optimal timing to begin posttransplant vaccination is 6 months after transplantation but should be individualized for each patient. Additional vaccines are required for SOT candidates or recipients with asplenia, persistent complement deficiencies, or at increased risk for meningococcal disease (college students, military personnel, and during outbreaks). In those scenarios, the SOT candidates and recipients should receive the meningococcal and Hib vaccines. An individualized evaluation should be done in travelers to foreign countries according to each patient's risks. In conclusion, the current evidence favors the use of live, attenuated vaccines before transplantation, and the inactivated vaccines could be safely used before or after transplantation.

REFERENCES

1. Chong PP, Avery RK. A comprehensive review of immunization practices in solid organ transplant and hematopoietic stem cell transplant recipients. Clin Ther 2017;39(8):1581–98.
2. Blumberg EA, Brozena SC, Stutman P, et al. Immunogenicity of pneumococcal vaccine in heart transplant recipients. Clin Infect Dis 2001;32(2):307–10.
3. Danziger-Isakov L, Kumar D. Vaccination in solid organ transplantation. Am J Transplant 2013;13(Suppl 4):311–7.
4. Cowan M, Chon WJ, Desai A, et al. Impact of immunosuppression on recall immune responses to influenza vaccination in stable renal transplant recipients. Transplantation 2014;97(8):846–53.
5. Felldin M, Andersson B, Studahl M, et al. Antibody persistence 1 year after pandemic H1N1 2009 influenza vaccination and immunogenicity of subsequent seasonal influenza vaccine among adult organ transplant patients. Transpl Int 2014;27(2):197–203.
6. Gerrits JH, van de Wetering J, Weimar W, et al. T-cell reactivity during tapering of immunosuppression to low-dose monotherapy prednisolone in HLA-identical living-related renal transplant recipients. Transplantation 2009;87(6):907–14.
7. Trubiano JA, Johnson D, Sohail A, et al. Travel vaccination recommendations and endemic infection risks in solid organ transplantation recipients. J Travel Med 2016;23(6) [pii:taw058].
8. Stark K, Gunther M, Neuhaus R, et al. Immunogenicity and safety of hepatitis A vaccine in liver and renal transplant recipients. J Infect Dis 1999;180(6):2014–7.
9. Mulley WR, Visvanathan K, Hurt AC, et al. Mycophenolate and lower graft function reduce the seroresponse of kidney transplant recipients to pandemic H1N1 vaccination. Kidney Int 2012;82(2):212–9.
10. Salles MJ, Sens YA, Boas LS, et al. Influenza virus vaccination in kidney transplant recipients: serum antibody response to different immunosuppressive drugs. Clin Transplant 2010;24(1):E17–23.
11. Orcurto A, Pascual M, Hoschler K, et al. Impact of anti-T-cell therapy in the immunogenicity of seasonal influenza vaccine in kidney transplant recipients. Transplantation 2012;94(6):630–6.

12. Kotton CN. Vaccination and immunization against travel-related diseases in immunocompromised hosts. Expert Rev Vaccines 2008;7(5):663–72.
13. Kotton CN, Hibberd PL. Travel medicine and the solid organ transplant recipient. Am J Transplant 2009;9(Suppl 4):S273–81.
14. Rubin LG, Levin MJ, Ljungman P, et al. 2013 IDSA clinical practice guideline for vaccination of the immunocompromised host. Clin Infect Dis 2014;58(3):309–18.
15. Rubin RH, Tolkoff-Rubin NE. Infection in the organ transplant patient; the Hegelian dialectic of transplantation. Trans Med Soc Lond 1994;111:81–90.
16. Peleg AY, Husain S, Kwak EJ, et al. Opportunistic infections in 547 organ transplant recipients receiving alemtuzumab, a humanized monoclonal CD-52 antibody. Clin Infect Dis 2007;44(2):204–12.
17. Issa NC, Fishman JA. Infectious complications of antilymphocyte therapies in solid organ transplantation. Clin Infect Dis 2009;48(6):772–86.
18. Nazi I. The effect of rituximab on vaccine responses in patients with immune thrombocytopenia. Blood 2013;122(11):1946–53.
19. Pandit A, Leblebjian H, Hammond SP, et al. Safety of live-attenuated measles-mumps-rubella and herpes zoster vaccination in multiple myeloma patients on maintenance lenalidomide or bortezomib after autologous hematopoietic cell transplantation. Bone Marrow Transplant 2018. [Epub ahead of print].
20. Schönermarck U, Kauke T, Jäger G, et al. Effect of apheresis for ABO and HLA desensitization on anti-measles antibody titers in renal transplantation. J Transplant 2011. Article ID 869065; 1–6.
21. Huebner RE, Schein MF, Bass JB Jr. The tuberculin skin test. Clin Infect Dis 1993; 17(6):968–75.
22. Verolet CM, Posfay-Barbe KM. Live virus vaccines in transplantation: friend or foe? Curr Infect Dis Rep 2015;17(4):472.
23. Croce E, Hatz C, Jonker EF, et al. Safety of live vaccinations on immunosuppressive therapy in patients with immune-mediated inflammatory diseases, solid organ transplantation or after bone-marrow transplantation - A systematic review of randomized trials, observational studies and case reports. Vaccine 2017; 35(9):1216–26.
24. Maluf DG, Stravitz RT, Cotterell AH, et al. Adult living donor versus deceased donor liver transplantation: a 6-year single center experience. Am J Transplant 2005;5(1):149–56.
25. Gruttadauria S, Vasta F, Mandala L, et al. Basiliximab in a triple-drug regimen with tacrolimus and steroids in liver transplantation. Transplant Proc 2005;37(6): 2611–3.
26. Ma Y, Wang GD, He XS, et al. Clinical and pathological analysis of acute rejection following orthotopic liver transplantation. Chin Med J 2009;122(12):1400–3.
27. Smith CK, McNeal MM, Meyer NR, et al. Rotavirus shedding in premature infants following first immunization. Vaccine 2011;29(45):8141–6.
28. Cortese MM, Parashar UD. Prevention of rotavirus gastroenteritis among infants and children: recommendations of the Advisory Committee on Immunization Practices (ACIP). MMWR Recomm Rep 2009;58(Rr-2):1–25.
29. Anderson EJ. Rotavirus vaccines: viral shedding and risk of transmission. Lancet Infect Dis 2008;8(10):642–9.
30. Center for Disease Control and Prevention. Altered immunocompetence. general best practice guidelines for immunization: best practices guidance of the advisory committee on immunization practices (ACIP). 2017. Available at: https://www.cdc.gov/vaccines/hcp/acip-recs/index.html. Accessed January 6, 2018.

31. DeVries AS, Harper J, Murray A, et al. Vaccine-derived poliomyelitis 12 years after infection in Minnesota. N Engl J Med 2011;364(24):2316–23.

32. Paralytic poliomyelitis–United States, 1980-1994. MMWR Morb Mortal Wkly Rep 1997;46(4):79–83.

33. Danerseau AM, Robinson JL. Efficacy and safety of measles, mumps, rubella and varicella live viral vaccines in transplant recipients receiving immunosuppressive drugs. World J Pediatr 2008;4(4):254–8.

34. Neu AM, Warady BA, Furth SL, et al. Antibody levels to diphtheria, tetanus, and rubella in infants vaccinated while on PD: a Study of the Pediatric Peritoneal Dialysis Study Consortium. Adv Perit Dial 1997;13:297–9.

35. Flynn JT, Frisch K, Kershaw DB, et al. Response to early measles-mumps-rubella vaccination in infants with chronic renal failure and/or receiving peritoneal dialysis. Adv peritoneal Dial Conf Peritoneal Dial 1999;15:269–72.

36. Turner A, Jeyaratnam D, Haworth F, et al. Measles-associated encephalopathy in children with renal transplants. Am J Transplant 2006;6(6):1459–65.

37. Rand EB, McCarthy CA, Whitington PF. Measles vaccination after orthotopic liver transplantation. J Pediatr 1993;123(1):87–9.

38. Shinjoh M, Miyairi I, Hoshino K, et al. Effective and safe immunizations with live-attenuated vaccines for children after living donor liver transplantation. Vaccine 2008;26(52):6859–63.

39. Kawano Y, Suzuki M, Kawada J, et al. Effectiveness and safety of immunization with live-attenuated and inactivated vaccines for pediatric liver transplantation recipients. Vaccine 2015;33(12):1440–5.

40. Olson AD, Shope TC, Flynn JT. Pretransplant varicella vaccination is cost-effective in pediatric renal transplantation. Pediatr Transplant 2001;5(1):44–50.

41. Donati M, Zuckerman M, Dhawan A, et al. Response to varicella immunization in pediatric liver transplant recipients. Transplantation 2000;70(9):1401–4.

42. Khan S, Erlichman J, Rand EB. Live virus immunization after orthotopic liver transplantation. Pediatr Transplant 2006;10(1):78–82.

43. Weinberg A, Horslen SP, Kaufman SS, et al. Safety and immunogenicity of varicella-zoster virus vaccine in pediatric liver and intestine transplant recipients. Am J Transplant 2006;6(3):565–8.

44. Posfay-Barbe KM, Pittet LF, Sottas C, et al. Varicella-zoster immunization in pediatric liver transplant recipients: safe and immunogenic. Am J Transplant 2012;12(11):2974–85.

45. Levitsky J, Te HS, Faust TW, et al. Varicella infection following varicella vaccination in a liver transplant recipient. Am J Transplant 2002;2(9):880–2.

46. Kraft JN, Shaw JC. Varicella infection caused by Oka strain vaccine in a heart transplant recipient. Arch Dermatol 2006;142(7):943–5.

47. Cohen JI. Strategies for herpes zoster vaccination of immunocompromised patients. J Infect Dis 2008;197(Suppl 2):S237–41.

48. U.S. Food and Drug administration. Shingrix. Vaccines Licensed for Use in the United States. 2017. Available at: https://www.fda.gov/BiologicsBloodVaccines/Vaccines/ApprovedProducts/ucm581491.htm. Accessed January 6, 2018.

49. Ison MG. Influenza prevention and treatment in transplant recipients and immunocompromised hosts. Influenza Other Respir Viruses 2013;7(Suppl 3):60–6.

50. Perez-Romero P, Bulnes-Ramos A, Torre-Cisneros J, et al. Influenza vaccination during the first 6 months after solid organ transplantation is efficacious and safe. Clin Microbiol Infect 2015;21(11):1040.e11-8.

51. Kumar D, Campbell P, Hoschler K, et al. Randomized controlled trial of adjuvanted versus nonadjuvanted influenza vaccine in kidney transplant recipients. Transplantation 2016;100(3):662–9.

52. Baluch A, Humar A, Eurich D, et al. Randomized controlled trial of high-dose intradermal versus standard-dose intramuscular influenza vaccine in organ transplant recipients. Am J Transplant 2013;13(4):1026–33.

53. Cordero E, Roca-Oporto C, Bulnes-Ramos A, et al. Two doses of inactivated influenza vaccine improve immune response in solid organ transplant recipients: results of TRANSGRIPE 1-2, a randomized controlled clinical trial. Clin Infect Dis 2017;64(7):829–38.

54. GiaQuinta S, Michaels MG, McCullers JA, et al. Randomized, double-blind comparison of standard-dose vs. high-dose trivalent inactivated influenza vaccine in pediatric solid organ transplant patients. Pediatr Transplant 2015;19(2):219–28.

55. Natori Y, Shiotsuka M, Slomovic J, et al. A double blind randomized trial of high dose vs. standard dose influenza vaccine in adult solid organ transplant recipients. Clin Infect Dis 2018;66(11):1698–704.

56. King JC Jr, Treanor J, Fast PE, et al. Comparison of the safety, vaccine virus shedding, and immunogenicity of influenza virus vaccine, trivalent, types A and B, live cold-adapted, administered to human immunodeficiency virus (HIV)-infected and non-HIV-infected adults. J Infect Dis 2000;181(2):725–8.

57. Halasa N, Englund JA, Nachman S, et al. Safety of live attenuated influenza vaccine in mild to moderately immunocompromised children with cancer. Vaccine 2011;29(24):4110–5.

58. Madeleine MM, Finch JL, Lynch CF, et al. HPV-related cancers after solid organ transplantation in the United States. Am J Transplant 2013;13(12):3202–9.

59. Grulich AE, van Leeuwen MT, Falster MO, et al. Incidence of cancers in people with HIV/AIDS compared with immunosuppressed transplant recipients: a meta-analysis. Lancet 2007;370(9581):59–67.

60. Kumar D, Unger ER, Panicker G, et al. Immunogenicity of quadrivalent human papillomavirus vaccine in organ transplant recipients. Am J Transplant 2013; 13(9):2411–7.

61. Kumar D, Humar A, Plevneshi A, et al. Invasive pneumococcal disease in solid organ transplant recipients–10-year prospective population surveillance. Am J Transplant 2007;7(5):1209–14.

62. Center for Disease Control and Prevention. Use of 13-valent pneumococcal conjugate vaccine and 23-valent pneumococcal polysaccharide vaccine for adults with immunocompromising conditions: recommendations of the Advisory Committee on Immunization Practices (ACIP). MMWR Morb Mortal Wkly Rep 2012; 61(40):816–9.

63. Center for Disease Control and Prevention. Use of 13-valent pneumococcal conjugate vaccine and 23-valent pneumococcal polysaccharide vaccine among children aged 6-18 years with immunocompromising conditions: recommendations of the Advisory Committee on Immunization Practices (ACIP). MMWR Morb Mortal Wkly Rep 2013;62(25):521–4.

64. Licensure of a 13-valent pneumococcal conjugate vaccine (PCV13) and recommendations for use among children - Advisory Committee on Immunization Practices (ACIP), 2010. MMWR Morb Mortal Wkly Rep 2010;59(9):258–61.

65. Kumar D, Rotstein C, Miyata G, et al. Randomized, double-blind, controlled trial of pneumococcal vaccination in renal transplant recipients. J Infect Dis 2003; 187(10):1639–45.

66. Kumar D, Chen MH, Wong G, et al. A randomized, double-blind, placebo-controlled trial to evaluate the prime-boost strategy for pneumococcal vaccination in adult liver transplant recipients. Clin Infect Dis 2008;47(7):885–92.

67. Enke BU, Bokenkamp A, Offner G, et al. Response to diphtheria and tetanus booster vaccination in pediatric renal transplant recipients. Transplantation 1997;64(2):237–41.

68. Ghio L, Pedrazzi C, Assael BM, et al. Immunity to diphtheria and tetanus in a young population on a dialysis regimen or with a renal transplant. J Pediatr 1997;130(6):987–9.

69. Sester M, Gartner BC, Girndt M, et al. Vaccination of the solid organ transplant recipient. Transplant Rev (Orlando) 2008;22(4):274–84.

70. Garcia Garrido HM, Wieten RW, Grobusch MP, et al. Response to hepatitis A vaccination in immunocompromised travelers. J Infect Dis 2015;212(3):378–85.

71. Gunther M, Stark K, Neuhaus R, et al. Rapid decline of antibodies after hepatitis A immunization in liver and renal transplant recipients. Transplantation 2001;71(3):477–9.

72. Michel ML, Tiollais P. Hepatitis B vaccines: protective efficacy and therapeutic potential. Pathol Biol (Paris) 2010;58(4):288–95.

73. Weinstein T, Chagnac A, Boaz M, et al. Improved immunogenicity of a novel third-generation recombinant hepatitis B vaccine in patients with end-stage renal disease. Nephron Clin Pract 2004;97(2):c67–72.

74. Jacobson IM, Jaffers G, Dienstag JL, et al. Immunogenicity of hepatitis B vaccine in renal transplant recipients. Transplantation 1985;39(4):393–5.

75. Villeneuve E, Vincelette J, Villeneuve JP. Ineffectiveness of hepatitis B vaccination in cirrhotic patients waiting for liver transplantation. Can J Gastroenterol 2000;14(Suppl B):59b–62b.

76. Kallinowski B, Benz C, Buchholz L, et al. Accelerated schedule of hepatitis B vaccination in liver transplant candidates. Transplant Proc 1998;30(3):797–9.

77. Center for Disease Control and Prevention. Hepatitis B information. 2016. Available at: https://www.cdc.gov/hepatitis/HBV/HBVfaq.htm. Accessed January 7, 2018.

78. Folaranmi T, Rubin L, Martin SW, et al. Use of serogroup b meningococcal vaccines in persons aged >/=10 years at increased risk for serogroup b meningococcal disease: recommendations of the advisory committee on immunization practices, 2015. MMWR Morb Mortal Wkly Rep 2015;64(22):608–12.

79. Wyplosz B, Derradji O, Hong E, et al. Low immunogenicity of quadrivalent meningococcal vaccines in solid organ transplant recipients. Transpl Infect Dis 2015;17(2):322–7.

80. Huzly D, Neifer S, Reinke P, et al. Routine immunizations in adult renal transplant recipients. Transplantation 1997;63(6):839–45.

81. Danzinger-Isakov L, Kumar D. Guidelines for vaccination of solid organ transplant candidates and recipients. Am J Transplant 2009;9(Suppl 4):S258–62.

82. WHO Publication. Cholera vaccines: WHO position paper-Recommendations. Vaccine 2010;28(30):4687–8.

83. World Health Organization. Japanese encephalitis vaccines: WHO position paper, February 2015-recommendations. Vaccine 2016;34(3):302–3.

84. Schuller E, Jilma B, Voicu V, et al. Long-term immunogenicity of the new Vero cell-derived, inactivated Japanese encephalitis virus vaccine IC51 Six and 12 month results of a multicenter follow-up phase 3 study. Vaccine 2008;26(34):4382–6.

85. Tauber E, Kollaritsch H, von Sonnenburg F, et al. Randomized, double-blind, placebo-controlled phase 3 trial of the safety and tolerability of IC51, an inactivated Japanese encephalitis vaccine. J Infect Dis 2008;198(4):493–9.

86. Cramer CH 2nd, Shieck V, Thomas SE, et al. Immune response to rabies vaccination in pediatric transplant patients. Pediatr Transplant 2008;12(8):874–7.

87. Rodriguez-Romo R, Morales-Buenrostro LE, Lecuona L, et al. Immune response after rabies vaccine in a kidney transplant recipient. Transpl Infect Dis 2011; 13(5):492–5.

88. Kuzmin IV, Bozick B, Guagliardo SA, et al. Bats, emerging infectious diseases, and the rabies paradigm revisited. Emerg Health Threats J 2011;4:7159.

89. WHO Publication. Rabies vaccines: WHO position paper–recommendations. Vaccine 2010;28(44):7140–2.

90. Vora NM, Orciari LA, Niezgoda M, et al. Clinical management and humoral immune responses to rabies post-exposure prophylaxis among three patients who received solid organs from a donor with rabies. Transpl Infect Dis 2015; 17(3):389–95.

91. Parry CM, Hien TT, Dougan G, et al. Typhoid fever. N Engl J Med 2002;347(22): 1770–82.

92. Jackson BR, Iqbal S, Mahon B. Updated recommendations for the use of typhoid vaccine–Advisory Committee on Immunization Practices, United States, 2015. MMWR Morb Mortal Wkly Rep 2015;64(11):305–8.

93. Wyplosz B, Burdet C, Francois H, et al. Persistence of yellow fever vaccine-induced antibodies after solid organ transplantation. Am J Transplant 2013; 13(9):2458–61.

94. Azevedo LS, Lasmar EP, Contieri FL, et al. Yellow fever vaccination in organ transplanted patients: is it safe? A multicenter study. Transpl Infect Dis 2012;14(3): 237–41.

95. Kengsakul K, Sathirapongsasuti K, Punyagupta S. Fatal myeloencephalitis following yellow fever vaccination in a case with HIV infection. J Med Assoc Thai 2002;85(1):131–4.

Strategies for Antimicrobial Stewardship in Solid Organ Transplant Recipients

Jonathan Hand, MD

KEYWORDS

- Antimicrobial stewardship • Solid organ transplant • Immunocompromised hosts
- Rapid diagnostics

KEY POINTS

- Complications of antimicrobial therapy, such as multidrug-resistant organisms and *C difficile*, commonly affect solid-organ transplant (SOT) recipients and have been associated with graft loss and mortality.
- Although published experience with antimicrobial stewardship program (ASP) interventions in SOT recipients is limited, opportunities exist to optimize timing, choice, dose, and duration of antibacterials, antifungals, and antivirals.
- A patient-centered, multidisciplinary strategy engaging frontline transplant providers and transplant infectious diseases specialists is essential for successful creation and implementation of ASP initiatives.
- Integration of the ASP with the laboratory is important when obtaining, implementing, and optimizing rapid technologies used in transplant recipients.
- Prioritization of global and local antimicrobial stewardship in the growing SOT population is needed.

INTRODUCTION

In the United States, antimicrobial stewardship programs (ASPs) are mandated by government regulations and the Centers for Disease Control and Prevention has proposed implementation guidance.[1] Global increases in multidrug-resistant organisms (MDROs) parallel increases of such infections within solid-organ transplant (SOT) recipients and have been associated with significant graft loss and mortality.[2,3] Early initiation of appropriate antimicrobials for infected SOT patients is associated with improved outcomes, although efficacy of empiric therapy is less likely for patients with MDR infections.[4,5] Similarly, the incidence of *Clostridium difficile* infection (CDI) in this population is rising and characterized by more severe disease, frequent

Disclosures: No commercial or financial conflicts of interest. No funding sources.
Department of Infectious Diseases, The University of Queensland School of Medicine, Ochsner Clinical School, Ochsner Medical Center, 1514 Jefferson Highway, New Orleans, LA 70121, USA
E-mail address: Jonathan.hand@ochsner.org

Infect Dis Clin N Am 32 (2018) 535–550
https://doi.org/10.1016/j.idc.2018.04.003
0891-5520/18/© 2018 Elsevier Inc. All rights reserved.

id.theclinics.com

recurrences, and graft loss.[6–8] There are limited treatment options for MDROs, and antibiotic exposure remains the principal risk factor for CDI. Therefore, transplant providers and programmatic interventions focusing on prevention are fundamental. Furthermore, the unrealized microbiome effects of dysbiosis, altering immune function, may predispose to allograft rejection.[9] To date, published literature related to safety and efficacy of antibiotic stewardship strategies in SOT recipients is limited, although implementation challenges in immunocompromised hosts have been described.[10] This review evaluates the evidence and best practices of antimicrobial stewardship in SOT and describes opportunities to optimize diagnostics and antimicrobial delivery, focused on improving patient outcomes.

DEFINITION AND STATE OF ANTIMICROBIAL STEWARDSHIP IN SOLID-ORGAN TRANSPLANTATION

Antimicrobial stewardship is defined in a multisociety consensus document as "coordinated interventions designed to improve and measure the appropriate use of [antibiotic] agents by promoting the selection of the optimal [antibiotic] drug regimen including dosing, duration of therapy, and route of administration."[11] A recent review by Dyar and colleagues[12] summarizes antimicrobial stewardship as "A coherent set of actions which promote using antimicrobials responsibly." Unfortunately, given the paucity of data on ASP interventions and outcomes in the SOT population, consensus guidelines only offer limited direction regarding these patients.[13] Similarly, in 2013 guidelines published by the American Society of Transplantation there was no mention of stewardship and clear implementation strategies were not defined.[14] Patient-level opportunities for ASPs in transplantation do exist and have been recently highlighted.[15] Although published studies are limited, 74% of transplant centers include adult SOT recipients in their institutional ASP activities.[16] **Table 1** highlights intervention strategies for ASPs in SOT.

DEFINING THE ANTIMICROBIAL STEWARDSHIP TEAM

ASPs are traditionally led by a physician and pharmacist with experience or interest in infectious diseases. A recently validated staffing calculator from the Veterans Health Administration system determined 1.0 clinical pharmacist full-time equivalent per 100 occupied beds was needed to perform activities of an ASP in the general hospitalized population.[17] This employee need calculation should be a minimum requirement for large transplant programs where transplant infectious diseases (TID) pharmacists may be needed. Although TID-specific pharmacists are rare and not mandated, involvement of a TID physician in the ASP may be beneficial given the team integration, SOT patient and provider familiarity, and clinical expertise. This relationship may lead to more in-person stewardship interventions. In a recent study by Messacar and colleagues[18] conducted in a pediatric hospital that cares for SOT recipients, investigators found in-person feedback, or "handshake stewardship," decreased antibiotic use and increased infectious diseases consultation. TID participation in SOT recipients' care has been associated with more stewardship-concordant therapy, decreased mortality, and lower readmission rates.[5,15] In a recent survey of mostly North American transplant centers, 36 of 42 programs reported a dedicated TID program, and the median ratio of SOT patients transplanted annually to faculty dedicated to TID was 72 (range, 15–259). TID providers involvement in ASPs were not evaluated.[19] Nursing ASP team members are also recommended and their involvement has been extensively described.[20] Transplant-unit nurses are

Table 1
Antimicrobial stewardship intervention strategies in solid-organ transplant recipients

Pharmacy and therapeutics committee involvement • Formulary review and restriction	Add new drugs for MDROs and CDI Manage shortages pertinent to SOT
Dose optimization	PK/PD strategies for antibiotics, antivirals, antifungals (TDM)
Agent selection • Antibiotic allergy delabeling	Transplant-specific antibiogram PCN skin testing or allergy assessment
Preauthorization and prospective audit and feedback	Most commonly used in transplant centers
Intravenous-to-oral conversion	Targeting antibiotic, antiviral, and antifungal drugs
Clinical practice guidelines for common infectious syndromes	Institution specific, treatment and prophylaxis, combining local epidemiology and published recommendations Assess adherence and provide feedback Implement EMR-based clinical decision support
Syndrome targets	*Staphylococcus aureus* bacteremia, candidemia, asymptomatic bacteriuria, surgical site infections, CMV (treatment and prophylaxis), viral respiratory pathogens
Education	Discuss local and published data and reasons for interventions with frontline providers
Metrics	Process and outcome measures specific to SOT population
Rapid diagnostics	Working closely with laboratory is imperative for implementation and rapid communication of results

Abbreviations: CMV, cytomegalovirus; EMR, electronic medical record; PCN, penicillin; PK/PD, pharmacokinetics/pharmacodynamics; TDM, therapeutic drug monitoring.

effectively positioned to apply these best practices in transplant recipients. **Fig. 1** provides suggested SOT ASP team members.

APPROACHING IMPLEMENTATION OF ANTIMICROBIAL STEWARDSHIP PROGRAMS IN SOLID-ORGAN TRANSPLANTATION

Prioritizing hospital leadership support for ASPs is essential.[21] But, participation of SOT practitioners involved with direct patient care (ie, physicians, midlevel providers, pharmacists, nurses) is critical for ASP success. Successful multidisciplinary approaches to define antimicrobial appropriateness have been described and included transplant patients.[22] Similarly, a change in management framework to implement stewardship-focused guidelines in immunocompromised hosts has been reported. The core design elements consisted of governance and leadership, stakeholder engagement, and work flow analysis and integration. Successful implementation required communication, training and education, and monitoring with evaluation.[23] At the heart of these initiatives is an understanding of institutional prescribing cultures within the context of transplantation. Therefore, programs should evaluate emotional and experiential behaviors that influence SOT providers' prescribing.[24] **Table 2** summarizes ASP strategy implementation examples and resources in SOT recipients.

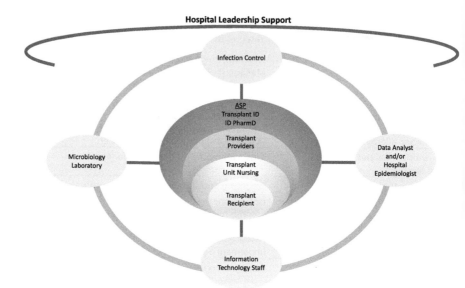

Fig. 1. The antimicrobial stewardship program team in solid-organ transplantation.

INTERVENTIONS
Formulary Review

ASP practitioners should be involved in institutional formulary review with direct pharmacy and therapeutics committee participation. Understanding MDROs that disproportionately affect this population and the costly, broad-spectrum new drugs recently approved to treat these infections enables ASPs to advocate for formulary changes. Moreover, ASPs in SOT are positioned to advocate for and identify specific formulary medications to restrict where needed. Formulary restriction is a common strategy and used in most transplant centers.[16] Involvement of pharmacy administration is needed to best manage critical shortages of drugs and vaccines affecting this population.[25]

Dose Optimization

Pharmacokinetics- and pharmacodynamics-based dosing strategies for certain drugs are recommended.[13] Dosing in complex transplant scenarios, such as critical illness, impaired renal function, or renal-replacement therapy, is still being studied.[26,27] Accounting for pathophysiologic differences in patients with cystic fibrosis or other end-stage organ disease in the pretransplant and post-transplant setting is not completely understood. Unpredictability of pharmacokinetics and pharmacodynamics parameters have shifted research to focus on individualized antimicrobial dosing strategies.[28] Importance of antiviral pharmacokinetics and pharmacodynamics has been recognized and dosing by these principles may lead to improved treatment response, decreased toxicities, and less resistant cytomegalovirus (CMV) infections.[29–31] ASP pharmacists are also important in managing antifungal drugs that have unclear clinically relevant therapeutic ranges, toxicities, drug-drug interactions, and high costs.[32] Evidence and guidance for antifungal therapeutic drug monitoring has been summarized previously and is associated with improved outcomes.[33] However, in-house triazole level testing is not standard at most transplant institutions.[16]

Table 2
Antimicrobial stewardship in solid-organ transplant recipients: strategy implementation examples and resources

Summary	References
Audits assessing ASP-concordant care	So et al,[15] 2016
Survey of ASP practices in SOT/HCT centers	Seo et al,[16] 2016
TID involvement in SOT patient care	Hamandi et al,[5] 2014
Survey of TID centers' program resources	Schaenman et al,[19] 2017
GCV/vGCV dosing optimization	Gagermeier et al,[29] 2014 Kiser et al,[30] 2012 Padulles et al,[31] 2016 Asberg et al,[46] 2007
Antifungal drug dosing optimization	Lempers et al,[32] 2015 Ashbee et al,[33] 2014 Hamdy et al,[47] 2017
Antibiograms	Rosa et al,[36] 2016 Korayem et al,[37] 2018
Antimicrobial allergy labels	Trubiano et al,[43] 2016 Khumra et al,[44] 2017
Prospective audit and feedback	So et al,[45] 2017
Institutional guidelines	Husain & So,[49] 2017
Asymptomatic bacteriuria and urinary complications	Origuen et al,[62] 2016 Patel et al,[64] 2017
Surgical site infection prevention	Frenette et al,[65] 2016 Anesi et al,[66] 2018
Respiratory viral infection management	Paulsen & Danziger-Isakov,[73] 2017
Microbiology laboratory and transplant care	Perez et al,[77] 2012
Procalcitonin-based antimicrobial management	Sandkovsky et al,[81] 2015 Sato et al,[82] 2016 Franeková et al,[84] 2017
Iron-related markers and infection	Chow et al,[83] 2017
Immune-monitoring strategies to predict infection	Fernandez-Ruiz et al,[85] 2014 Mian et al,[86] 2018
CMV cell-mediated immunity monitoring	Kumar et al,[69] 2017 San-Juan et al,[70] 2015 Lisboa et al,[71] 2012 Manuel et al,[72] 2013
Fungal biomarkers	Singh & Husain,[88] 2013 Husain et al,[89] 2016 Ambasta et al,[90] 2015 Levesque et al,[94] 2015 Singh et al,[95] 2015

Abbreviations: CMV, cytomegalovirus; GCV/vGCV, ganciclovir/valganciclovir; HCT, hematopoietic cell transplantation; TID, transplant infectious diseases.

Antimicrobial Agent Selection

Inadequate therapy for transplant patients infected with MDROs is common and has been associated with a 3.5-fold increase in mortality (See Michele Bartoletti and colleagues' article, "Multidrug Resistant Bacterial Infections in Solid Organ Transplant Candidates and Recipients," in this issue).[4,34] Mortality remains high even when appropriate empiric therapy is used, increasing the importance of adequate, early treatment.[35] Antibiograms, detailing hospital and unit-specific antimicrobial susceptibility patterns, remain instrumental in selecting appropriate therapy. Although transplant unit-specific antibiograms are infrequently created, they may report significantly more resistant gram-negative isolates when compared with hospital-wide antibiograms.[16,36] Similarly, urine-specific antibiograms for kidney transplant recipients have demonstrated variance from institutional resistance patterns.[37]

Antibiotic Allergy Assessment

Antibiotic allergy labeling, specifically β-lactam allergy labels, have been associated with poor patient outcomes.[38–41] Consequently, allergy assessments and penicillin skin testing are recommended for patients with such labels.[13] Poor outcomes in immunocompromised patients with β-lactam allergy labels have also been reported and are disproportionately high in SOT patients.[42,43] Similarly, in a small cohort of liver transplant recipients antibiotic allergy labeling rates were high and associated with a nonsignificant increase in MDROs and CDI. A total of 23% of these patients had their antibiotic allergy label quickly delabeled suggesting allergy assessments should be consistently performed to potentially prevent poor patient outcomes.[44]

Preauthorization and Prospective Audit and Feedback

Antimicrobial preauthorization requires approval of restricted antibiotics by ASP practitioners before administration. Prospective audit and feedback involves evaluation of the antimicrobial prescribed with subsequent ASP optimization if warranted. Both strategies are the most common interventions used in SOT centers.[16] Although evaluation of their efficacy in SOT is limited, general advantages and disadvantages have been summarized.[13] So and colleagues[45] presented results of prospective audit and feedback in transplant patients demonstrating increases in ASP-concordant care.

Intravenous to Oral Antimicrobial Conversion

Intravenous-to-oral conversion can help patients avoid complications of intravenous catheters, reducing length of stay and costs.[13] Although 59% of transplant centers routinely perform this intervention, there are no studies assessing the feasibility or efficacy in this population.[16] Data gleaned from the VICTOR trial informed more routine use of oral valganciclovir (vGCV) for treatment of nonsevere CMV disease.[46] Guidelines suggest antifungal agents should also be converted from intravenous-to-oral when possible and there is ample opportunity at transplant centers to optimize this practice.[47,48]

Clinical Practice Guidelines

Institution-specific guidelines for common infectious syndromes inform practitioners of evidence and local epidemiology-based prescribing recommendations.[13] Guideline development is common in centers caring for SOT recipients.[16] This process should involve pertinent stakeholders and implementation requires education. An institutional guideline for infections in SOT has been created as an online resource by a Canadian transplant center.[49] This institution reported ASP concordant prescribing in 70% of SOT recipients and was higher when TID consultation was provided (78.5% vs 59.6%; $P = .03$). Inappropriate management was most commonly related to failure to de-escalate, unnecessarily broad-spectrum treatment, and needlessly prolonged duration.[15] Prophylaxis for opportunistic infections is another example of a commonly used clinical practice guideline. Computerized clinical decision support and surveillance systems are helpful for guideline implementation, but are currently used in only 37% of SOT centers with ASPs.[13,16] Vaccination of the general population is an additional tool to prevent MDRO infections and should be applied in the context of ASP in SOT.[50]

Infectious Diseases Syndrome Targets

Optimizing care bundles and other process interventions for Staphylococcus aureus bacteremia, candidemia, and MDR bloodstream infections in SOT patients may not only improve process measures, but also mortality.[51–53] Antifungal stewardship programs have been successful, and establishing yeast susceptibility testing and tracking through an "antifungigram" may enhance candidemia management.[54–57]

With the reported rise of MDR urinary isolates and their associated complications in kidney transplant recipients, asymptomatic bacteriuria is an opportune clinical syndrome to target in this population.[58–60] Retrospective reports have suggested limited benefit in treating asymptomatic bacteriuria in this population.[61] Additionally, a recent prospective, single-center study enrolled patients greater than 2 months after kidney transplant and compared outcomes of patients randomized to receive antibiotic treatment of asymptomatic bacteriuria to those not treated with antibiotics. Investigators found no difference in multiple outcomes including symptomatic urinary tract infection, allograft function and rejection, and mortality.[62] Multicenter European studies aiming to answer a similar question are ongoing.[63] Other nonantimicrobial strategies, such as early ureteral stent removal after kidney transplant, could also be considered with bundled protocol development.[64]

Rates of surgical site infections in SOT are organ dependent and likely preventable. In a single-center study in abdominal transplant recipients, a series of infection control interventions, combined with ASP audit and feedback, significantly decreased surgical site infections.[65] A recent review summarizes evidence-based perioperative antimicrobial strategies to prevent surgical site infections in SOT.[66]

Common Viral Syndrome Targets

Common therapies for CMV, ganciclovir and vGCV, may cause neutropenia, which is associated with poor outcomes and therapy discontinuation in SOT.[67–69] Studies using CMV cell-mediated immune (CMI) guidance have shown postoperative delay of vGCV prophylaxis is safe and associated with a trend toward less CMV disease.[70] Furthermore, CMV-CMI monitoring may guide preemptive CMV management, withholding drug in patients with adequate CMV-CMI response.[71] In centers using universal CMV prophylaxis, CMV-CMI may predict those patients in whom prolongation of vGCV is needed.[72] In a study by Kumar and colleagues[69] secondary prophylaxis was safely discontinued in patients with a positive CMV-CMI response.

Molecular diagnosis is recommended for viral respiratory pathogens and multiplex polymerase chain reaction (PCR) panels are routinely used.[16,73] Prolonged viral shedding is common in immunocompromised hosts and application of viral panel testing in ASPs supporting this population has not been well defined.[73,74] No consensus exists for optimal treatment of respiratory syncytial virus infection in SOT recipients, particularly lung transplant. Yet opportunities exist to create institutional protocols to avoid inappropriate use of costly and potentially toxic ribavirin therapy, intravenous immunoglobulin, and corticosteroids.[73]

Metrics

Although meaningful SOT-specific process and outcome measures related to ASP have not been defined, examples of metrics used to evaluate program interventions have been described.[13] Transplant centers report most frequently monitoring rates of CDI and antimicrobial cost and use, with 23% of centers measuring no specific outcome.[16] Challenges and shortcomings facing interpretations of commonly used process and outcome metrics have led investigators to create and validate new, more nuanced approaches to antimicrobial appropriateness and clinical impact, like the desirability of outcome ranking and the response adjusted for days of antibiotic risk.[75]

THE MICROBIOLOGY LABORATORY: INTEGRATION AND COLLABORATION

The microbiology laboratory is the cornerstone of the ASP and dedicated laboratory space and personnel to care for transplant-specific tests may be needed.[76] Staff with expertise in bacteriology and mycobacteriology, virology, mycology, parasitology, and serologic testing are central to successful programs. Additionally, laboratories must help monitor the needs of the transplant population, evaluating rapidly advancing technologies that require significant capital and justification.[76,77] Occasionally internal validation of nonclinical laboratory technology and methods is needed. Frequent meetings of the ASP team and microbiology laboratory improve relationships and optimize rapid communication of results.[76,78] Appropriate diagnostic test ordering, execution, and result reporting or, "diagnostic stewardship", is necessary to avoid potential harms of inappropriate diagnoses and overtreatment.[79] TID and ASP providers' close work with the laboratory, coupling antimicrobial and diagnostic stewardship, is paramount in the rapidly changing, molecular testing landscape relevant to transplant patients.[80]

RAPID DIAGNOSTICS
Host Biomarkers

The clinical utility of procalcitonin in transplant patients is unclear. Although it has been used successfully, difficulties with interpretation in each specific organ transplanted, lack of clinically relevant defined cutoff values, and unknown optimal test timing challenge its routine use. Higher values have been reported after antithymocyte globulin administration and allograft rejection.[81,82] Unsurprisingly, given these issues, SOT providers reported procalcitonin to be of limited clinical use.[16] Other host biomarkers, such as presepsin, hepcidin, and other iron markers, have also been evaluated in SOT recipients but do not yet have indications for routine use.[83,84] Host immune monitoring strategies to stratify SOT recipients' risk for viral, fungal, and bacterial infections have been studied but their role in ASPs have not been determined.[85,86]

Fungal Biomarkers

The galactomannan (GM) and (1–3)-beta-D-glucan (BDG) assays identify cell wall components and are routinely used to aid in diagnosis and management of invasive aspergillosis (IA) in patients with hematologic disorders. However, in the SOT population serum screening with GM and BDG is not routinely recommended because GM sensitivity is low (approximately 22%) and has a high false-positive rate.[87,88] Similarly, routine use of BDG for IA in SOT is not recommended given suboptimal performance and numerous factors that interfere with the assay.[87–89] In lung transplant recipients bronchoalveolar lavage (BAL) GM for IA seems to be more useful and reliable but variable sensitivity and specificity have been reported.[90] BAL GM is used in preemptive antifungal treatment strategies after cardiothoracic transplant.[89] Additionally, diagnostic performance may improve when serum BDG is combined with BAL GM.[91] Exhaled breath condensate sampling to detect GM in lung transplant recipients has also lacked correlation with IA.[92] Although in-house BDG and GM testing is infrequent,

88% of ASPs involved in hematopoietic cell transplant and SOT considered serum and BAL GM testing to be the most useful.[16] The BDG assay is an adjunctive diagnostic tool to diagnose invasive candidiasis and *Pneumocystis jirovecii* pneumonia. However, data on utility and accuracy in SOT patients are limited and conflicting with poor overall sensitivity and specificity.[93–95]

Culture-Based Molecular Methods

Matrix-assisted laser desorption/ionization time-of-flight mass spectrometry (MALDI TOF MS) can identify bacterial and fungal species from growth in blood cultures or solid media and has been studied in immunocompromised populations.[96] MALDI-TOF MS combined with ASP interventions for patients, including SOT, with bacteremia or candidemia decreased time to optimal antimicrobial therapy.[97] Peptide nucleic acid fluorescent *in situ* hybridization is able to identify bacteria and *Candida* species from positive blood cultures but similar to other rapid diagnostic platforms, may be limited when used in the absence of ASP action.[98,99] Multiplex molecular PCR assays, such as the BioFire FilmArray (BioFire Diagnostics, Salt Lake City, UT) and the Nanosphere Verigene (Nanosphere, Inc, Northbrook, IL) systems, used to detect a variety of blood culture pathogens and resistance markers, have not been specifically evaluated in transplant recipients but seem promising for ASPs. However, it is unclear how detected resistance markers should be interpreted phenotypically and how this affects drug choice. These multiplex panels are available at multiple transplant centers and are perceived as useful.[16] Promising, cost-effective platforms for rapid identification are being investigated.[100]

Nonculture-Based Molecular Methods

The use and effectiveness of PCR testing for *Aspergillus* and *Candida* on blood and BAL specimens in SOT is debated and should be performed on an individual basis and interpreted in conjunction with other diagnostic tests.[48,87,89] Studies evaluating serum *Candida* PCR that have included transplant patients demonstrated high diagnostic accuracy for invasive candidiasis.[48] Ultimately studies are limited by lack of standardization, difficulty in distinguishing colonization from invasive disease, and lack of experience with use in SOT.[48,87,89]

The T2Candida panel (T2 Biosystems, Lexington, MA), combining PCR with nuclear magnetic resonance spectroscopy, can detect five *Candida* species from whole blood with high sensitivity and negative predictive value.[101] It has recently been shown to improve time to appropriate antifungal therapy and decrease unnecessary therapy.[102,103] This technology is also being studied for bacterial detection and identification.[104]

FUTURE DIRECTIONS

New molecular rapid diagnostic testing is on the horizon and understanding limitations and clinical benefit for transplant patients is imperative.[105] Future studies of ASP in SOT recipients should also aim to develop metrics of clinical relevance. Additionally, the role of new, nontraditional treatments in ASP and SOT has not been determined.[106] Eventually, National Healthcare Safety Network antibiotic use and resistance benchmarking should be refined, enabling SOT centers to compare and improve antimicrobial prescribing. In the meantime, centers caring for SOT recipients should continue to publish their experience with ASP interventions in these patients. Further support and position statements from relevant governing bodies and professional societies involved in SOT care are needed to establish antimicrobial stewardship as a priority.

SUMMARY

Given their complexity, SOT patients stand to gain the most from antimicrobial optimization strategies. Although stewardship activities and principles used in the general patient population can and should be applied to SOT recipients, not all are optimally suited for copy-paste implementation. This affords an opportunity to identify nuanced and individualized approaches to protect patients and the antimicrobials they may need in the future. Ultimately, to improve ASPs in SOT, TID providers should be directly involved in these activities facilitating the "handshake", multidisciplinary care structure needed in transplantation medicine.

REFERENCES

1. CDC. Core elements of hospital antibiotic stewardship programs. Atlanta (GA): US Department of Health and Human Services, CDC; 2014. Available at: http://www.cdc.gov/getsmart/healthcare/implementation/core-elements.html. Accessed January 15, 2018.
2. Roca I, Akova M, Baquero F, et al. The global threat of antimicrobial resistance: science for intervention. New Microbes New Infect 2015;6:22–9.
3. Cervera C, van Delden C, Gavalda J, et al. Multidrug-resistant bacteria in solid organ transplant recipients. Clin Microbiol Infect 2014;20(Suppl 7):49–73.
4. Hamandi B, Holbrook AM, Humar A, et al. Delay of adequate empiric antibiotic therapy is associated with increased mortality among solid-organ transplant patients. Am J Transplant 2009;9(7):1657–65.
5. Hamandi B, Husain S, Humar A, et al. Impact of infectious disease consultation on the clinical and economic outcomes of solid organ transplant recipients admitted for infectious complications. Clin Infect Dis 2014;59(8):1074–82.
6. Dubberke ER, Burdette SD, AST Infectious Diseases Community of Practice. *Clostridium difficile* infections in solid organ transplantation. Am J Transplant 2013;13(Suppl 4):42–9.
7. Paudel S, Zacharioudakis IM, Zervou FN, et al. Prevalence of Clostridium difficile infection among solid organ transplant recipients: a meta-analysis of published studies. PLoS One 2015;10(4):e0124483.
8. Cusini A, Beguelin C, Stampf S, et al. *Clostridium difficile* infection is associated with graft loss in solid organ transplant recipients. Am J Transplant 2018. https://doi.org/10.1111/ajt.14640.
9. Nellore A, Fishman JA. The microbiome, systemic immune function, and allotransplantation. Clin Microbiol Rev 2016;29(1):191–9.
10. Abbo LM, Ariza-Heredia EJ. Antimicrobial stewardship in immunocompromised hosts. Infect Dis Clin North Am 2014;28(2):263–79.
11. Society for Healthcare Epidemiology of America, Infectious Diseases Society of America, Pediatric Infectious Diseases Society. Policy statement on antimicrobial stewardship by the Society for Healthcare Epidemiology of America (SHEA), the Infectious Diseases Society of America (IDSA), and the Pediatric Infectious Diseases Society (PIDS). Infect Control Hosp Epidemiol 2012;33(4):322–7.
12. Dyar OJ, Huttner B, Schouten J, et al. What is antimicrobial stewardship? Clin Microbiol Infect 2017;23(11):793–8.

13. Barlam TF, Cosgrove SE, Abbo LM, et al. Implementing an antibiotic steward-ship program: guidelines by the infectious diseases society of America and the Society for Healthcare Epidemiology of America. Clin Infect Dis 2016; 62(10):e51–77.
14. Aitken SL, Palmer HR, Topal JE, et al. Call for antimicrobial stewardship in solid organ transplantation. Am J Transplant 2013;13(9):2499.
15. So M, Yang DY, Bell C, et al. Solid organ transplant patients: are there opportunities for antimicrobial stewardship? Clin Transplant 2016;30(6):659–68.
16. Seo SK, Lo K, Abbo LM. Current state of antimicrobial stewardship at solid organ and hematopoietic cell transplant centers in the United States. Infect Control Hosp Epidemiol 2016;37(10):1195–200.
17. Echevarria K, Groppi J, Kelly AA, et al. Development and application of an objective staffing calculator for antimicrobial stewardship programs in the Veterans Health Administration. Am J Health Syst Pharm 2017;74(21):1785–90.
18. Messacar K, Campbell K, Pearce K, et al. A handshake from antimicrobial stewardship opens doors for infectious disease consultations. Clin Infect Dis 2017; 64(10):1449–52.
19. Schaenman JM, Kumar D, Kotton CN, et al. Transplant center support for infectious diseases. Transpl Infect Dis 2017;19:e12746.
20. Olans RN, Olans RD, DeMaria A Jr. The critical role of the staff nurse in antimicrobial stewardship: unrecognized, but already there. Clin Infect Dis 2016;62(1): 84–9.
21. Spellberg B, Bartlett JG, Gilbert DN. How to pitch an antibiotic stewardship program to the hospital C-suite. Open Forum Infect Dis 2016;3(4):ofw210.
22. Dresser LD, Bell CM, Steinberg M, et al. Use of a structured panel process to define antimicrobial prescribing appropriateness in critical care. J Antimicrob Chemother 2018;73(1):246–9.
23. So M, Husain S, Nakamachi Y, et al. Implementing antimicrobial stewardship-oriented guidelines using a change management approach: the example of febrile neutropenia. Journal of Antimicrobial Stewardship 2017;1(1):38–48.
24. Pakyz AL, Moczygemba LR, VanderWielen LM, et al. Facilitators and barriers to implementing antimicrobial stewardship strategies: results from a qualitative study. Am J Infect Control 2014;42(10 Suppl):S257–63.
25. Gross AE, Johannes RS, Gupta V, et al. The effect of a piperacillin/tazobactam shortage on antimicrobial prescribing and Clostridium difficile risk in 88 US Medical Centers. Clin Infect Dis 2017;65(4):613–8.
26. Roberts JA, Kumar A, Lipman J. Right dose, right now: customized drug dosing in the critically ill. Crit Care Med 2017;45(2):331–6.
27. Roberts JA, Lefrant JY, Lipman J. What's new in pharmacokinetics of antimicrobials in AKI and RRT? Intensive Care Med 2017;43(6):904–6.
28. Sime FB, Roberts MS, Roberts JA. Optimization of dosing regimens and dosing in special populations. Clin Microbiol Infect 2015;21(10):886–93.
29. Gagermeier JP, Rusinak JD, Lurain NS, et al. Subtherapeutic ganciclovir (GCV) levels and GCV-resistant cytomegalovirus in lung transplant recipients. Transpl Infect Dis 2014;16(6):941–50.
30. Kiser TH, Fish DN, Zamora MR. Evaluation of valganciclovir pharmacokinetics in lung transplant recipients. J Heart Lung Transplant 2012;31(2):159–66.
31. Padulles A, Colom H, Bestard O, et al. Contribution of population pharmacokinetics to dose optimization of ganciclovir-valganciclovir in solid-organ transplant patients. Antimicrob Agents Chemother 2016;60(4):1992–2002.

32. Lempers VJ, Martial LC, Schreuder MF, et al. Drug-interactions of azole anti-fungals with selected immunosuppressants in transplant patients: strategies for optimal management in clinical practice. Curr Opin Pharmacol 2015;24: 38–44.

33. Ashbee HR, Barnes RA, Johnson EM, et al. Therapeutic drug monitoring (TDM) of antifungal agents: guidelines from the British Society for Medical Mycology. J Antimicrob Chemother 2014;69(5):1162–76.

34. Qiao B, Wu J, Wan Q, et al. Factors influencing mortality in abdominal solid organ transplant recipients with multidrug-resistant gram-negative bacteremia. BMC Infect Dis 2017;17(1):171.

35. Candel FJ, Grima E, Matesanz M, et al. Bacteremia and septic shock after solid-organ transplantation. Transplant Proc 2005;37(9):4097–9.

36. Rosa R, Simkins J, Camargo JF, et al. Solid organ transplant antibiograms: an opportunity for antimicrobial stewardship. Diagn Microbiol Infect Dis 2016; 86(4):460–3.

37. Korayem GB, Zangeneh TT, Matthias KR. Recurrence of urinary tract infections and development of urinary-specific antibiogram for kidney transplant recipients. J Glob Antimicrob Resist 2018;12:119–23.

38. Blumenthal KG, Ryan EE, Li Y, et al. The impact of a reported penicillin allergy on surgical site infection risk. Clin Infect Dis 2018;66(3):329–36.

39. Charneski L, Deshpande G, Smith SW. Impact of an antimicrobial allergy label in the medical record on clinical outcomes in hospitalized patients. Pharmaco-therapy 2011;31(8):742–7.

40. MacFadden DR, LaDelfa A, Leen J, et al. Impact of reported beta-lactam allergy on inpatient outcomes: a multicenter prospective cohort study. Clin Infect Dis 2016;63(7):904–10.

41. Macy E, Contreras R. Health care use and serious infection prevalence associated with penicillin "allergy" in hospitalized patients: a cohort study. J Allergy Clin Immunol 2014;133(3):790–6.

42. Huang K-HG, Cluzet V, Hamilton K, et al. The impact of reported beta-lactam allergy in hospitalized patients with hematologic malignancies requiring antibiotics. Clin Infect Dis 2018. https://doi.org/10.1093/cid/ciy037.

43. Trubiano JA, Chen C, Cheng AC, et al. Antimicrobial allergy 'labels' drive inappropriate antimicrobial prescribing: lessons for stewardship. J Antimicrob Chemother 2016;71(6):1715–22.

44. Khumra S, Chan J, Urbancic K, et al. Antibiotic allergy labels in a liver transplant recipient study. Antimicrob Agents Chemother 2017;61(5) [pii:e00078-17].

45. So M, Morris A, Bell C, et al. Academic detailing with prescribers as an antimicrobial stewardship intervention in solid organ transplant patients [abstract]. Am J Transplant 2017;17(suppl 3). Available at: http://atcmeetingabstracts.com/abstract/effect-of-academic-detailing-with-prescribers-as-an-antimicrobial-stewardship-intervention-in-solid-organ-transplant-patients/.

46. Asberg A, Humar A, Rollag H, et al. Oral valganciclovir is noninferior to intravenous ganciclovir for the treatment of cytomegalovirus disease in solid organ transplant recipients. Am J Transplant 2007;7(9):2106–13.

47. Hamdy RF, Zaoutis TE, Seo SK. Antifungal stewardship considerations for adults and pediatrics. Virulence 2017;8(6):658–72.

48. Pappas PG, Kauffman CA, Andes DR, et al. Clinical practice guideline for the management of candidiasis: 2016 update by the Infectious Diseases Society of America. Clin Infect Dis 2016;62(4):e1–50.

49. Husain S, So M. Empiric management of common infections in solid organ transplant patients. Available at: http://www.antimicrobialstewardship.com/sites/default/files/article_files/mot_protocol_-_aug_2017_final_dated_secured.pdf. Accessed January 14, 2018.
50. Jansen KU, Knirsch C, Anderson AS. The role of vaccines in preventing bacterial antimicrobial resistance. Nat Med 2018;24(1):10–9.
51. Gouliouris T, Micallef C, Yang H, et al. Impact of a candidaemia care bundle on patient care at a large teaching hospital in England. J Infect 2016;72(4):501–3.
52. Molina J, Penalva G, Gil-Navarro MV, et al. Long-term impact of an educational antimicrobial stewardship program on hospital-acquired candidemia and multidrug-resistant bloodstream infections: a quasi-experimental study of interrupted time-series analysis. Clin Infect Dis 2017;65(12):1992–9.
53. Malinis MF, Mawhorter SD, Jain A, et al. Staphylococcus aureus bacteremia in solid organ transplant recipients: evidence for improved survival when compared with nontransplant patients. Transplantation 2012;93(10):1045–50.
54. Pfaller MA, Diekema DJ. Progress in antifungal susceptibility testing of Candida spp. by use of Clinical and Laboratory Standards Institute broth microdilution methods, 2010 to 2012. J Clin Microbiol 2012;50(9):2846–56.
55. Shah DN, Yau R, Weston J, et al. Evaluation of antifungal therapy in patients with candidaemia based on susceptibility testing results: implications for antimicrobial stewardship programmes. J Antimicrob Chemother 2011;66(9):2146–51.
56. Micallef C, Aliyu SH, Santos R, et al. Introduction of an antifungal stewardship programme targeting high-cost antifungals at a tertiary hospital in Cambridge, England. J Antimicrob Chemother 2015;70(6):1908–11.
57. Mondain V, Lieutier F, Hasseine L, et al. A 6-year antifungal stewardship programme in a teaching hospital. Infection 2013;41(3):621–8.
58. Brakemeier S, Taxeidi SI, Zukunft B, et al. Extended-spectrum beta-lactamase-producing enterobacteriaceae-related urinary tract infection in kidney transplant recipients: risk factors, treatment, and long-term outcome. Transplant Proc 2017;49(8):1757–65.
59. Delmas-Frenette C, Dorais M, Tavares-Brum A, et al. Epidemiology and outcome of antimicrobial resistance to gram-negative pathogens in bacteriuric kidney transplant recipients. Transpl Infect Dis 2017. https://doi.org/10.1111/tid.12722.
60. Origuen J, Fernandez-Ruiz M, Lopez-Medrano F, et al. Progressive increase of resistance in Enterobacteriaceae urinary isolates from kidney transplant recipients over the past decade: narrowing of the therapeutic options. Transpl Infect Dis 2016;18(4):575–84.
61. El Amari EB, Hadaya K, Buhler L, et al. Outcome of treated and untreated asymptomatic bacteriuria in renal transplant recipients. Nephrol Dial Transplant 2011;26(12):4109–14.
62. Origuen J, Lopez-Medrano F, Fernandez-Ruiz M, et al. Should asymptomatic bacteriuria be systematically treated in kidney transplant recipients? Results from a randomized controlled trial. Am J Transplant 2016;16(10):2943–53.
63. Coussement J, Hazzan M, Weekers L, et al. The Bacteriuria In Renal Transplantation (BIRT) study: a prospective, randomized, parallel-group, multicenter, open-label, superiority trial comparing antibiotics versus no treatment in the prevention of symptomatic urinary tract infection in kidney transplant recipients with asymptomatic bacteriuria. ClinicalTrials.gov identifier: NCT01871753 (ongoing study, recruiting – protocol published by The Lancet). 2014; Available at: https://clinicaltrials.gov/show/NCT01871753. Accessed January 21, 2018.

64. Patel P, Rebollo-Mesa I, Ryan E, et al. Prophylactic ureteric stents in renal transplant recipients: a multicenter randomized controlled trial of early versus late removal. Am J Transplant 2017;17(8):2129–38.

65. Frenette C, Sperlea D, Leharova Y, et al. Impact of an infection control and antimicrobial stewardship program on solid organ transplantation and hepatobiliary surgical site infections. Infect Control Hosp Epidemiol 2016;37(12):1468–74.

66. Anesi JA, Blumberg EA, Abbo LM. Perioperative antibiotic prophylaxis to prevent surgical site infections in solid organ transplantation. Transplantation 2018;102(1):21–34.

67. Alraddadi B, Nierenberg NE, Price LL, et al. Characteristics and outcomes of neutropenia after orthotopic liver transplantation. Liver Transpl 2016;22(2): 217–25.

68. Hurst FP, Belur P, Nee R, et al. Poor outcomes associated with neutropenia after kidney transplantation: analysis of United States Renal Data System. Transplantation 2011;92(1):36–40.

69. Kumar D, Mian M, Singer L, et al. An interventional study using cell-mediated immunity to personalize therapy for cytomegalovirus infection after transplantation. Am J Transplant 2017;17(9):2468–73.

70. San-Juan R, Navarro D, Garcia-Reyne A, et al. Effect of delaying prophylaxis against CMV in D+/R- solid organ transplant recipients in the development of CMV-specific cellular immunity and occurrence of late CMV disease. J Infect 2015;71(5):561–70.

71. Lisboa LF, Kumar D, Wilson LE, et al. Clinical utility of cytomegalovirus cell-mediated immunity in transplant recipients with cytomegalovirus viremia. Transplantation 2012;93(2):195–200.

72. Manuel O, Husain S, Kumar D, et al. Assessment of cytomegalovirus-specific cell-mediated immunity for the prediction of cytomegalovirus disease in high-risk solid-organ transplant recipients: a multicenter cohort study. Clin Infect Dis 2013;56(6):817–24.

73. Paulsen GC, Danziger-Isakov L. Respiratory viral infections in solid organ and hematopoietic stem cell transplantation. Clin Chest Med 2017;38(4):707–26.

74. Mercuro N, Kenney RM, Tibbetts R, et al. Role of respiratory virus panels in antimicrobial stewardship in immunocompromised patients. Open Forum Infect Dis 2016;3(suppl_1):1866.

75. Evans SR, Rubin D, Follmann D, et al. Desirability of outcome ranking (DOOR) and response adjusted for duration of antibiotic risk (RADAR). Clin Infect Dis 2015;61(5):800–6.

76. LaRocco MT, Burgert SJ. Infection in the bone marrow transplant recipient and role of the microbiology laboratory in clinical transplantation. Clin Microbiol Rev 1997;10(2):277–97.

77. Perez JL, Ayats J, de Ona M, et al. The role of the clinical microbiology laboratory in solid organ transplantation programs. Enferm Infecc Microbiol Clin 2012; 30(Suppl 2):2–9.

78. MacVane SH, Hurst JM, Steed LL. The role of antimicrobial stewardship in the clinical microbiology laboratory: stepping up to the plate. Open Forum Infect Dis 2016;3(4):ofw201.

79. Morgan DJ, Malani P, Diekema DJ. Diagnostic stewardship-leveraging the laboratory to improve antimicrobial use. JAMA 2017;318(7):607–8.

80. Messacar K, Parker SK, Todd JK, et al. Implementation of rapid molecular infectious disease diagnostics: the role of diagnostic and antimicrobial stewardship. J Clin Microbiol 2017;55(3):715–23.

81. Sandkovsky U, Kalil AC, Florescu DF. The use and value of procalcitonin in solid organ transplantation. Clin Transplant 2015;29(8):689–96.
82. Sato A, Kaido T, Iida T, et al. Bundled strategies against infection after liver transplantation: lessons from multidrug-resistant *Pseudomonas aeruginosa*. Liver Transpl 2016;22(4):436–45.
83. Chow JKL, Ganz T, Ruthazer R, et al. Iron-related markers are associated with infection after liver transplantation. Liver Transpl 2017;23(12):1541–52.
84. Franeková J, Sečník P, Lavríková P, et al. Serial measurement of presepsin, procalcitonin, and C-reactive protein in the early postoperative period and the response to antithymocyte globulin administration after heart transplantation. Clin Transplant 2017;31:e12870.
85. Fernandez-Ruiz M, Kumar D, Humar A. Clinical immune-monitoring strategies for predicting infection risk in solid organ transplantation. Clin Transl Immunology 2014;3(2):e12.
86. Mian M, Natori Y, Ferreira V, et al. Evaluation of a novel global immunity assay to predict infection in organ transplant recipients. Clin Infect Dis 2018;66(9):1392–7.
87. Patterson TF, Thompson GR 3rd, Denning DW, et al. Practice guidelines for the diagnosis and management of aspergillosis: 2016 update by the Infectious Diseases Society of America. Clin Infect Dis 2016;63(4):e1–60.
88. Singh N, Husain S, American Society of Transplantation Infectious Diseases Community of Practice. Aspergillosis in solid organ transplantation. Am J Transplant 2013;13(Suppl 4):228–41.
89. Husain S, Sole A, Alexander BD, et al. The 2015 International Society for Heart and Lung Transplantation Guidelines for the management of fungal infections in mechanical circulatory support and cardiothoracic organ transplant recipients: executive summary. J Heart Lung Transplant 2016;35(3):261–82.
90. Ambasta A, Carson J, Church DL. The use of biomarkers and molecular methods for the earlier diagnosis of invasive aspergillosis in immunocompromised patients. Med Mycol 2015;53(6):531–57.
91. Lahmer T, Neuenhahn M, Held J, et al. Comparison of 1,3-beta-d-glucan with galactomannan in serum and bronchoalveolar fluid for the detection of *Aspergillus* species in immunosuppressed mechanical ventilated critically ill patients. J Crit Care 2016;36:259–64.
92. Bhimji A, Bhaskaran A, Singer LG, et al. *Aspergillus* galactomannan detection in exhaled breath condensate compared to bronchoalveolar lavage fluid for the diagnosis of invasive aspergillosis in immunocompromised patients. Clin Microbiol Infect 2017. https://doi.org/10.1016/j.cmi.2017.09.018.
93. Angebault C, Lanternier F, Dalle F, et al. Prospective evaluation of serum beta-glucan testing in patients with probable or proven fungal diseases. Open Forum Infect Dis 2016;3(3):ofw128.
94. Levesque E, El Anbassi S, Sitterle E, et al. Contribution of (1,3)-beta-D-glucan to diagnosis of invasive candidiasis after liver transplantation. J Clin Microbiol 2015;53(3):771–6.
95. Singh N, Winston DJ, Limaye AP, et al. Performance characteristics of galactomannan and beta-d-glucan in high-risk liver transplant recipients. Transplantation 2015;99(12):2543–50.
96. Egli A, Osthoff M, Goldenberger D, et al. Matrix-assisted laser desorption/ionization time-of-flight mass spectrometry (MALDI-TOF) directly from positive blood culture flasks allows rapid identification of bloodstream infections in immunosuppressed hosts. Transpl Infect Dis 2015;17(3):481–7.

97. Huang AM, Newton D, Kunapuli A, et al. Impact of rapid organism identification via matrix-assisted laser desorption/ionization time-of-flight combined with antimicrobial stewardship team intervention in adult patients with bacteremia and candidemia. Clin Infect Dis 2013;57(9):1237–45.

98. Cosgrove SE, Li DX, Tamma PD, et al. Use of PNA FISH for blood cultures growing gram-positive cocci in chains without a concomitant antibiotic stewardship intervention does not improve time to appropriate antibiotic therapy. Diagn Microbiol Infect Dis 2016;86(1):86–92.

99. Heil EL, Daniels LM, Long DM, et al. Impact of a rapid peptide nucleic acid fluorescence in situ hybridization assay on treatment of *Candida* infections. Am J Health Syst Pharm 2012;69(21):1910–4.

100. Ao W, Klonoski J, Berlinghoff E, et al. Rapid detection and differentiation of clinically relevant candida species simultaneously from blood culture by use of a novel signal amplification approach. J Clin Microbiol 2018. https://doi.org/10.1128/JCM.00982-17.

101. Mylonakis E, Clancy CJ, Ostrosky-Zeichner L, et al. T2 magnetic resonance assay for the rapid diagnosis of candidemia in whole blood: a clinical trial. Clin Infect Dis 2015;60(6):892–9.

102. Wilson NM, Alangaden G, Tibbetts RJ, et al. T2 magnetic resonance assay improves timely management of candidemia. Journal of Antimicrobial Stewardship 2017;1(1):12–8.

103. Turner OD, Hayes JF, McCarty TP, et al. Relationship of T2 candida panel to disease severity, mortality and time to therapy in patients with candidemia. Open Forum Infect Dis 2017;4(suppl_1):S609.

104. Neely L, Plourde D, Suchocki A, et al. T2Bacteria: rapid and sensitive detection and identification of sepsis pathogens in whole blood specimens by T2MR [presentation abstract]. Paper presented at: Association of Molecular Pathology Annual Meeting. Austin, Texas, November 5–7, 2015.

105. Simner PJ, Miller S, Carroll KC. Understanding the promises and hurdles of metagenomic next-generation sequencing as a diagnostic tool for infectious diseases. Clin Infect Dis 2018;66(5):778–88.

106. Tse BN, Adalja AA, Houchens C, et al. Challenges and opportunities of nontraditional approaches to treating bacterial infections. Clin Infect Dis 2017;65(3):495–500.

Multidrug-Resistant Bacterial Infections in Solid Organ Transplant Candidates and Recipients

Michele Bartoletti, MD, PhD*, Maddalena Giannella, MD, PhD,
Sara Tedeschi, MD, Pierluigi Viale, MD

KEYWORDS

- Multidrug-resistant pathogens • Solid organ transplantation
- Extended-spectrum β-lactamase-producing enterobacteriaceae
- Carbapenem-resistant gram-negative bacilli
- Methicillin-resistant *Staphylococcus aureus* • Vancomycin-resistant enterococci
- Donor-derived infections

KEY POINTS

- The magnitude of the challenge of multidrug-resistant pathogens is huge; this problem affects several aspects of the management of transplant candidates and recipients.
- Areas of uncertainty are predominant in this field concerning selection of candidates, infection prevention, infection control policies, and treatment.
- In addition, continually updated recommendations are needed to face the ever-present and evolving epidemiology of bacterial infection in this setting.

INTRODUCTION

The advancements in surgical techniques, immunosuppressive therapies, and infection control and prophylaxis, along with significant changes in the policy of graft recruitment and allocation altered dramatically the characteristics of patients undergoing solid organ transplantation (SOT) in recent years. In fact, an increasing rate of patients being transplanted in critical condition, directly transferred from intensive care units (ICUs), often receiving marginal organs, is commonly observed.

As a whole, these variations have increased the graft availability and improved the accessibility to organ transplantation; however, they have also changed, and

Infectious Diseases Unit, Department of Medical and Surgical Sciences, Sant'Orsola-Malpighi Hospital, University of Bologna, Via Massarenti 11, Bologna 40138, Italy
* Corresponding author.
E-mail address: michele.bartoletti4@unibo.it

Infect Dis Clin N Am 32 (2018) 551–580
https://doi.org/10.1016/j.idc.2018.04.004
0891-5520/18/© 2018 Elsevier Inc. All rights reserved.

id.theclinics.com

increased, the infectious risk. In the current era, ruled by an alarming evolution of anti-microbial resistances, SOT recipients seem one of the patient categories most prone to develop infection caused by multidrug-resistant (MDR) pathogens.[1–3] Not surprisingly, infections caused by MDR pathogens are found more frequently in SOT recipients than in the non-SOT population.[4]

The current major challenges of MDR pathogens are the following. First, MDR infections in transplant recipients are frequently associated with graft complication, and their treatment is often hampered by an ominous lack of effective drugs, resulting in an overall poor outcome. Second, MDR pathogens are frequently associated with outbreaks. This factor is related to the ability of these pathogens, especially Gram-negative bacilli, to spread among a frail population. Third, donor-derived infections (DDI) caused by MDR pathogens are increasingly reported with significant impact on recipients' outcomes.[5]

In light of a clear need of updating the body of knowledge of the infectious risk in the transplanted populations, the current review emphasizes the epidemiologic trends, old and new risk factors, and pretransplant and posttransplant clinical management of MDR-related infection in SOT recipients. We focus on infections owing to methicillin-resistant *Staphylococcus aureus* (MRSA), vancomycin-resistant Enterococci (VRE), extended spectrum β-lactamase (ESBL)-producing, and carbapenem-resistant Enterobacteriaceae (CRE), MDR *Pseudomonas aeruginosa*, and carbapenem-resistant *Acinetobacter baumannii* (CR-AB).

EPIDEMIOLOGY OF MULTIDRUG-RESISTANT PATHOGENS AMONG SOLID ORGAN TRANSPLANT RECIPIENTS

The prevalence, risk factors, and mortality of infection caused by MDR pathogens in the setting of organ transplant are summarized in **Table 1**. Significant differences are present between different pathogens. Furthermore, the prevalence and incidence of infections may vary among different centers located in different countries and between American and European centers.

Methicillin-Resistant Staphylococcus aureus

S aureus is a major cause of invasive infection in the general population, being the second most common bacterial species after *Escherichia coli*.[6] Among all *S aureus* infections, those owing to MRSA represent 21% to 24% of cases in Europe and 31% to 39% in the United States.[7,8] However, in recent years, the incidence of MRSA infection has had a significant downward trend observed in both the United States and Europe, owing to the widespread use of specific infection prevention and control measures.[7,9] In SOT recipients, a similar decrease in MRSA infection may be hypothesized when comparing recent epidemiologic studies with older reports.[10–12]

Overall, the incidence of MRSA infection seems to be higher in lung and liver transplant recipients (0.2–5.7 cases per 100 transplant-years for the former, 0.1 cases per 100 transplant-years the latter) with respect to other kinds of transplants. Most MRSA infections occur in the early posttransplant period, after a median of 7 to 29 days after liver and lung transplantation.[12–14] A longer time frame between transplant and infection is reported among kidney transplant recipients in a recent study.[15] The most frequent sources of infection are pneumonia, bloodstream infection (BSI), vascular catheters, and the surgical site itself, with surgical site infections (SSIs) found mostly in heart and lung transplant recipients. Risk factors for infection found in previous studies are pretransplant and posttransplant nasal colonization, ICU stay, mechanical ventilation for more than 5 days, and cytomegalovirus primary infection in

Table 1
Summary of prevalence, risk factors, and outcome of infection caused by MDR pathogens in solid organ transplant recipients

Microorganism or Group	Organ Transplanted	Prevalence	Risk Factors	Mortality
All MDR pathogens[21,64,131–134]	Liver	15%	Abdominal infection episodes, reoperation, acute rejection, use of pretransplant broad-spectrum antibiotics and prolonged (≥72 h) endotracheal intubation	6-mo mortality 39%
	Kidney	14%	Age >50 y, HCV infection, double kidney-pancreas transplantation, posttransplant RRT, surgical reoperation, nephrostomy	19%
	Lung	37%–51%[a]	ICU stay >14 d, presence of a tracheostomy, previous exposure to broad-spectrum antibiotics	14%
	Heart	25%	NA	NA
MRSA[10,12,14,16–19]	Liver	1.4%–23%	ICU stay, CMV primary coinfection	30-d mortality 21%–25%
	Kidney	0.8%–2%	NA	In-hospital mortality 0%–10%
	Lung	10%–60%	Mechanical ventilation >5 d; MRSA nasal carriage; MRSA in recipient sterile cultures	30-d mortality 17%
	Heart	30%	NA	NA
VRE[24,26]	Liver	2%–11%	Biliary leak, reoperation	In hospital 9%–48% 1-y mortality 56%–80%
	Kidney	0%[b]		
ESBL[41,44,135]	Liver	7%	Pretransplant ESBL fecal carriage, MELD >25, reoperation	30-d mortality 15%–26%
	Kidney	3%–11%	Double kidney/pancreas transplantation, previous use of antibiotics, posttransplant dialysis requirement, posttransplant urinary obstruction	30-d mortality 14%
	Lung	2%	NA	30-d mortality 17%
	Heart	5%	NA	30-d mortality 14%

(continued on next page)

Table 1
(continued)

Microorganism or Group	Organ Transplanted	Prevalence	Risk Factors	Mortality
CRE[47,48,51,53,136,137]	Liver	5%–19%	RRT, mechanical ventilation >48 h; HCV recurrence, colonization at any time with CR-KP	In-hospital mortality 18%
	Kidney	2%–26%	Multiorgan transplantation, the use of a ureteral stent	In-hospital mortality 33%–41%
	Lung	0.4%–20.0%	NA	30-d mortality 26%; 1-y mortality 53%
	Heart	5%–17%	NA	50%
Carbapenem-resistant *Acinetobacter baumannii*[55-57]	Liver	8%–29%	Prolonged cold ischemia, post-LT dialysis, LT owing to fulminant hepatitis	60-d mortality 42%
	Kidney	3%	NA	30-d mortality 39%
	Lung	21%	NA	30-d mortality 62%
	Heart	7%	NA	NA
MDR-*Pseudomonas aeruginosa*[60-62,131,132]	Liver	4%	Previous transplantation	37%–38%
	Kidney	6%–9%	Hospital-acquired BSI	NA
	Lung	14%	ICU admission in the previous year	1-y mortality 27%
	Heart	19%	Septic shock	NA

Abbreviations: BSI, bloodstream infection; CMV, cytomegalovirus; CRE, carbapenem-resistant Enterobacteriaceae; CR-KP, carbapenem-resistant *Klebsiella pneumoniae*; ESBL-E, extended spectrum β-lactamase-producing Enterobacteriaceae; HCV, hepatitis C virus; ICU, intensive care unit; LT, liver transplantation; MDR, multidrug-resistant; MELD, model for end-stage liver disease; MRSA, methicillin resistant *Staphylococcus aureus*; NA, not available; RRT, renal replacement therapy; VRE, vancomycin-resistant Enterobacteriaceae.

[a] Study on MDR organisms in lung transplant patients evaluated mostly airway colonization and respiratory tract infection rather than other types of infection.

[b] One study evaluated 38 kidney transplanted patients colonized with VRE. No one developed VRE-related infection.[86]

cytomegalovirus-seronegative recipients. The mortality for infection caused by MRSA ranges between 14% and 36%.[10,12,14,16–19]

Vancomycin-Resistant Enterococci

Enterococcus spp infection is common after abdominal SOT. The prevalence of *Enterococcus* spp infection is reported in up to 15% of SOT recipients, mainly liver transplant recipients.[20] *Enterococcus* spp is the causative pathogen of 6% to 15% of BSIs in SOT recipients. This rate can reach 20% in hospital-acquired BSI.[21–23] Among all enterococcal infections, the impact of VRE is extremely variable between countries. Centers in North America reported a prevalence of 2% to 11% of VRE infection in liver transplant recipients,[24–26] whereas nearly no infections were reported in studies conducted in Europe.[20,21] This marked disparity may be related to the differing use of vancomycin between American and European hospitals.[27]

VRE infections occur mainly in liver transplant recipients, probably as a consequence of the high prevalence of colonized or infected patients before transplantation.[28,29] In a case-control study, liver transplantation was found to be an independent risk factor for VRE BSI.[30] Infections occur within an average of 29 to 48 days after transplantation. The main types of infection are bacteremia, peritonitis, SSI, and urinary and biliary tract infections.[28,31,32] In an epidemiologic study focused on SSI after liver transplantation, VRE accounted for 23% of all culture-positive superficial and deep SSI. Risk factors for deep VRE SSI were pretransplant VRE colonization, renal failure requiring hemodialysis, bile leak, and male gender.[33] Other kinds of infections, such as endocarditis and mediastinitis, have been reported.[34] Last, VRE in heart transplant recipients have been described mostly in patients with a VRE left ventricular assist device infection in the pretransplant period.[35] Overall, crude mortality for VRE infection represents 9% to 48% of cases, but can reach 56% to 80% during the 1-year of follow-up period.[25,26,31,32]

Extended Spectrum β-Lactamase–Producing Enterobacteriaceae

ESBL production in gram-negative bacteria, especially Enterobacteriaceae, has emerged in past decade and became a global health concern in the general patient population. Despite being initially found mainly during outbreaks in hospitalized patients, throughout the years ESBL-producing strains have become common in the community.[36,37]

Similarly, the prevalence of ESBL-producing strains among transplant patients has increased dramatically in recent years. A study analyzing the etiology of BSI occurring among transplant recipients in a center in Spain in the first year posttransplant, an increasing rate of ESBL-producing strains was found, principally *Klebsiella pneumoniae*, from 7% in 2007 to 2008 to 34% in 2015 to 2016.[38] Another study performed in China evaluating 350 consecutive liver and kidney transplants found a prevalence of 12% of infection caused by ESBL-producing Enterobacteriaceae.[39]

Most infections in patients receiving liver, lung, and heart allografts occur early in the posttransplant period.[40–42] However, longer delays between transplantation and infection have been observed in kidney transplant recipients (28–864 days).[40,43] Urinary tract infections (UTI) are a type of infection commonly associated with ESBL isolation as well as BSI, intraabdominal infection, and pneumonia with differences among different kinds of transplants. More specifically, ESBL-producing Enterobacteriaceae cause mostly UTI in kidney transplant recipients and pneumonia in lung transplant recipients. Mortality associated with infection owing to ESBL-producing strains may vary from 8% to 26% of cases.[40,41] In addition, a significant rate of recurrent infection has been observed (21%–41% of cases). In particular, recurrent UTI in kidney transplant recipients are frequently reported.[41,43,44]

Carbapenem-Resistant Enterobacteriaceae

Nowadays the global emergence of CRE is a major health challenge. The SOT population seems particularly at risk to develop CRE infections. SOT recipients are characterized by a high propensity to develop bacterial infections in the initial posttransplant period. Consequently, the antimicrobial pressure owing to both antibiotic treatment and prophylaxis is very high in this setting. Thus, in studies analyzing CRE BSI episodes in the general patient population, SOT patients are involved in 14% to 37% of cases.[45,46] In addition, a multicenter study conducted in SOT recipients in Italy shows that the prevalence of carbapenem resistance was 26% among all isolated Enterobacteriaceae and 49% among all isolated *Klebsiella* spp.[47]

Overall, in endemic areas, the incidence of CRE infection after SOT is approximately 5%; CRE infection commonly occurs in the initial posttransplant period (on average 11–36 days).[48–50] Infections associated with CRE are usually BSI, including catheter-related BSI, pneumonia, UTI, intraabdominal infections, and SSIs. Posttransplant renal replacement therapy, CRE rectal colonization, HCV recurrence in liver transplant recipients, bile leak, and prolonged mechanical ventilation are risk factors for CRE during the early posttransplant period.[37,48] The CRE-associated crude mortality rates vary from 25% to 71%, with differences reported between *K pneumoniae* carbapenemase (KPC)-producing CRE and KPC-negative CRE.[50–54]

Carbapenem-resistant Acinetobacter baumannii

CR-AB is commonly reported to affect 9% to 29% of SOT patients. This variability is primarily related to the distinctive propensity of CR-AB to generate outbreaks.[55–57] Epidemiologic studies of BSI in SOT patients report a rate of CR-AB of 2% to 6%.[21] Most infections occur in liver and lung transplant recipients, commonly during the ICU stay in the early posttransplant period. The most common infections are SSI, pneumonia, and BSI, with a mortality rate after 30 days of 57% to 62%.[55,56] Factors associated with poor prognosis are ICU admission, treatment with mechanical ventilation, transplantation for fulminant hepatitis, re-transplantation, prolonged cold ischemia time, and longer surgical time.[56] Despite the high reported mortality rate, the role of CR-AB in determining the prognosis in SOT recipients is under debate and some authors have raised the question whether CR-AB represents a marker of severity of illness rather than a factor associated with poor prognosis. In fact, in a study evaluating a series of 49 infections caused by *A baumannii* in liver and kidney transplant recipients, carbapenem resistance did not negatively affect the prognosis of patients.[58]

Multidrug-Resistant Pseudomonas aeruginosa

P aeruginosa is involved in 6% to 13% of BSI after SOT, being a leading pathogen in lung transplant patients[23,38,59] The prevalence of drug resistance among *P aeruginosa* strains may vary significantly between centers. Among the infections caused by *P aeruginosa*, 44% to 55% of cases were caused by an MDR strain.[59,60] Moreover, a single-center study found a worrisome rate of 63% of extensively drug-resistant (XDR) strains among all *P aeruginosa* BSI cases.[61] There are also concerns regarding *P aeruginosa* infections and colonization among lung transplant candidates, especially those affected by cystic fibrosis. Studies conducted in this population showed close to 50% of lung transplant candidates harboring pandrug-resistant *P aeruginosa* in the airways.[62] Colonization and/or infection by *P aeruginosa* after lung transplantation is associated with a higher risk of developing bronchiolitis obliterans syndrome and death.[63] Finally, MDR P aeruginosa is frequently found among recurrent cases of UTI among kidney transplant recipients.[64]

Outside the lung transplantation setting, the most common sources of MDR/XDR P aeruginosa BSI are the urinary tract, central venous catheters and the abdomen. About one-half of infections occur during the first 90 days and one-quarter during the first 2 weeks after the transplant.[60,61] Retransplantation, nosocomial BSI, septic shock, and prior ICU admission were found to be risk factors for MDR/XDR P aeruginosa infection. Infection caused by MDR/XDR P aeruginosa are associated with a recurrence rate of 21%, and a higher rate of ICU admission and renal impairment when compared with infections caused by other pathogens, as well as a 30-day mortality rate of 38%.[61]

PRETRANSPLANT SCREENING AND MANAGEMENT OF COLONIZED PATIENTS

Infection or colonization by MDR is common in patients awaiting transplantation (Table 2). In fact, patients with end-stage diseases treatable with transplantation share several risk factors for infections caused by MDR, including variable levels of immune system impairment, frequent health care contacts, ICU admission, greater susceptibility to infection, and subsequently increased exposure to broad-spectrum antibiotics.

Infection is a leading cause of morbidity and mortality in patients with end-stage liver disease. About one-third of patients admitted for an episode of acute decompensation of liver disease develops a bacterial or fungal infection.[65] In addition, infection seems to accelerate the course of the disease, being the most important event triggering the acute-on-chronic liver failure syndrome.[66] Thus, it is not surprising that approximately 20% of patients undergo transplantation during the course of an infectious episode.[67] MDR in this setting causes approximately 30% to 46% of infections and is associated with inadequate empirical therapy and increased mortality.[29,68,69]

Table 2
Incidence and etiology of MDR pathogens among infectious episodes in patients with underlying transplant-treatable diseases

Disease/ Condition	Rate of MDR Pathogens Among Episodes of Infections/ Colonization	Main Isolated Pathogens	Comments/Notes
Liver cirrhosis[68,69,138]	25%–47%	MRSA 3%–7% ESBL-E 12%–15% CRE 3%–8% VRE 0%–7%	Major infections are spontaneous bacterial peritonitis, BSI, UTI, and pneumonia
End-stage renal disease[73,74]	12%–25%	MRSA 0%–14% VRE 2%–21% ESBL-E 12%–25%	Most of infections studied are hemodialysis catheter-related BSIs
Cystic fibrosis[76,139]	48%	MRSA 17%–36% MDR Pseudomonas aeruginosa 21%–52% ESBL-E 4%	Studies collected mostly culture (surveillance or diagnostic) samples rather than Infectious episodes

Abbreviations: BSI, bloodstream infection; CRE, carbapenem-resistant Enterobacteriaceae; ESBL-E, extended spectrum β-lactamase-producing Enterobacteriaceae; MDR, multidrug-resistant; MRSA, methicillin resistant Staphylococcus aureus; UTI, urinary tract infection; VRE, vancomycin-resistant Enterococci.

Infectious biliary complications such as recurrent cholangitis or infected bilomas in liver transplant recipients may be an indication for retransplantation.[70,71] In this case, candidates for retransplantation may be at risk for infection with colonizing MDR pathogens. In fact, the management of this condition may consist in prolonged and/or recurrent antibiotic treatment while awaiting transplantation,[71] which is the ultimate cure for such infections. Thus, transplantation should not be delayed in hopes of curing such infections.

Patients with end-stage kidney disease receiving hemodialysis are at increased risk of developing hemodialysis catheter-related BSI or local access-related infections. Although these infections are typically associated with a low mortality rate, severe complications such as endocarditis and metastatic localizations are not unusual. Outpatients receiving hemodialysis are commonly considered a group of patients at risk of infection caused by MDR pathogens. In addition, colonization with MDR pathogens is frequent. In a study evaluating surveillance cultures of patients receiving outpatient hemodialysis, the rates of MDR gram-negative bacteria, VRE, and MRSA isolation were 16%, 13%, and 5%, respectively.[72] Among episodes of infections, grampositive cocci are prevalent, with MRSA and VRE isolated in 0% to 14% and 2% to 21% of cases, respectively.[73,74] In addition, recent studies have reported an increased rate of ESBL-producing Enterobacteriaceae in 12% to 25% of cases.[73,74]

Chronic respiratory infections remain a significant cause of morbidity and mortality in patients with cystic fibrosis. P aeruginosa is commonly isolated in the respiratory tract of 41% to 60% of these patients.[75,76] Although studies have shown a trend toward a decrease in the number of cases of Pseudomonas spp isolation over the past decade, the rate of MDR/XDR and pandrug-resistant (PDR) P aeruginosa strains seems to have increased.[76] A similar trend is observed for other pathogens such us MRSA, CR-AB, Stenotrophomonas maltophilia, and Achromobacter xylosoxidans.[75,76]

SCREENING FOR SPECIFIC PATHOGENS
Methicillin-Resistant Staphylococcus aureus

Different studies focused on the role and necessity of active pretransplant and posttransplant screening and treatment of MRSA nasal carriers. Pretransplant MRSA colonization is common in liver transplant candidates. In a study conducted in a single liver transplant unit, 22% of patients were found to be pretransplant carriers, developing an MRSA infection in 31% of cases during the posttransplant period.[77] Similarly, pretransplant nasal carriage was found to be a risk factor for posttransplant MRSA infection in several other studies.[10,14,24] Posttransplant colonization was also found in 9% to 22% of liver transplant recipients in studies performed in Brazil and Japan. Factors associated with posttransplant colonization were advanced age (>60 years), indwelling urinary catheter for greater than 5 days, postoperative bleeding at the surgical site, renal replacement therapy, prolonged ICU stay, and preoperative (but not postoperative) use of fluoroquinolones. In patients who experienced postoperative colonization, an increased number of MRSA infection was observed and, in a postoperative study, MRSA contraction was an independent predictor of infection.[78–80] A recent metanalysis of 17 published studies found that both pretransplant and posttransplant colonization had increased the risk of MRSA infection during the posttransplant period.[81]

Nasal mupirocin is commonly used in the preoperative period to reduce the risk of postoperative MRSA infection. However, in liver transplant recipients, a lack of mupirocin efficacy is reported. In a study conducted in a center characterized by a high prevalence of MRSA colonization among liver transplant candidates (44%), mupirocin was initially effective in decolonizing 86% of carriers. However, 37% of decolonized patients experienced recolonization and most of methicillin-susceptible *S aureus* carriers eventually became MRSA carriers.[82] In a second study performed in the same center, the application of a more aggressive infection control bundle that included surveillance cultures, cohorting, and contact precaution for all MRSA-colonized or -infected patients plus mupirocin treatment for carriers, was effective in reducing the rate of new MRSA acquisition from 46% to 10% and of MRSA infection from 40% to 4% of patients.[83]

Vancomycin-Resistant Enterococci

Outbreaks of VRE are described in transplant units and in most cases were associated with extensive environmental contamination in addition to human-to-human spread.[84,85]

Pretransplant fecal colonization can reach 44% of cases in liver transplant candidates. In a single-center study, risk factors for pretransplant VRE colonization were central venous catheterization, third-generation cephalosporine use, antianarobes treatment, rifaximin, neomycin or proton pump inhibitor use, paracentesis or endoscopic retrograde cholangiopancreatography, and admission to the liver unit.[28] Posttransplant colonization is also common in liver and kidney transplant patients and occurs in 13% to 18% of cases.[26,86] In 1 study, posttransplant VRE colonization was independently associated with reoperation and antianarobes treatment.[26] Both pretransplant and posttransplant VRE colonization is associated with increased risk of subsequent VRE infection.[81]

Enterobacteriaceae

Similarly to other MDR pathogens, ESBL-producing Enterobacteriaceae fecal colonization is frequent in liver and kidney transplant candidates during the pretransplant phase (4%–31% of subjects) and was found to be independently associated with posttransplant infection.[42,87]

Similarly, the prevalence of CRE fecal carriers before liver transplantation is reported at between 5% and 18% of cases. Studies evaluating the impact of pretransplant colonization on posttransplant infection risk report conflicting results.[48,50] Thus, the management of pretransplant CRE rectal colonization remains controversial, regarding both the transplant indication and the rationale for specific pharmacologic prophylaxis. In an Italian study of 237 liver transplant recipients, carriers at the time of liver transplantation developed CRE infection in the posttransplant period in 18% of cases, whereas those acquiring CRE colonization during the posttransplant period developed a clinically significant infection in 47% of cases.[48] In a second study performed in Brazil and evaluating 386 consecutive liver transplant recipients, those identified as carriers before transplantation (16% of cases) developed an invasive infection in 40% of cases.[50] This important difference in terms of invasive infection risk may be related to different epidemiologic features (eg, different carbapenemase types were detected in these studies) and differing definition of carriers. In fact, in the study by Giannella and colleagues,[48] only rectal swabs were used to identify carriers, whereas in the study by Freire and colleagues,[50] any CRE-positive surveillance or clinical specimen culture defined a patient as a CRE carrier, resulting in selection bias. In both studies, CRE colonization was found to be a risk factor for CRE infection. However, both studies were characterized by a small number of events, and additional large-scale studies are needed to have generalizable results.

Carbapenem-Resistant Nonfermentative Gram-Negative Bacilli

The extent and the clinical role of *P aeruginosa* colonization are poorly evaluated in settings other than lung transplantation. As stated, the impact of drug-resistant *P aeruginosa* lung colonization is a major concern in patients with cystic fibrosis and/or severe bronchiectasis awaiting lung transplantation. In this setting, however, the presence of MDR or even PDR *P aeruginosa* strains before transplantation do not affect short- or long-term survival.[88] In later studies, a significant increase in the prevalence of *S maltophilia* and *A xylosoxidans* has been observed. None of these pathogens constitute an exclusion criterion for lung transplantation. However, major concerns were raised for patients colonized by MDR *Burkholderia cepacia* complex; particularly subspecies *cenocepacia*, because this organism was associated with an unacceptable rate of futile transplants.[89,90]

Similarly, pretransplant CR-AB colonization seems to increase the risk of posttransplant infection. In a study conducted among 196 liver transplant recipients, pretransplant identification of CR-AB in both clinical samples or surveillance cultures was found to increase the risk of posttransplant infection. The study, however, was conducted during a clonal outbreak of CR-AB that involved one-third of the included patients and, therefore, the results may be disproportionally influenced. Another interesting finding of this study was that the adaptation of surgical prophylaxis to CR-AB–positive surveillance cultures with use of polymyxins for colonized patients did not lead to a decrease in the subsequent rate of infection. In addition, an increase in the rate of polymyxin-resistant strains was observed in patients receiving prophylaxis with polymyxins.[55]

Currently, the most comprehensive guidelines focusing on the management of MDR in SOT candidates and recipients are those of the American Society of Transplantation, published in 2013, those of the European society of Clinical Microbiology and Infectious Diseases, published in 2014 and the recently published consensus produced by the Spanish Transplantation Infection Study Group. Recommendations on screening and prevention management are summarized in **Tables 3** and **4**.[5,91–94]

DONOR-DERIVED INFECTIONS

One crucial issue in the management of MDR pathogens in transplantation is to avoid the transmission of possibly difficult-to-treat pathogens from donors to recipients, especially in cases of deceased-donor transplantation. Deceased donors are often typically critically ill patients admitted in the ICU and have several risk factors for developing and acquiring MDR pathogen-related colonization or infection. Approximately 5% of donors are bacteremic during organ procurement and, thus, microbiological data may not be available at the time of transplantation.[95] Thus, with the recent spread of MDR pathogens that are typically resistant to the standard antibiotic prophylaxis or preemptive therapy, transmission of MDR pathogens from donors to recipients has been reported increasingly.

The most exhaustive experience on the risk of DDI caused by MDR pathogens describes an Italian series of 30 transplants using patients with colonization or infection caused by carbapenem-resistant *K pneumoniae* (CR-KP) or CR-AB as donors, including 14 cases of undiagnosed donor BSIs at the time of transplant. Proven transmission occurred only when donor infection was underestimated or miscommunicated to caregivers, which occurred in 4 of the 14 bacteremic cases. In addition, infection occurred only when the donor was infected or colonized by CR-KP, but not when the donor was infected or colonized by CR-AB (15 cases)[96]

Table 3
Summary of recommendations of different guidelines or expert consensus on the pretransplant and posttransplant management of Gram-positive MDR pathogens

Scientific Society	AST[93,94]	ESCMID[5]
Year issued	2013	2014
Universal nasal or skin screening of transplant candidate for MRSA	Not recommended routinely. Consider in facilities with unacceptable high rate of MRSA transmission. Colonized patients can be identified with nasal or skin surveillance cultures.	Nasal screening is recommended in areas with low/moderate prevalence of MRSA.
Universal screening of transplant candidate for VRE	Not recommended routinely but should be implemented during outbreaks.	Not recommended routinely but should be implemented during outbreaks.
Antibiotic prophylaxis in MRSA carriers	MRSA-active preoperative prophylaxis.	Topic not discussed.
Antibiotic prophylaxis in VRE carriers	Consider adjusting perioperative prophylaxis.	Topic not discussed.
Decolonization for MRSA carriers and timing	Consider pretransplant decolonization with intranasal application of 2% topical mupirocin twice daily for 5 d combined with chlorhexidine baths for 7 d.	Recommended selective decolonization with mupirocin and chlorhexidine bath in areas with low/moderate prevalence of MRSA and universal decolonization in areas with high MRSA prevalence during the ICU stay, after transplantation.
Decolonization for VRE carriers	Not recommended.	Not recommended.
Other preventive measures for MRSA and VRE	Implement antimicrobial stewardship programs. Contact precautions for all carriers and infected patients. Use dedicated equipment. Environmental cleaning, Monitor compliance with hand hygiene.	Recommended isolation or cohorting of carriers, contact precautions, and environmental cleaning.

Abbreviations: AST, American Society of Transplantation; ESCMID, European Society of Clinical Microbiology and Infectious Disease; ICU, intensive care unit; MDR, multidrug-resistant; MRSA, methicillin-resistant *Staphylococcus aureus*; VRE, vancomycin-resistant Enterococci.

Cases of possible/probable DDI caused by MDR pathogens and reported in the literature are summarized in **Table 5**. The 34 cases of MDR pathogen transmission identified (33 infection, 1 airway colonization in a lung transplant recipient) include 8 CR-KP infections, 7 MDR *P aeruginosa* infections, 5 ESBL-producing Enterobacteriaceae, 1 CR-AB infection, 1 CR-KP airway colonization, 8 MRSA, and 4 VRE infections. In 22 of 34 cases, the results of donor culture were either not available, negative at the time of transplantation, or the results were not adequately communicated to the caregiver. In 5 additional cases, the information was underestimated. In

Table 4
Summary of recommendations of different guidelines or expert consensus on the pretransplant and posttransplant management of Gram-negative MDR pathogens

Scientific Society	AST[92]	ESCMID[5]	GESITRA- EIMC/REIPI[91]
Year issued	2013	2014	2018
Universal screening of transplant candidate for ESBL-producing Enterobacteriaceae	Not recommended	Not recommended in endemic areas, recommended during outbreaks	Not recommended
Universal screening of transplant candidate/ recipients for CRE	Not recommended	Not recommended in endemic areas, recommended during outbreaks	Recommended at transplantation After transplantation, in accordance with institutional policy
Universal screening of transplant candidate for MDR nonfermenters	Not recommended	Not recommended in endemic areas, recommended during outbreaks Recommended screening of respiratory samples in lung transplant candidates	Not recommended routinely
Delist carriers of GN-MDR	Decision on case-by-case basis	Decision on case-by-case basis for lung transplant candidates colonized by nonfermenting MDR/XDR rods	Not recommended in any case

Accept donor with MDR Enterobacteriaceae-positive cultures	Topic not discussed	Topic not discussed	Accept ESBL-E carriers Accept donor with nonbacteremic, non–graft-related CRE infection. In this case, donor should receive a 7-d CRE treatment at minimum Reject kidney from donor with CRE-UTI or lung from donor with CRE pneumonia
Accept donor with MDR nonfermenting positive cultures	Topic not discussed	Topic not discussed	Accept organs with positive MDR-*Pseudomonas aeruginosa* only in exceptional cases Accept donor with CR-AB Reject CR-AB colonized lungs and kidneys from donor with CR-AB
Antibiotic prophylaxis in ESBL carriers	Standard prophylaxis not exceeding 48 h of duration, with exception for lung transplant recipients	Topic not discussed	Specific prophylaxis is recommended Avoid carbapenem when possible Consider nebulized antibiotic in colonized lung transplant recipients, or recipients of colonized graft
Antibiotic prophylaxis in other GN-MDR	Standard prophylaxis	Topic not discussed	Adopt surgical prophylaxis in accordance with local patterns Lung transplant recipients should receive prophylaxis driven by pretransplant cultures Colonized lung candidate or recipients should receive nebulized colistin perioperatively

(continued on next page)

Table 4
(continued)

Scientific Society	AST[92]	ESCMID[5]	GESITRA- EIMC/REIPI[91]
Decolonization for ESBL carriers	Not recommended	Not recommended	Not recommended
Decolonization for GN-MDR carriers	Not recommended	Not recommended	Not recommended
Other preventive measures for ESBL carriers	Same as other GN-MDR	Isolation of carriers of ESBL-producing *Escherichia coli* is not recommended Contact precautions and isolation of patients with other ESBL-producing Enterobacteriaceae are recommended	Screening for ESBL-E may be useful; handwashing or disinfection with alcohol-based gels are recommended in all cases Contact precautions are strongly recommended for ESBL- producing *K pneumoniae* and weakly recommended for ESBL-producing *E coli*
Other preventive measures for GN-MDR carriers	Reduce/avoid the unneeded antibiotic exposure in the pretransplant and posttransplant period Reduce the exposure to indwelling devices and reduce the duration of endotracheal intubation Promote hand hygiene Use of contact precautions: separate carriers in private room or cohort patients with same GN-MDR	Placement of patients in single-bed isolation Use of contact precautions and environmental cleaning	Perform surveillance cultures in the posttransplant period Promote and monitor compliance of hand hygiene Contact precautions is recommended for infected and colonized patients HCW should wear goggles and face mask when performing procedures on CR-AB colonized/infected patients Staff cohorting and active screening during outbreaks

Abbreviations: AST, American Society of Transplantation; CR-AB, carbapenem-resistant *Acinetobacter baumannii*; CRE, carbapenem-resistant enterobacteriaceae; EIMC, Spanish Society of Infectious Diseases and Clinical Microbiology; ESBL-E, extended spectrum β-lactamase enterobacteriaceae; ESCMID, European Society of Clinical Microbiology and Infectious Disease; GESITRA, Group for Study of Infection in Transplantation; GN-MDR, gram-negative multidrug resistant; HCW, health care workers; REIPI, Spanish Network for Research in Infectious Diseases; UTI, urinary tract infection; XDR, extensively drug-resistant.

Table 5
Cases of donor-derived infection involving MDR pathogens

Strain	Donor Infection/ Colonization	Recipients' Organ(s)	Posttransplant Infection	Information Available Before Infection Development	Prophylaxis/ Preemptive Treatment of Recipient	Outcome	Confirmation of Transmission with Genotyping
CR-KP[140]	Lung colonization	Liver	BSI	No	Standard prophylaxis	Survived at 1 y posttransplant	No
CR-KP[141]	Meningitis and pneumonia	Liver and kidney	Intraabdominal	Yes	Targeted with tigecycline	Alive 5 mo after transplantation	No
CR-KP[142]	Lung and rectal colonization	Kidney-pancreas	IAI	No	Colistin, meropenem and tigecycline	Died 6 mo after transplant	Yes (PFGE)
CR-KP[96]	BSI	Right lobe split liver	SSI	Yes	Meropenem	Alive at 18-mo follow-up	Yes (PFGE)
		Lungs	Airway colonization	Yes	Meropenem	Alive	Yes (PFGE)
CR-KP[96]	Blood, urine, and BAL	Liver	SSI – intraabdominal collection	Yes	3 d of meropenem and gentamicin	Alive 6 mo after transplant	Yes (PFGE)
CR-KP[96]	CR-KP urine	Kidney	Perigraft collection	No	Standard prophylaxis	Died 2 mo after transplant	Yes (PFGE)
CR-KP[143]	Unknown	Kidney	BSI	No	Standard prophylaxis	Lost to follow-up	Yes (PFGE and MLSG)[a]
		Liver	IAI	No	Standard prophylaxis	Alive 6 mo after transplant	

(continued on next page)

Table 5
(continued)

Strain	Donor Infection/ Colonization	Recipients' Organ(s)	Posttransplant Infection	Information Available Before Infection Development	Prophylaxis/ Preemptive Treatment of Recipient	Outcome	Confirmation of Transmission with Genotyping
ESBL-producing *Escherichia coli*[144]	UTI	Kidney	UTI complicated with pseudoaneurysm	No	Standard prophylaxis	Survived but underwent nephrectomy	No
		Kidney	Pyelonephritis	No	Standard prophylaxis	Survived but underwent nephrectomy	No
ESBL-producing *Klebsiella pneumoniae*[145]	Unknown	Liver	IAI	No	Standard prophylaxis	Died within 3 mo after transplant	No[a]
ESBL-producing *K pneumoniae*[145]	Unknown	Liver	IAI	No	Standard prophylaxis	Alive 3 mo after transplant	No[a]
ESBL-producing *Enterobacter aerogenes*[145]	Unknown	Liver	BSI	No	Standard prophylaxis	Alive after 3 mo form transplant	No[a]
CR-AB[146]	Lung	Lung	Tracheobronchitis	No	Standard prophylaxis	Died 65 d after transplant	Yes (PFGE and RAPD)
MDR *Pseudomonas aeruginosa*[147]	Pneumonia	Kidney	SSI and brain mycotic aneurysm	No	Standard prophylaxis	Died	No
		Kidney	BSI	No	Standard prophylaxis	Died	No
MDR *P aeruginosa*[148]	Urine and peritoneal fluid	Kidney	SSI-Perigraft collection	No	Standard prophylaxis	Alive 1 y after transplant	Yes (PFGE)

MDR *P aeruginosa*[149]	Peritoneal fluid	Heart	Empyema	Yes	Standard prophylaxis	Alive	No
		Liver	Cholangitis	Yes	Meropenem	Died 38 d after transplant	No
		Kidney	SSI	Yes	Meropenem	Died	No
		Kidney	SSI	Yes	Unknown	Lost to follow-up	No
MRSA[150]	Mitral valve endocarditis	Liver	BSI	Yes	Vancomycin	Alive 1 y after transplant	Yes (WGS)
MRSA[151]	Nasal carrier	Living-donor-liver	Pneumonia	No	Standard prophylaxis	Deceased	Yes (PFGE)
MRSA[152]	BSI	Heart	Myocarditis	No	Standard prophylaxis	Died	Yes
MRSA[153]	Endocarditis	Liver	Recurrent BSI	Yes	Daptomycin	Alive	Yes (PFGE)
MRSA[154]	Endotracheal tube colonization	Liver	BSI with disseminated localizations	No	Standard prophylaxis	Alive	Yes
		Kidney	BSI	No	Vancomycin	Alive	Yes
MRSA[155]	Endocarditis	Liver	BSI	Yes	Daptomycin	Alive	Yes (WGS)
		Lung	Pneumonia	Yes	Vancomycin	Alive	Yes (WGS)
VRE[156]	Unknown	Liver	IAI	No	Standard prophylaxis	Deceased after 7 mo	Yes (WGS)[b]
		Kidney	Perigraft collection	No	Standard prophylaxis	Alive	Yes (WGS)[b]
		Kidney	UTI	No	Standard prophylaxis	Alive	Yes (WGS)[b]
VRE[157]	BSI	Liver	IAI	No	Standard prophylaxis	Alive	Yes (WGS)

Abbreviations: BAL, bronchoalveolar lavage; BSI, bloodstream infection; CR-AB, carbapenem-resistant *Acinetobacter baumannii*; CR-KP, Carbapenem-resistant *Klebsiella pneumoniae*; MDR multidrug-resistant; ESBL, extended spectrum β-lactamase; IAI, intraabdominal infection; MLSG, multilocus sequence genotyping; MRSA, methicillin-resistant *Staphylococcus aureus*; PFGE, pulsed-field gel electrophoresis; RAPD, random amplification of polymorphic DNA; SSI, surgical site infection; UTI, urinary tract infection; VRE, vancomycin-resistant Enterobacteriaceae; WGS, whole-genome sequencing.

[a] The strain was not recovered in the donor. However, the recipients undergoing transplantation in different hospitals acquired an identical strain and the hypothesis of donor-derived infection is likely. Contamination during the harvesting procedure may have occurred.

[b] In this report, the same teicoplanin-resistant VRE was recovered from 3 different recipients receiving an organ from the same donor. Whole-genome sequencing confirmed the identity of the strains.

all of these cases (27 of 34), patients did not receive adequate preemptive treatment. Preemptive therapy or prophylaxis failed to prevent DDI in 5 of the 8 reported cases of MRSA transmission and in 2 cases of MDR *P aeruginosa* transmission. Mortality was reported in 11 cases, 9 of which did not receive preemptive antibiotics. Two kidney transplant recipients experienced graft loss; neither received preemptive treatment.

TREATMENT

Treatment of MDR pathogens in SOT recipients is extremely challenging for several reasons. First, the diagnosis may be difficult or delayed. In fact, multiple simultaneous conditions such as infection and graft rejection or multiple infectious processes may overlap. For instance, viral replication (eg, cytomegalovirus) or opportunistic infections may be diagnosed together with bacterial infections. Second, the wide differences of the epidemiology between centers and the varying risk factors found in different studies may hamper the ability to identify those patients who may need broader spectrum empirical treatment. Third, most patients have indwelling devices (eg, urinary catheters or ureteral stents in kidney transplantation) that may be responsible for recurrence of infection even after adequate treatment. In addition, infection source control may be more challenging than in non-SOT patients owing to surgical complexity. Fourth, drug comparative studies in SOT recipients are limited and most data come from mixed populations that comprise both transplant and nontransplant patients. Finally, drug–drug interactions may occur between immunosuppressive drugs and antimicrobials, altering the drugs' pharmacokinetics and pharmacodynamics and potentially worsening the clinical course of patients. Thus, several aspects should be kept in mind when choosing empirical antimicrobial treatment. Regarding the risk for MDR organisms, the most important factors are by far prior antibiotic exposure, and prior infection or colonization with an MDR organism.

Treatment of Gram-Positive Multidrug-Resistant Pathogens

Vancomycin is considered the treatment of choice for MRSA infection in most cases. Although the superiority of other drugs versus vancomycin was poorly demonstrated in clinical trials, observational studies suggest that alternative regimens could be associated with improved outcomes under specific situations.[97,98] More specifically, with the spread of strains with reduced susceptibility to vancomycin, treatment failure with this drug was reported.[99] In a metaanalysis including 22 studies, higher mortality was reported in infections caused by MRSA strains with vancomycin a minimum inhibitory concentration of 2 mg/mL or greater, especially in case of BSI.[100] In 1 case-control study, the use of daptomycin was associated with an improved outcome compared with vancomycin.[97] According to the Infectious Diseases Society of America guidelines, MRSA pneumonia should be treated with either vancomycin or linezolid.[101] In a randomized trial enrolling patients with nosocomial pneumonia caused by MRSA, patients treated with linezolid achieved a better clinical and microbiological cure and a lower rate of nephrotoxicity when compared with those treated with vancomycin.[102]

Although vancomycin-resistant *Enterococcus faecalis* may be susceptible to ampicillin, most of vancomycin resistant enterococcus infections have been attributed to *Enterococcus faecium*.

Options for treating vancomycin-resistant enterococcus infections are linezolid, daptomycin, or tigecycline. Well-designed comparative studies are not available to assess the best treatment for VRE. However, a metanalysis of 10 retrospective studies comparing outcome of patients treated with linezolid or daptomycin for VRE bacteremia found an increased risk of mortality in patients receiving daptomycin.[103]

Treatment of Gram-Negative Multidrug-Resistant Pathogens

Although ESBL-producing gram-negative bacteria emerged as a major global public health concern more than 2 decades ago, issues concerning the best treatment choices continue to be unresolved.[104] The major challenge regards the right place in therapy of carbapenems and β-lactam β-lactamase inhibitors (BLBLI) combinations: the efficacy of carbapenems is well-recognized, however, carbapenem overuse can induce several resistance pathways, including the selection of carbapenemases. Therefore, efforts toward the use of carbapenem-sparing regimens whenever an alternative exists should be encouraged.

The role of BLBLI combinations for ESBL-Enterobacteriaceae infections is controversial. Observational studies suggest that BLBLI may be an alternative to carbapenems in infections originated from the urinary tract or with adequate source control; for other sites, treatment failures may occur mainly when the minimum inhibitory concentrations are above a minimum level.[105,106] A recent study showed that when susceptible in vitro, treatment other than with a BLBLI for ESBL-E infections such as aminoglycosides or fluoroquinolones is not associated with worse outcome compared with carbapenems[107]

Although tigecycline does not feature in vitro activity against P aeruginosa or certain Enterobacteriaceae (Proteus spp., Serratia spp., Morganella morganii, Providencia stuartii), it is still an option for complicated intraabdominal infections because of its favorable pharmacokinetics in the abdominal organs and in vitro activity against anaerobic organisms, enterococci, several ESBLs, and some strains of carbapenemase-producing Enterobacteriaceae.[108,109] However, because of poor plasma concentration, tigecycline performs poorly in bacteremic patients, with a much higher risk of failure to clear bacteremia.[110] Similarly, tigecycline shows poor urine concentration with standard dosage. Therefore, tigecycline should not be considered as a first-line therapy in patients with health care–associated pneumonia, bacteremia, and UTI when other effective drugs are available. In addition, reported experience in an SOT setting is limited.[111]

The recent challenges in the management of gram-negative MDR organism infections, especially in critically ill patients, have revived the clinical use of polymyxins, fosfomycin, and minocycline.[112,113] There remain open questions about the need for combination therapy and the role of carbapenems, administered at high doses and by extended infusions, in the treatment of infections with CRE. In large observational trials, combination treatment including high-dose carbapenems and colistin or aminoglycosides were associated with better outcomes, especially in critically ill patients.[114,115]

Ceftolozane/tazobactam and ceftazidime/avibactam have recently been approved in some national agencies for the treatment of complicated UTIs, intraabdominal infections, and nosocomial pneumonia.[116,117]

Ceftolozane/tazobactam is a new antibiotic that has been approved for treatment of complicated intraabdominal infections (in combination with metronidazole), including infection by ESBLs and P aeruginosa, and may be valuable for treating infections caused by gram-negative MDR organisms to preserve carbapenems.[118,119] It may be useful as empirical therapy to preserve the use of carbapenems for use in critical patients with risk factors for ESBL isolation or as targeted therapy in patients with isolation of a susceptible ESBL-producing Enterobacteriaceae or MDR P aeruginosa. It should be pointed out that, in some countries, the production of metallo-β-lactamase enzymes that are not inactivated by ceftolozane/tazobactam may be one of the mechanisms of carbapenem resistance in *P aeruginosa*.

Ceftazidime-avibactam (CAZ-AVI) is a novel drug that combines a third-generation cephalosporin with an inhibitor of β-lactamase.[120,121] Despite the settings of registration trials, a greater interest for CAZ-AVI is due to the activity of avibactam in inactivating a large number of β-lactamase enzymes, including carbapenemase KPC and most OXA-48, representing the first β-lactam antibiotic combination showing this characteristic.[122]

Recent case series have reported on the use of CAZ-AVI in patients with CRE infection.[123–125] Although reporting efficacy in a variety of clinical situations, first-line therapy, and compassionate use, the overall success rates ranged from 45% to 74%, with relapse rates of up to 23%. Three observational studies have reported higher rates of clinical success and lower mortality with CAZ-AVI compared with other regimens for CRE infection.[46,126,127] In the clinical studies on CRE infection, CAZ-AVI was used in combination in 27% to 63% of cases.[46,123,124,126,127] There was great variety in the combination antibiotics, with aminoglycosides, carbapenems, and tigecycline used most frequently. However, direct comparisons between monotherapy and combination therapy, and between different kinds of combinations, were not performed.[46,123,124,126,127] In a study by Shields and colleagues,[123] where SOT recipients constituted 21% of the population, CAZ-AVI was predominantly used as monotherapy, and approximately 30% of patients received combination regimens, primarily with aminoglycosides as the second agent. There was an alarmingly high rate (24%) of CRE relapse after completion of therapy. Most relapsing patients had received monotherapy (7 of 10), and 3 of them (8% of the entire cohort) developed reinfection by a strain that had developed resistance (minimum inhibitory concentration of ≥ 16 μg/mL) to CAZ-AVI after only 10 to 19 days of therapy. Whether combination therapy can be used to prevent the emergence of resistance to CAZ-AVI in CRE is not known.

Vaborbactam is another novel β-lactamase inhibitor that shows an important activity against KPC producers. Unfortunately, it has no activity against OXA-48 or metallo-β-lactamase enzymes.[128] Vaborbactam was evaluated in combination with meropenem in a phase III randomized study and was compared with piperacillin-tazobactam for treatment of complicated UTIs. Meropenem-vaborbactam was statistically superior to piperacillin-tazobactam in clinical cure and eradication of baseline pathogen.[129] Meropenem-vaborbactam was also evaluated in a small phase III trial including 70 patients with CRE infection randomized (2:1) to receive meropenem-vaborbactam (2 g and 2 g every 8 hours) or best available treatment. The latter consisted of monotherapy (26%), dual therapy (46.7%), triple therapy (6.7%), and therapy with 4 or more drugs (13.3%). Overall, meropenem-vaborbactam showed higher clinical cure (57.1% vs 26.7%; absolute difference, 30.5%; 95% confidence interval, 1.5%–59.4%) and a lower rate of nephrotoxicity. Despite these promising results, the study was characterized by important heterogeneity of treatment administered in the comparator arm, limiting direct comparison between regimens.[130]

SUMMARY

The magnitude of the challenge of MDR pathogens is huge; this problem affects several aspects of the management of transplant candidates and recipients. Areas of uncertainty are predominant in this field concerning selection of candidates, infection prevention, infection control policies, and treatment. In addition, continually updated recommendations are needed to face the ever-present and evolving epidemiology of bacterial infection in this setting.

REFERENCES

1. Laxminarayan R, Duse A, Wattal C, et al. Antibiotic resistance-the need for global solutions. Lancet Infect Dis 2013;13(12):1057–98.
2. Abouna GM. Organ shortage crisis: problems and possible solutions. Transplant Proc 2008;40(1):34–8.
3. Karvellas CJ, Lescot T, Goldberg P, et al. Liver transplantation in the critically ill: a multicenter Canadian retrospective cohort study. Crit Care 2013;17(1):R28.
4. Camargo LF, Marra AR, Pignatari AC, et al. Nosocomial bloodstream infections in a nationwide study: comparison between solid organ transplant patients and the general population. Transpl Infect Dis 2015;17(2):308–13.
5. Cervera C, van Delden C, Gavalda J, et al. Multidrug-resistant bacteria in solid organ transplant recipients. Clin Microbiol Infect 2014;20(Suppl 7):49–73.
6. Laupland KB, Gregson DB, Flemons WW, et al. Burden of community-onset bloodstream infection: a population-based assessment. Epidemiol Infect 2007;135(6):1037–42.
7. Landrum ML, Neumann C, Cook C, et al. Epidemiology of Staphylococcus aureus blood and skin and soft tissue infections in the us military health system, 2005-2010. JAMA 2012;308(1):50–9.
8. de Kraker ME, Jarlier V, Monen JC, et al. The changing epidemiology of bacteraemias in Europe: trends from the European Antimicrobial Resistance Surveillance System. Clin Microbiol Infect 2013;19(9):860–8.
9. Dantes R, Mu Y, Belflower R, et al. National burden of invasive methicillin-resistant Staphylococcus aureus infections, United States, 2011. JAMA Intern Med 2013;173(21):1970–8.
10. Singh N, Paterson DL, Chang FY, et al. Methicillin-resistant Staphylococcus aureus: the other emerging resistant gram-positive coccus among liver transplant recipients. Clin Infect Dis 2000;30(2):322–7.
11. Karvellas CJ, McPhail M, Pink F, et al. Bloodstream infection after elective liver transplantation is associated with increased mortality in patients with cirrhosis. J Crit Care 2011;26(5):468–74.
12. Florescu DF, McCartney AM, Qiu F, et al. Staphylococcus aureus infections after liver transplantation. Infection 2012;40(3):263–9.
13. Bert F, Larroque B, Paugam-Burtz C, et al. Microbial epidemiology and outcome of bloodstream infections in liver transplant recipients: an analysis of 259 episodes. Liver Transpl 2010;16(3):393–401.
14. Shields RK, Clancy CJ, Minces LR, et al. Staphylococcus aureus infections in the early period after lung transplantation: epidemiology, risk factors, and outcomes. J Heart Lung Transplant 2012;31(11):1199–206.
15. Florescu DF, Qiu F, West SB, et al. Staphylococcus aureus infections in kidney transplantation: a matched case controlled study. Scand J Infect Dis 2012; 44(6):427–32.
16. Schneider CR, Buell JF, Gearhart M, et al. Methicillin-resistant Staphylococcus aureus infection in liver transplantation: a matched controlled study. Transplant Proc 2005;37(2):1243–4.
17. Hsu RB, Fang CT, Chang SC, et al. Infectious complications after heart transplantation in Chinese recipients. Am J Transplant 2005;5(8):2011–6.
18. Oliveira-Cunha M, Bowman V, di Benedetto G, et al. Outcomes of methicillin-resistant Staphylococcus aureus infection after kidney and/or pancreas transplantation. Transplant Proc 2013;45(6):2207–10.

19. Gupta MR, Valentine VG, Walker JE Jr, et al. Clinical spectrum of gram-positive infections in lung transplantation. Transpl Infect Dis 2009;11(5):424–31.

20. Bucheli E, Kralidis G, Boggian K, et al. Impact of enterococcal colonization and infection in solid organ transplantation recipients from the swiss transplant cohort study. Transpl Infect Dis 2014;16(1):26–36.

21. Bodro M, Sabe N, Tubau F, et al. Risk factors and outcomes of bacteremia caused by drug-resistant escape pathogens in solid-organ transplant recipients. Transplantation 2013;96(9):843–9.

22. Berenger BM, Doucette K, Smith SW. Epidemiology and risk factors for nosocomial bloodstream infections in solid organ transplants over a 10-year period. Transpl Infect Dis 2016;18(2):183–90.

23. Moreno A, Cervera C, Gavalda J, et al. Bloodstream infections among transplant recipients: results of a nationwide surveillance in Spain. Am J Transplant 2007; 7(11):2579–86.

24. Russell DL, Flood A, Zaroda TE, et al. Outcomes of colonization with MRSA and VRE among liver transplant candidates and recipients. Am J Transplant 2008; 8(8):1737–43.

25. Newell KA, Millis JM, Arnow PM, et al. Incidence and outcome of infection by vancomycin-resistant enterococcus following orthotopic liver transplantation. Transplantation 1998;65(3):439–42.

26. McNeil SA, Malani PN, Chenoweth CE, et al. Vancomycin-resistant enterococcal colonization and infection in liver transplant candidates and recipients: a prospective surveillance study. Clin Infect Dis 2006;42(2):195–203.

27. Bonten MJ, Willems R, Weinstein RA. Vancomycin-resistant enterococci: why are they here, and where do they come from? Lancet Infect Dis 2001;1(5): 314–25.

28. Banach DB, Peaper DR, Fortune BE, et al. The clinical and molecular epidemiology of pre-transplant vancomycin-resistant enterococci colonization among liver transplant recipients. Clin Transplant 2016;30(3):306–11.

29. Tandon P, Delisle A, Topal JE, et al. High prevalence of antibiotic-resistant bacterial infections among patients with cirrhosis at a us liver center. Clin Gastroenterol Hepatol 2012;10(11):1291–8.

30. Bhavnani SM, Drake JA, Forrest A, et al. A nationwide, multicenter, case-control study comparing risk factors, treatment, and outcome for vancomycin-resistant and -susceptible enterococcal bacteremia. Diagn Microbiol Infect Dis 2000; 36(3):145–58.

31. Gearhart M, Martin J, Rudich S, et al. Consequences of vancomycin-resistant enterococcus in liver transplant recipients: a matched control study. Clin Transplant 2005;19(6):711–6.

32. Orloff SL, Busch AM, Olyaei AJ, et al. Vancomycin-resistant enterococcus in liver transplant patients. Am J Surg 1999;177(5):418–22.

33. Viehman JA, Clancy CJ, Clarke L, et al. Surgical site infections after liver transplantation: emergence of multidrug-resistant bacteria and implications for prophylaxis and treatment strategies. Transplantation 2016;100(10):2107–14.

34. Forrest GN, Arnold RS, Gammie JS, et al. Single center experience of a vancomycin resistant enterococcal endocarditis cohort. J Infect 2011;63(6):420–8.

35. Simon D, Fischer S, Grossman A, et al. Left ventricular assist device-related infection: treatment and outcome. Clin Infect Dis 2005;40(8):1108–15.

36. Paterson DL, Singh N, Rihs JD, et al. Control of an outbreak of infection due to extended-spectrum beta-lactamase–producing Escherichia coli in a liver transplantation unit. Clin Infect Dis 2001;33(1):126–8.

37. Harris PN, Tambyah PA, Paterson DL. Beta-lactam and beta-lactamase inhibitor combinations in the treatment of extended-spectrum beta-lactamase producing enterobacteriaceae: time for a reappraisal in the era of few antibiotic options? Lancet Infect Dis 2015;15(4):475–85.

38. Oriol I, Sabe N, Simonetti AF, et al. Changing trends in the aetiology, treatment and outcomes of bloodstream infection occurring in the first year after solid organ transplantation: a single-centre prospective cohort study. Transpl Int 2017; 30(9):903–13.

39. Men TY, Wang JN, Li H, et al. Prevalence of multidrug-resistant gram-negative bacilli producing extended-spectrum beta-lactamases (ESBLs) and ESBL genes in solid organ transplant recipients. Transpl Infect Dis 2013;15(1):14–21.

40. Aguiar EB, Maciel LC, Halpern M, et al. Outcome of bacteremia caused by extended-spectrum beta-lactamase-producing enterobacteriaceae after solid organ transplantation. Transplant Proc 2014;46(6):1753–6.

41. Bui KT, Mehta S, Khuu TH, et al. Extended spectrum beta-lactamase-producing enterobacteriaceae infection in heart and lung transplant recipients and in mechanical circulatory support recipients. Transplantation 2014;97(5):590–4.

42. Bert F, Larroque B, Paugam-Burtz C, et al. Pretransplant fecal carriage of extended-spectrum beta-lactamase-producing enterobacteriaceae and infection after liver transplant, France. Emerg Infect Dis 2012;18(6):908–16.

43. Espinar MJ, Miranda IM, Costa-de-Oliveira S, et al. Urinary tract infections in kidney transplant patients due to Escherichia coli and Klebsiella pneumoniae-producing extended-spectrum beta-lactamases: risk factors and molecular epidemiology. PLoS One 2015;10(8):e0134737.

44. Pilmis B, Scemla A, Join-Lambert O, et al. ESBL-producing enterobacteriaceae-related urinary tract infections in kidney transplant recipients: incidence and risk factors for recurrence. Infect Dis (Lond) 2015;47(10):714–8.

45. Giannella M, Graziano E, Marconi L, et al. Risk factors for recurrent carbapenem resistant Klebsiella pneumoniae bloodstream infection: a prospective cohort study. Eur J Clin Microbiol Infect Dis 2017;36(10):1965–70.

46. Shields RK, Nguyen MH, Chen L, et al. Ceftazidime-avibactam is superior to other treatment regimens against carbapenem-resistant Klebsiella pneumoniae bacteremia. Antimicrob Agents Chemother 2017;61(8) [pii:e00883-17].

47. Lanini S, Costa AN, Puro V, et al. Incidence of carbapenem-resistant gram negatives in Italian transplant recipients: a nationwide surveillance study. PloS one 2015;10(4):e0123706.

48. Giannella M, Bartoletti M, Morelli MC, et al. Risk factors for infection with carbapenem-resistant Klebsiella pneumoniae after liver transplantation: the importance of pre- and posttransplant colonization. Am J Transplant 2015; 15(6):1708–15.

49. Cicora F, Mos F, Paz M, et al. Infections with blakpc-2-producing Klebsiella pneumoniae in renal transplant patients: a retrospective study. Transplant Proc 2013;45(9):3389–93.

50. Freire MP, Oshiro IC, Pierrotti LC, et al. Carbapenem-resistant enterobacteriaceae acquired before liver transplantation: impact on recipient outcomes. Transplantation 2017;101(4):811–20.

51. Kalpoe JS, Sonnenberg E, Factor SH, et al. Mortality associated with carbapenem-resistant Klebsiella pneumoniae infections in liver transplant recipients. Liver Transpl 2012;18(4):468–74.

52. Lubbert C, Becker-Rux D, Rodloff AC, et al. Colonization of liver transplant recipients with kpc-producing Klebsiella pneumoniae is associated with high

infection rates and excess mortality: a case-control analysis. Infection 2014; 42(2):309–16.

53. Bergamasco MD, Barroso Barbosa M, de Oliveira Garcia D, et al. Infection with Klebsiella pneumoniae carbapenemase (kpc)-producing k. Pneumoniae in solid organ transplantation. Transpl Infect Dis 2012;14(2):198–205.

54. Clancy CJ, Chen L, Shields RK, et al. Epidemiology and molecular characterization of bacteremia due to carbapenem-resistant Klebsiella pneumoniae in transplant recipients. Am J Transplant 2013;13(10):2619–33.

55. Freire MP, Pierrotti LC, Oshiro IC, et al. Carbapenem-resistant Acinetobacter baumannii acquired before liver transplantation: impact on recipient outcomes. Liver Transpl 2016;22(5):615–26.

56. Liu H, Ye Q, Wan Q, et al. Predictors of mortality in solid-organ transplant recipients with infections caused by Acinetobacter baumannii. Ther Clin Risk Manag 2015;11:1251–7.

57. Biderman P, Bugaevsky Y, Ben-Zvi H, et al. Multidrug-resistant Acinetobacter baumannii infections in lung transplant patients in the cardiothoracic intensive care unit. Clin Transplant 2015;29(9):756–62.

58. de Gouvea EF, Martins IS, Halpern M, et al. The influence of carbapenem resistance on mortality in solid organ transplant recipients with Acinetobacter baumannii infection. BMC Infect Dis 2012;12:351.

59. Husain S, Chan KM, Palmer SM, et al. Bacteremia in lung transplant recipients in the current era. Am J Transplant 2006;6(12):3000–7.

60. Johnson LE, D'Agata EM, Paterson DL, et al. Pseudomonas aeruginosa bacteremia over a 10-year period: multidrug resistance and outcomes in transplant recipients. Transpl Infect Dis 2009;11(3):227–34.

61. Bodro M, Sabe N, Tubau F, et al. Extensively drug-resistant Pseudomonas aeruginosa bacteremia in solid organ transplant recipients. Transplantation 2015; 99(3):616–22.

62. Hadjiliadis D, Steele MP, Chaparro C, et al. Survival of lung transplant patients with cystic fibrosis harboring panresistant bacteria other than Burkholderia cepacia, compared with patients harboring sensitive bacteria. J Heart Lung Transplant 2007;26(8):834–8.

63. Gregson AL, Wang X, Weigt SS, et al. Interaction between Pseudomonas and cxc chemokines increases risk of bronchiolitis obliterans syndrome and death in lung transplantation. Am J Respir Crit Care Med 2013;187(5):518–26.

64. Linares L, Cervera C, Cofan F, et al. Epidemiology and outcomes of multiple antibiotic-resistant bacterial infection in renal transplantation. Transplant Proc 2007;39(7):2222–4.

65. Jalan R, Fernandez J, Wiest R, et al. Bacterial infections in cirrhosis: a position statement based on the EASL special conference 2013. J Hepatol 2014;60(6): 1310–24.

66. Fernandez J, Acevedo J, Wiest R, et al. Bacterial and fungal infections in acute-on-chronic liver failure: prevalence, characteristics and impact on prognosis. Gut 2017. https://doi.org/10.1136/gutjnl-2017-314240.

67. Bertuzzo VR, Giannella M, Cucchetti A, et al. Impact of preoperative infection on outcome after liver transplantation. Br J Surg 2017;104(2):E172–81.

68. Bartoletti M, Giannella M, Caraceni P, et al. Epidemiology and outcomes of bloodstream infection in patients with cirrhosis. J Hepatol 2014;61(1):51–8.

69. Bartoletti M, Giannella M, Lewis R, et al. A prospective multicentre study of the epidemiology and outcomes of bloodstream infection in cirrhotic patients. Clin Microbiol Infect 2017. https://doi.org/10.1016/j.cmi.2017.08.001.

70. Safdar N, Said A, Lucey MR, et al. Infected bilomas in liver transplant recipients: clinical features, optimal management, and risk factors for mortality. Clin Infect Dis 2004;39(4):517–25.

71. van Delden C. Bacterial biliary tract infections in liver transplant recipients. Curr Opin Organ Transplant 2014;19(3):223–8.

72. Pop-Vicas A, Strom J, Stanley K, et al. Multidrug-resistant gram-negative bacteria among patients who require chronic hemodialysis. Clin J Am Soc Nephrol 2008;3(3):752–8.

73. Worth LJ, Spelman T, Holt SG, et al. Epidemiology of infections and antimicrobial use in Australian haemodialysis outpatients: findings from a Victorian surveillance network, 2008-2015. J Hosp Infect 2017;97(1):93–8.

74. Melzer M, Santhakumaran T, Welch C. The characteristics and outcome of bacteraemia in renal transplant recipients and non-transplant renal patients. Infection 2016;44(5):617–22.

75. Razvi S, Quittell L, Sewall A, et al. Respiratory microbiology of patients with cystic fibrosis in the United States, 1995 to 2005. Chest 2009;136(6):1554–60.

76. Rutter WC, Burgess DR, Burgess DS. Increasing incidence of multidrug resistance among cystic fibrosis respiratory bacterial isolates. Microb Drug Resist 2017;23(1):51–5.

77. Desai D, Desai N, Nightingale P, et al. Carriage of methicillin-resistant Staphylococcus aureus is associated with an increased risk of infection after liver transplantation. Liver Transpl 2003;9(7):754–9.

78. Hashimoto M, Sugawara Y, Tamura S, et al. Acquisition of methicillin-resistant Staphylococcus aureus after living donor liver transplantation: a retrospective cohort study. BMC Infect Dis 2008;8:155.

79. Hashimoto M, Sugawara Y, Tamura S, et al. Impact of new methicillin-resistant Staphylococcus aureus carriage postoperatively after living donor liver transplantation. Transplant Proc 2007;39(10):3271–5.

80. Santoro-Lopes G, de Gouvea EF, Monteiro RC, et al. Colonization with methicillin-resistant Staphylococcus aureus after liver transplantation. Liver Transpl 2005;11(2):203–9.

81. Ziakas PD, Pliakos EE, Zervou FN, et al. MRSA and VRE colonization in solid organ transplantation: a meta-analysis of published studies. Am J Transplant 2014;14(8):1887–94.

82. Paterson DL, Rihs JD, Squier C, et al. Lack of efficacy of mupirocin in the prevention of infections with Staphylococcus aureus in liver transplant recipients and candidates. Transplantation 2003;75(2):194–8.

83. Singh N, Squier C, Wannstedt C, et al. Impact of an aggressive infection control strategy on endemic Staphylococcus aureus infection in liver transplant recipients. Infect Control Hosp Epidemiol 2006;27(2):122–6.

84. Herrera S, Sorli L, Perez-Saez MJ, et al. Characterization and rapid control of a vancomycin-resistant Enterococcus faecium (VREF) outbreak in a renal transplant unit in Spain: the environment matters. Enferm Infecc Microbiol Clin 2017;35(1):5–11.

85. Bakir M, Bova JL, Newell KA, et al. Epidemiology and clinical consequences of vancomycin-resistant enterococci in liver transplant patients. Transplantation 2001;72(6):1032–7.

86. Freitas MC, Pacheco-Silva A, Barbosa D, et al. Prevalence of vancomycin-resistant enterococcus fecal colonization among kidney transplant patients. BMC Infect Dis 2006;6:133.

87. Alevizakos M, Kallias A, Flokas ME, et al. Colonization with extended-spectrum beta-lactamase-producing enterobacteriaceae in solid organ transplantation: a meta-analysis and review. Transpl Infect Dis 2017;19(4). https://doi.org/10.1111/tid.12718.

88. Aris RM, Gilligan PH, Neuringer IP, et al. The effects of panresistant bacteria in cystic fibrosis patients on lung transplant outcome. Am J Respir Crit Care Med 1997;155(5):1699–704.

89. Alexander BD, Petzold EW, Reller LB, et al. Survival after lung transplantation of cystic fibrosis patients infected with Burkholderia cepacia complex. Am J Transplant 2008;8(5):1025–30.

90. De Soyza A, Meachery G, Hester KL, et al. Lung transplantation for patients with cystic fibrosis and Burkholderia cepacia complex infection: a single-center experience. J Heart Lung Transplant 2010;29(12):1395–404.

91. Aguado JM, Silva JT, Fernandez-Ruiz M, et al. Management of multidrug resistant gram-negative bacilli infections in solid organ transplant recipients: SET/GESITRA-SEIMC/REIPI recommendations. Transplant Rev (Orlando) 2018; 32(1):36–57.

92. van Duin D, van Delden C. Multidrug-resistant gram-negative bacteria infections in solid organ transplantation. Am J Transplant 2013;13(Suppl 4):31–41.

93. Garzoni C, Vergidis P. Methicillin-resistant, vancomycin-intermediate and vancomycin-resistant Staphylococcus aureus infections in solid organ transplantation. Am J Transplant 2013;13(Suppl 4):50–8.

94. Patel G, Snydman DR. Vancomycin-resistant enterococcus infections in solid organ transplantation. Am J Transplant 2013;13(Suppl 4):59–67.

95. Lumbreras C, Sanz F, Gonzalez A, et al. Clinical significance of donor-unrecognized bacteremia in the outcome of solid-organ transplant recipients. Clin Infect Dis 2001;33(5):722–6.

96. Mularoni A, Bertani A, Vizzini G, et al. Outcome of transplantation using organs from donors infected or colonized with carbapenem-resistant gram-negative bacteria. Am J Transplant 2015;15(10):2674–82.

97. Moore CL, Osaki-Kiyan P, Haque NZ, et al. Daptomycin versus vancomycin for bloodstream infections due to methicillin-resistant Staphylococcus aureus with a high vancomycin minimum inhibitory concentration: a case-control study. Clin Infect Dis 2012;54(1):51–8.

98. Claeys KC, Zasowski EJ, Casapao AM, et al. Daptomycin improves outcomes regardless of vancomycin MIC in a propensity-matched analysis of methicillin-resistant Staphylococcus aureus bloodstream infections. Antimicrob Agents Chemother 2016;60(10):5841–8.

99. Soriano A, Marco F, Martinez JA, et al. Influence of vancomycin minimum inhibitory concentration on the treatment of methicillin-resistant Staphylococcus aureus bacteremia. Clin Infect Dis 2008;46(2):193–200.

100. van Hal SJ, Lodise TP, Paterson DL. The clinical significance of vancomycin minimum inhibitory concentration in Staphylococcus aureus infections: a systematic review and meta-analysis. Clin Infect Dis 2012;54(6):755–71.

101. Kalil AC, Metersky ML, Klompas M, et al. Management of adults with hospital-acquired and ventilator-associated pneumonia: 2016 clinical practice guidelines by the Infectious Diseases Society of America and the American Thoracic Society. Clin Infect Dis 2016;63(5):e61–111.

102. Wunderink RG, Niederman MS, Kollef MH, et al. Linezolid in methicillin-resistant Staphylococcus aureus nosocomial pneumonia: a randomized, controlled study. Clin Infect Dis 2012;54(5):621–9.

103. Balli EP, Venetis CA, Miyakis S. Systematic review and meta-analysis of linezolid versus daptomycin for treatment of vancomycin-resistant enterococcal bacteremia. Antimicrob Agents Chemother 2014;58(2):734–9.
104. Viale P, Giannella M, Bartoletti M, et al. Considerations about antimicrobial stewardship in settings with epidemic extended-spectrum beta-lactamase-producing or carbapenem-resistant enterobacteriaceae. Infect Dis Ther 2015; 4(Suppl 1):65–83.
105. Gutierrez-Gutierrez B, Perez-Galera S, Salamanca E, et al. A multinational, preregistered cohort study of beta-lactam/beta-lactamase inhibitor combinations for treatment of bloodstream infections due to extended-spectrum-beta-lactamase-producing enterobacteriaceae. Antimicrob Agents Chemother 2016;60(7):4159–69.
106. Rodriguez-Bano J, Navarro MD, Retamar P, et al. Beta-lactam/beta-lactam inhibitor combinations for the treatment of bacteremia due to extended-spectrum beta-lactamase-producing Escherichia coli: a post hoc analysis of prospective cohorts. Clin Infect Dis 2012;54(2):167–74.
107. Palacios-Baena ZR, Gutierrez-Gutierrez B, Calbo E, et al. Empiric therapy with carbapenem-sparing regimens for bloodstream infections due to extended-spectrum beta-lactamase-producing enterobacteriaceae: results from the increment cohort. Clin Infect Dis 2017;65(10):1615–23.
108. Montravers P, Dupont H, Bedos JP, et al. Tigecycline use in critically ill patients: a multicentre prospective observational study in the intensive care setting. Intensive Care Med 2014;40(7):988–97.
109. Eckmann C, Montravers P, Bassetti M, et al. Efficacy of tigecycline for the treatment of complicated intra-abdominal infections in real-life clinical practice from five European observational studies. J Antimicrob Chemother 2013;68(Suppl 2): 25–35.
110. McGovern PC, Wible M, El-Tahtawy A, et al. All-cause mortality imbalance in the tigecycline phase 3 and 4 clinical trials. Int J Antimicrob Agents 2013;41(5): 463–7.
111. Mouloudi E, Massa E, Piperidou M, et al. Tigecycline for treatment of carbapenem-resistant Klebsiella pneumoniae infections after liver transplantation in the intensive care unit: a 3-year study. Transplant Proc 2014;46(9): 3219–21.
112. Falagas ME, Rafailidis PI. Re-emergence of colistin in today's world of multidrug-resistant organisms: personal perspectives. Expert Opin Investig Drugs 2008;17(7):973–81.
113. Zayyad H, Eliakim-Raz N, Leibovici L, et al. Revival of old antibiotics: needs, the state of evidence and expectations. Int J Antimicrob Agents 2017;49(5):536–41.
114. Gutierrez-Gutierrez B, Salamanca E, de Cueto M, et al. Effect of appropriate combination therapy on mortality of patients with bloodstream infections due to carbapenemase-producing enterobacteriaceae (increment): a retrospective cohort study. Lancet Infect Dis 2017;17(7):726–34.
115. Tumbarello M, Trecarichi EM, De Rosa FG, et al. Infections caused by kpc-producing Klebsiella pneumoniae: differences in therapy and mortality in a multicentre study. J Antimicrob Chemother 2015;70(7):2133–43.
116. Eckmann C, Solomkin J. Ceftolozane/tazobactam for the treatment of complicated intra-abdominal infections. Expert Opin Pharmacother 2015;16(2):271–80.
117. Goodlet KJ, Nicolau DP, Nailor MD. Ceftolozane/tazobactam and ceftazidime/avibactam for the treatment of complicated intra-abdominal infections. Ther Clin Risk Manag 2016;12:1811–26.

118. Popejoy MW, Paterson DL, Cloutier D, et al. Efficacy of ceftolozane/tazobactam against urinary tract and intra-abdominal infections caused by ESBL-producing Escherichia coli and Klebsiella pneumoniae: a pooled analysis of phase 3 clinical trials. J Antimicrob Chemother 2017;72(1):268–72.

119. Tamma PD, Rodriguez-Bano J. The use of noncarbapenem beta-lactams for the treatment of extended-spectrum beta-lactamase infections. Clin Infect Dis 2017; 64(7):972–80.

120. Wagenlehner FM, Sobel JD, Newell P, et al. Ceftazidime-avibactam versus doripenem for the treatment of complicated urinary tract infections, including acute pyelonephritis: recapture, a phase 3 randomized trial program. Clin Infect Dis 2016;63(6):754–62.

121. Mazuski JE, Gasink LB, Armstrong J, et al. Efficacy and safety of ceftazidime-avibactam plus metronidazole versus meropenem in the treatment of complicated intra-abdominal infection: results from a randomized, controlled, double-blind, phase 3 program. Clin Infect Dis 2016;62(11):1380–9.

122. Sharma R, Park TE, Moy S. Ceftazidime-avibactam: a novel cephalosporin/beta-lactamase inhibitor combination for the treatment of resistant gram-negative organisms. Clin Ther 2016;38(3):431–44.

123. Shields RK, Potoski BA, Haidar G, et al. Clinical outcomes, drug toxicity, and emergence of ceftazidime-avibactam resistance among patients treated for carbapenem-resistant enterobacteriaceae infections. Clin Infect Dis 2016; 63(12):1615–8.

124. Temkin E, Torre-Cisneros J, Beovic B, et al. Ceftazidime-avibactam as salvage therapy for infections caused by carbapenem-resistant organisms. Antimicrob Agents Chemother 2017;61(2) [pii:e01964-16].

125. King M, Heil E, Kuriakose S, et al. Multicenter study of outcomes with ceftazidime-avibactam in patients with carbapenem-resistant enterobacteriaceae infections. Antimicrob Agents Chemother 2017;61(7) [pii:e00449-17].

126. Caston JJ, Lacort-Peralta I, Martin-Davila P, et al. Clinical efficacy of ceftazidime/avibactam versus other active agents for the treatment of bacteremia due to carbapenemase-producing enterobacteriaceae in hematologic patients. Int J Infect Dis 2017;59:118–23.

127. van Duin D, Lok JJ, Earley M, et al. Colistin versus ceftazidime-avibactam in the treatment of infections due to carbapenem-resistant enterobacteriaceae. Clin Infect Dis 2018;66(2):163–71.

128. Rodriguez-Bano J, Gutierrez-Gutierrez B, Machuca I, et al. Treatment of infections caused by extended-spectrum-beta-lactamase-, AMPC-, and carbapenemase-producing enterobacteriaceae. Clin Microbiol Rev 2018;31 [pii:e00079-17].

129. Bidair M, Zervos M, Sagan O, et al. Clinical outcomes in adults with complicated urinary tract infections (cuti), including acute pyelonephritis (ap) in tango 1, a phase 3 randomized, double-blind, double-dummy trial comparing meropenem-vaborbactam (m-v) with piperacillin-tazobactam (p-t), poster p1289. European Congress of Clinical Microbiology and Infectious Disease. Vienna (Austria), April 22–25, 2017.

130. Kaye KS, Vazquez J, Mathers A, et al. Clinical outcomes of serious infections due to carbapenem-resistant enterobacteriaceae (CRE) in tango ii, a phase 3, randomized, multi-national, open-label trial of meropenem-vaborbactam (m-v) versus best available therapy (bat). Poster 1862. San Diego (CA): IDWeek; 2017.

131. Tebano G, Geneve C, Tanaka S, et al. Epidemiology and risk factors of multidrug-resistant bacteria in respiratory samples after lung transplantation. Transpl Infect Dis 2016;18(1):22–30.

132. Shi SH, Kong HS, Xu J, et al. Multidrug resistant gram-negative bacilli as pre-dominant bacteremic pathogens in liver transplant recipients. Transpl Infect Dis 2009;11(5):405–12.
133. Dudau D, Camous J, Marchand S, et al. Incidence of nosocomial pneumonia and risk of recurrence after antimicrobial therapy in critically ill lung and heart-lung transplant patients. Clin Transplant 2014;28(1):27–36.
134. Zhong L, Men TY, Li H, et al. Multidrug-resistant gram-negative bacterial infec-tions after liver transplantation - spectrum and risk factors. J Infect 2012;64(3): 299–310.
135. Linares L, Cervera C, Cofan F, et al. Risk factors for infection with extended-spectrum and ampc beta-lactamase-producing gram-negative rods in renal transplantation. Am J Transplant 2008;8(5):1000–5.
136. Freire MP, Abdala E, Moura ML, et al. Risk factors and outcome of infections with Klebsiella pneumoniae carbapenemase-producing k. Pneumoniae in kidney transplant recipients. Infection 2015;43(3):315–23.
137. Raviv Y, Shitrit D, Amital A, et al. Multidrug-resistant Klebsiella pneumoniae acquisition in lung transplant recipients. Clin Transplant 2012;26(4):E388–94.
138. Bartoletti M, Giannella M, Lewis RE, et al. Bloodstream infections in patients with liver cirrhosis. Virulence 2016;7(3):309–19.
139. Salsgiver EL, Fink AK, Knapp EA, et al. Changing epidemiology of the respira-tory bacteriology of patients with cystic fibrosis. Chest 2016;149(2):390–400.
140. Mills JP, Wilck MB, Weikert BC, et al. Successful treatment of a disseminated infection with extensively drug-resistant Klebsiella pneumoniae in a liver trans-plant recipient with a fosfomycin-based multidrug regimen. Transpl Infect Dis 2016;18(5):777–81.
141. Ariza-Heredia EJ, Patel R, Blumberg EA, et al. Outcomes of transplantation us-ing organs from a donor infected with Klebsiella pneumoniae carbapenemase (kpc)-producing k. Pneumoniae. Transpl Infect Dis 2012;14(3):229–36.
142. Varotti G, Dodi F, Marchese A, et al. Fatal donor-derived carbapenem-resistant Klebsiella pneumoniae infection in a combined kidney-pancreas transplanta-tion. Case Rep Transplant 2016;2016:7920951.
143. Giani T, Conte V, Mandala S, et al. Cross-infection of solid organ transplant re-cipients by a multidrug-resistant Klebsiella pneumoniae isolate producing the oxa-48 carbapenemase, likely derived from a multiorgan donor. J Clin Microbiol 2014;52(7):2702–5.
144. Transmission of multidrug-resistant Escherichia coli through kidney transplantation–California and Texas, 2009. Am J Transplant 2011;11(3):628–32.
145. Ye QF, Zhou W, Wan QQ. Donor-derived infections among Chinese donation af-ter cardiac death liver recipients. World J Gastroenterol 2017;23(31):5809–16.
146. Martins N, Martins IS, de Freitas WV, et al. Severe infection in a lung transplant recipient caused by donor-transmitted carbapenem-resistant Acinetobacter baumannii. Transpl Infect Dis 2012;14(3):316–20.
147. Orlando G, Di Cocco P, Gravante G, et al. Fatal hemorrhage in two renal graft recipients with multi-drug resistant Pseudomonas aeruginosa infection. Transpl Infect Dis 2009;11(5):442–7.
148. Simkins J, Muggia V. Favorable outcome in a renal transplant recipient with donor-derived infection due to multidrug-resistant Pseudomonas aeruginosa. Transpl Infect Dis 2012;14(3):292–5.
149. Watkins AC, Vedula GV, Horan J, et al. The deceased organ donor with an "open abdomen": proceed with caution. Transpl Infect Dis 2012;14(3):311–5.

150. Altman DR, Sebra R, Hand J, et al. Transmission of methicillin-resistant Staphylococcus aureus via deceased donor liver transplantation confirmed by whole genome sequencing. Am J Transplant 2014;14(11):2640–4.
151. Obed A, Schnitzbauer AA, Bein T, et al. Fatal pneumonia caused by pantonvalentine leucocidine-positive methicillin-resistant Staphylococcus aureus (PVL-MRSA) transmitted from a healthy donor in living-donor liver transplantation. Transplantation 2006;81(1):121–4.
152. Coll P, Montserrat I, Ballester M, et al. Epidemiologic evidence of transmission of donor-related bacterial infection through a transplanted heart. J Heart Lung Transplant 1997;16(4):464–7.
153. Miceli MH, Gonulalan M, Perri MB, et al. Transmission of infection to liver transplant recipients from donors with infective endocarditis: lessons learned. Transpl Infect Dis 2015;17(1):140–6.
154. Johnston L, Chui L, Chang N, et al. Cross-Canada spread of methicillin-resistant Staphylococcus aureus via transplant organs. Clin Infect Dis 1999;29(4):819–23.
155. Wendt JM, Kaul D, Limbago BM, et al. Transmission of methicillin-resistant Staphylococcus aureus infection through solid organ transplantation: confirmation via whole genome sequencing. Am J Transplant 2014;14(11):2633–9.
156. Holmes NE, Ballard SA, Lam MM, et al. Genomic analysis of teicoplanin resistance emerging during treatment of vanb vancomycin-resistant Enterococcus faecium infections in solid organ transplant recipients including donor-derived cases. J Antimicrob Chemother 2013;68(9):2134–9.
157. Bashir A, Attie O, Sullivan M, et al. Genomic confirmation of vancomycin-resistant enterococcus transmission from deceased donor to liver transplant recipient. PLoS One 2017;12(3):e0170449.

Prevention and Treatment of Cytomegalovirus Infections in Solid Organ Transplant Recipients

Christine E. Koval, MD

KEYWORDS

- CMV • Cytomegalovirus • Herpesvirus infection • Solid organ transplantation
- CMV prophylaxis • CMV treatment

KEY POINTS

- Cytomegalovirus (CMV) prophylaxis and preemptive monitoring have reduced the incidence of early CMV disease in solid organ transplantation, but late disease has emerged as a significant problem.
- CMV-specific cell-mediated immunity (CMI) is required to control CMV in the absence of antiviral therapy, and achieving strong CMI without coincident allograft rejection is the ultimate goal of CMV management strategies.
- Measurement of CMV-specific CMI may help refine CMV prophylaxis and preemptive monitoring strategies.
- Valganciclovir remains the mainstay of CMV treatment but comes at the cost of frequent myelosuppression.
- Letermovir is a newly approved antiviral with strong activity against CMV and minimal side effects and may change the landscape of CMV management.

Human cytomegalovirus (CMV) is a double-stranded DNA virus and member of the herpes virus family. Infection prevalence reaches 60% to 80% by adulthood in the United States and nearly 100% in many parts of the world.[1,2] First recognized as a major complication of solid organ transplantation (SOT) 50 years ago, it remains the most common viral infection encountered after SOT and can occur as a primary infection, secondary infection, or reactivation from a latent reservoir.[3] Although humans have evolved to live a lifetime with persistent asymptomatic infection, recipients of SOT

Disclosure Statement: The author has no commercial or financial conflicts of interest and declares no funding sources that would create a conflict of interest.
Department of Infectious Diseases, Cleveland Clinic Foundation, 9500 Euclid Avenue, Box G21, Cleveland, OH 44195, USA
E-mail address: kovalc@ccf.org

Infect Dis Clin N Am 32 (2018) 581–597
https://doi.org/10.1016/j.idc.2018.04.008
0891-5520/18/© 2018 Elsevier Inc. All rights reserved.

id.theclinics.com

are challenged to adapt to and control CMV infection while deliberately impairing immune recognition of their allograft.

CYTOMEGALOVIRUS INFECTION AND THE IMMUNE RESPONSE

Primary infection in immunocompetent individuals is most often asymptomatic and transmitted via secretions of an infected individual. CMV disseminates from the respiratory epithelium, most commonly via mononuclear cells and polymorphonuclear cells to endothelial, epithelial, and fibroblast of tissues and organs.[1] Prolonged shedding in saliva and urine after primary infection provides evidence for coincident chronic viral replication in some sites but emergence of latency elsewhere.

The innate immune system provides initial antiviral activity until the adaptive immune response can exert more definitive control of infection. Both CD4 and CD8 T-cell responses are instrumental for control of CMV and guard against replication and infection of new cells.[4,5] CMV establishes lifelong latency in endothelium, epithelium, smooth muscle, and fibroblasts by evading immune detection.[5,6] Infections with CMV variants and intermittent viral replication from latency expand the breadth of CMV recognition over a lifetime.[1,7] Although humoral immunity may restrict viral dissemination early in the primary infection and with reinfection, its role beyond this is debated.[4,8,9] CMV immunoglobulin G (IgG), however, is reflective of past infection.

Cytomegalovirus in Solid Organ Transplant Recipients

Immunologic recognition of acute CMV infection and control of latent infection require many of the same mechanisms that are disabled by the immunosuppression that prevents allograft rejection. **Fig. 1** depicts the evolution of CMV infection in the normal host and the impact of transplantation.

RISK FACTORS FOR CYTOMEGALOVIRUS DISEASE

Risk for CMV disease is associated with past CMV infection, new CMV exposure, the degree of T-cell impairment, and the type of organ being transplanted (**Table 1**).

Cytomegalovirus Immunoglobulin G Donor/Recipient Status

About 20% to 30% of adult transplant recipients are CMV IgG negative and are at greatest risk for primary infection. The donor organ is the most common source for primary infection, but it can also occur through blood products and community exposures (eg, healthy children with salivary shedding). CMV IgG results can be falsely positive or negative. Direct testing for CMV-specific cell-mediated immunity (CMI) is more sensitive and more specific than antibody testing at identifying those with latent infection but is not practical in the transplant donation process and is not currently recommended as a screening tool for recipients.[10] False-positive CMV IgG is most often due to passive antibodies via blood products, usually intravenous immunoglobulin (IVIG). False-negative CMV IgG testing can occur rarely from waning antibody over time or from insensitive testing methods.[10]

Type and Degree of Immunosuppression

T-cell depleting agents are highly associated with CMV disease. High doses of steroids and higher levels of calcineurin inhibitors, mycophenolic acid, and azathioprine are also associated with CMV disease. CMV uses mammalian target of rapamycin (mTOR) pathways for viral replication, and the use of mTOR inhibitors have been associated with a lower risk for CMV infection and CMV syndrome (but not consistently

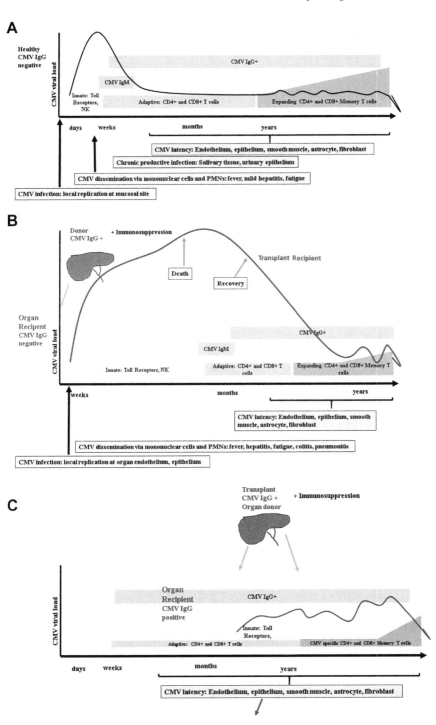

Fig. 1. (*A*) Immune response from CMV infection to latency in the healthy host. (*B*) Immunologic effects of typical immunosuppressive drugs and CMV infection after SOT in CMV D+/R− and (*C*) CMV D+/R+.

Table 1
Risk factors for cytomegalovirus disease

	High Risk	Intermediate Risk	Lower Risk	Comments
CMV serostatus	CMV IgG D+/R−	CMV IgG D+/R+, CMV IgG D−/R+	CMV IgG D−/R−	Falsely positive (blood products, IVIG) Falsely negative (loss of antibody, CVID) Equivocal results in donor: interpret as positive Equivocal results in recipient: interpret as negative Not all serologic testing products equivalent
Immunosuppression	Antilymphocyte antibodies (thymoglobulin, alemtuzumab, OKT3)	MMF, azathioprine, tacrolimus, cyclosporine, high-dose steroids	Maintenance steroids mTOR inhibitors	Increased risk for all agents, with higher doses
Organ transplanted	Lung Pancreas Intestine	Heart composite tissue	Liver Kidney	Burden of latently infected cells Higher levels of immunosuppression
CMV-specific cell-mediated immunity	Low	Intermediate	High	Data limited May be useful at guiding prophylaxis and preemptive prevention strategies

Abbreviations: CVID, common variable immunodeficiency; IVIG, intravenous immune globulin; MMF, mycophenolate mofetil; mTOR, mammalian target of rapamycin; OKT3, anti-CD3 antibody.

CMV disease).[11,12] Guidelines weakly recommend transition to mTOR inhibitors in patients with challenging CMV infection.[13]

Organ Transplanted

Lung, pancreas, and intestinal transplant recipients seem to be at greater risk for CMV disease than other organs. This circumstance may be, in part, due to the use of more aggressive immunosuppression for these transplants. CMV pneumonitis is particularly prevalent in the lung allograft and enteritis is particularly problematic in intestinal transplantation, suggesting a rich source of latent virus at risk for active infection[14–16]; the data are supported by murine models of CMV latency.[17]

CLINICAL MANIFESTATIONS

In the absence of prevention, CMV infection and disease typically occur in the first 3 months after transplantation, the peak period of immunosuppression.[3,18] CMV infection represents the period of CMV viral replication before the onset of significant symptoms (**Fig. 2**). CMV disease includes both CMV syndrome and tissue invasive disease. CMV syndrome is characterized by fever, malaise, leukopenia, and/or thrombocytopenia and is the most common presentation of symptomatic CMV infection.

Tissue-invasive CMV disease has a predilection for the allograft itself, a possible consequence of D+ allografts or disordered immune response within the allograft. Disease also occurs as colitis or enteritis, pneumonitis, hepatitis, and less commonly nephritis, myocarditis, pancreatitis, retinitis, meningoencephalitis, or polyneuritis. Because of the low incidence of retinitis, it not recommended to pursue retinal examination in the absence of visual symptoms.

CMV disease has been associated with a variety of secondary outcomes, including bacterial and fungal infections and posttransplant lymphoproliferative disorder.[19,20] An association with manifestations of chronic allograft rejection, including bronchiolitis

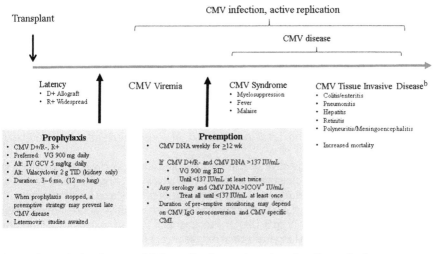

Fig. 2. The typical trajectory of CMV replication to tissue invasive disease in the organ transplant recipient. Insets depict the CMV prevention strategies available. Alt, alternative; GCV ganciclovir; ICOV, internal cutoff value; IV, intravenous; VG valganciclovir. [a] ICOV for initiating treatment decided at transplant program or center. [b] CMV tissue invasive disease can occur without CMV viremia. (*Courtesy of* Dr .Eric Cober.)

obliterans syndrome, chronic allograft vasculopathy, and vanishing bile duct syndrome, has also been made; but data are not consistent.[18,21,22] Most importantly, CMV infection has been associated with graft loss and increased mortality.[3,22,23]

DIAGNOSTICS

CMV infection is detected in blood by antigen detection with pp65 or with quantitative CMV DNA detection by polymerase chain reaction (PCR). Given the logistical limitations to performing antigen testing, most centers are now using CMV DNA detection by PCR. There are several commercial assays for CMV DNA detection, and many laboratories have developed their own home brew assays. Development of the World Health Organization's first CMV international standard based on international units, available since October 2010, allows laboratories to standardize results for comparison with those obtained at other laboratories using the same standard.[24] Not all laboratories use the standard (reported as international units per milliliter).

CMV syndrome is diagnosed by detecting CMV infection and having compatible clinical findings of malaise, and/or fever, leukopenia, and/or thrombocytopenia. CMV antibodies (IgG and IgM) are not typically used to diagnose acute infection in organ transplantation.

A definitive diagnosis of tissue-invasive CMV disease is made with histopathologic evidence of CMV (inclusion bodies or viral antigens by immunohistochemistry) with or without virus culture of the tissue. Diagnosis of tissue-invasive disease can be made presumptively in the setting of CMV viremia and compatible signs, symptoms (diarrhea, hepatitis, and so forth), and laboratory findings. If not appropriately responsive to antiviral therapy, a tissue diagnosis should be sought. Tissue-invasive disease can occur in the absence of CMV viremia, particularly in patients who are recipient CMV IgG positive (CMV R+), and requires tissue biopsy to diagnose.

PREVENTION

Preventive strategies are intended to avoid CMV disease as well as improve longer-term outcomes. **Fig. 2** highlights the different strategies used for CMV prevention.[25] Both strategies have greatly reduced the incidence of early CMV disease.[19] Many programs use a combined strategy for at-risk patients of prophylaxis followed by preemptive monitoring. An ongoing randomized, prospective, multicenter trial comparing prophylaxis with preemptive management in donor CMV IgG positive (CMV D+)/R− liver transplant recipients may help to answer many outlying questions (https://clinicaltrials.gov/ct2/show/study/NCT01552369?cond=CMV+liver+transplant+AND+%22Cytomegalovirus+Infections%22&rank=2). The ideal combination of these strategies has not been established.

Prophylaxis entails giving antivirals (intravenous ganciclovir, oral valganciclovir or, in select kidney transplant recipients, high dose valacyclovir) during the peak period of immunosuppression. Data support at least 3 months of prophylaxis for most organs.[26] Longer courses (6 months) have been shown to be more effective at preventing CMV, particularly in high-risk (CMV IgG D+/R−) recipients.[20] Prophylaxis with 12 months compared with 3 months in lung transplant recipients seems to be even more effective in these patients.[27,28] Prophylaxis is also associated with reduced incidence of opportunistic infections, graft loss, and mortality.[20,27] Consensus guidelines recommended prophylaxis for most at-risk recipients for most organs.[14,23] There are particular concerns for valganciclovir prophylaxis in liver transplant recipients due to data that indicate inferior efficacy to oral ganciclovir.[29]

Longer courses of prophylaxis may be attractive, but there are costs to the strategy. One concern is that prophylaxis delays effective immunologic control. Late CMV infection (beyond 6 months) has emerged as a significant cause of morbidity and mortality in transplantation.[30] Other concerns include myelosuppression, antiviral resistance, and the high cost of antivirals. It is acknowledged that in studies supporting the benefits of prophylaxis, many randomized effectively, the comparator group is not a concurrent preemptive monitoring group.

Preemptive monitoring entails testing blood routinely for early CMV replication and treating the infection before it progresses to symptomatic disease. There is no established threshold of CMV DNA viral load at which one should treat with antiviral agents and no established lower threshold at which one should stop this treatment. Each center is currently responsible for establishing its own practice. However, lower thresholds for initiating and stopping treatment would be appropriate for those at greatest risk for progression to CMV disease (CMV D+/R− with recent exposure to lymphocyte depleting antibody). Those with CMV R+ and no lymphocyte depletion may warrant higher thresholds. Antiviral therapy is continued until the viral load reaches the lower limit threshold measured once or twice separated by a week. Preemptive prevention of CMV disease requires the resources for obtaining and responding to laboratory results in a rapid fashion. It also requires that patients be adherent to laboratory testing and available to start treatment. Preemptive monitoring has been evaluated by multiple studies and in retrospective meta-analyses and has been shown to reduce the risk for CMV disease but does not seem to have the same beneficial effects on allograft outcomes and patient mortality as universal prophylaxis.[31]

TREATMENT

Treatment of CMV early after transplant is challenging. Assessing the immunosuppression strategy for each patient is important to predicting the duration and intensity of T-cell impairment. It is unlikely that adaptive immunity will occur in the setting of recent lymphocyte-depleting agents. Consideration can sometimes be given to reducing tacrolimus trough concentration, reducing or stopping mycophenolate mofetil, and lowering prednisone dosing when appropriate. Changes, when done, to immunosuppressive medications should be made *only* by the transplant team to avoid rejection, as therapy for rejection will invariably make CMV management even more challenging while having deleterious effects on graft function.

Ganciclovir, valganciclovir, foscarnet, and cidofovir target viral replication at the step of DNA polymerization. The drug letermovir is the first drug approved for CMV that acts at the level of viral packaging. Dosing and indications for the available antivirals are listed in **Table 2**. Treatment is generally recommended for at least 2 weeks for tissue-invasive disease and until CMV DNA is less than the lowest limit of detection on 2 separate measurements separated by at least 1 week. Continuing a maintenance (or secondary prophylaxis) dose for weeks to a few months (until adaptive immune response improves) may be warranted depending on the risk for recurrent infection (CMV D+/R−, recent lymphocyte-depleting agent).

Ganciclovir and valganciclovir are the recommended first-line antivirals for CMV infection and disease. Valganciclovir is converted to ganciclovir by hydrolysis before reaching the systemic circulation and can provide drug exposure similar to that of intravenous ganciclovir. Although Asberg and colleagues demonstrated noninferior treatment outcomes with valganciclovir compared with intravenous ganciclovir, their study comprised mostly kidney transplant recipients with non–life-threatening CMV disease.[32] Thus, when drug absorption is uncertain or disease severity warrants,

Table 2
Antivirals available for treatment of cytomegalovirus infection or disease

	Indication	Dosage	Side Effects	Comments
Valganciclovir Oral High dose	CMV infection • CMV DNA <1 × 10⁵ IU/mL[a] CMV disease GCV resistance (<5× GCV EC50)	900 mg twice daily 1350–1800 mg twice daily	Leukopenia Anemia Thrombocytopenia	Dose adjust for renal impairment Consider adequacy of GI absorption Oral option after initial therapy with IV ganciclovir
Ganciclovir Intravenous High dose	CMV infection • CMV DNA >1 × 10⁵ IU/mL[a] CMV disease requiring hospital admit[a] GCV resistance (<5 × GCV EC50)	5 mg/kg every 12 h 7.5–10.0 mg/kg every 12 h	Leukopenia Anemia Thrombocytopenia	Dose adjust for renal impairment Can change to oral valganciclovir to complete course
Foscarnet Intravenous	CMV infection or disease with GCV resistance (≥5× GCV EC50)	90 mg/kg every 12 h	Nephrotoxicity Electrolyte wasting Cytopenias	Dose adjust for renal impairment Hospital admission usually required for hydration, initial monitoring of renal function, K, Mg, Ca, P
Cidofovir Intravenous	CMV infection or disease refractory and resistant to GCV and FOS	5 mg/kg weekly ×2 then every 2 wk	Highly nephrotoxic	Alternative lower doses used
Letermovir Oral Intravenous	Primary CMV infection? Secondary CMV infection? CMV disease? CMV with GCV and/or FOS resistance	480 mg daily (240 mg daily with CSA)	Peripheral edema Headache Nausea Diarrhea	CYP3A4 inhibitor Increases concentration of CSA Increased concentration by CSA May increase concentration of tacrolimus Not active against HSV or VZV

Abbreviations: Ca, calcium; CSA, cyclosporine; EC50, 50% effective concentration; FOS, foscarnet; GCV, ganciclovir; GI, gastrointestinal; HSV, herpes simplex virus; IV, intravenous; K, potassium; Mg, magnesium; P, phosphorus; VZV, varicella zoster virus.

[a] Valganciclovir may suffice for less severe infection, clinically assessed, but with stronger consideration only when CMV DNA <1 × 10⁵ IU/mL. Otherwise intravenous ganciclovir may be more reliable. There is no established cutoff.

intravenous ganciclovir is recommended.[33] Dose reductions are recommended for reduced creatinine clearance. Because of fluctuations in creatinine concentrations with acute illness and volume depletion, it may be preferred to err on the higher side of dosing early when disease severity warrants rather than trying to catch up, because late eradication of CMV DNA is associated with antiviral resistance.[34] Judicious use of granulocyte colony-stimulating factor may be required to allow for fully effective therapy.[22]

Foscarnet is the second-line agent for CMV disease or infection that is refractory or resistant to ganciclovir therapy.[35] It is active against ganciclovir-resistant strains harboring only UL97 mutations. Foscarnet generally requires hospital admission to initiate intravenous therapy (with insertion of a central venous catheter) for adequate hydration and initial monitoring of creatinine and electrolytes. Most patients will require planned oral electrolyte repletion before discharge on intravenous foscarnet.

Cidofovir is an intravenous antiviral agent with activity against CMV, other herpes viruses, adenovirus, and polyoma viruses. Its use is limited by frequent and possibly severe nephrotoxicity particularly in the setting of calcineurin inhibitor therapy. There is also the potential for cross-resistance to ganciclovir with certain UL54/pol gene mutations, so it may not be an option for some patients failing ganciclovir. Cidofovir has been used successfully in SOT recipients with refractory CMV disease, with high rates of renal injury or failure.[36,37]

Letermovir blocks the terminase complex of CMV, preventing cleavage and packaging of viral DNA.[38] It has high potency and is active against strains resistant to ganciclovir, cidofovir, and foscarnet. It has no activity against herpes simplex virus or varicella zoster virus and, thus, may require coadministration with an acyclovir derivative.[39] In clinical trials, the safety profile of letermovir is excellent with no myelosuppression or nephrotoxicity.[40,41] It was FDA approved in November 2017 for CMV prophylaxis in stem cell transplant recipients.[42] It is unclear how it will be used in the SOT setting; but given its favorable safety profile, it has the potential to significantly change CMV management strategies. In a phase 2b clinical trial of preemptive management of CMV infection in 27 kidney or kidney pancreas transplant recipients in Germany, letermovir demonstrated similar outcomes to valganciclovir.[43] It has been used successfully under compassionate provision for a lung transplant recipient with drug-resistant CMV refractory to other available antivirals.[44] Because of metabolism by CYP3A4, dose adjustments are required in the setting of calcineurin inhibitors.[45] For both treatment and prevention, it was observed that, although effective, the rate of viral load decline was slower than expected for letermovir possibly reflecting its mechanism of action and should be considered with future use.

Use of CMV hyperimmune globulin and IVIG preparations as part of CMV prophylaxis and therapy remain controversial and only weakly recommended in clinical guidelines.[14,22,46] Nevertheless, it remains widely used for prophylaxis in intestinal transplantation and for salvage therapy for CMV-refractory disease.[16,37] Data remain inconclusive for its clinical benefits in the era of more potent direct antiviral agents. Randomized data from the 1990s provide evidence for its role in prophylaxis for D+/R− cardiac transplant recipients.[46,47] Data for its purported benefit in the setting of severe CMV pneumonitis have not consistently been demonstrated.[48,49] Secondary hypogammaglobulinemia in the posttransplant setting has been associated with CMV disease, but it is unclear that this is a direct effect of low antibody and not a downstream effect of cell-mediated immune impairment.[50]

Leflunomide is a disease-modifying drug used to treat rheumatoid arthritis that has coincident anti-CMV activity. Cases and case series have been reported, and it may improve CMV disease in the setting of resistance to standard antivirals; but outcomes are varied, and it has not been formally studied.[51–53] It takes several weeks to achieve the target blood level, has a very long half-life, and has the potential for hepatotoxicity and irreversible peripheral neuropathy, particularly at the higher doses used to treat CMV and is not recommended unless other more proven therapies are not available.[13,22]

The last option for managing severe CMV disease, open only to intestinal and kidney transplant recipients, is stopping immunosuppression completely and allowing for allograft failure, often with allograft removal.

The investigational drugs brincidofovir, an oral lipid conjugate of cidofovir, and maribavir, an oral benzimidazole L-riboside that inhibits the UL97 viral protein kinase of CMV, hold some promise as alternative agents of CMV prophylaxis and treatment of refractory/resistant CMV. Neither is currently approved for use in the United States.

One published case[53] reported efficacy of the antimalarial drug artesunate in treating ganciclovir- and foscarnet-resistant CMV, but a subsequent case report[54] did not corroborate this experience.

CYTOMEGALOVIRUS-SPECIFIC CELL-MEDIATED IMMUNITY

The CMV-specific immunity may be the most direct measure of CMV infection risk and may help stratify the risk for CMV recurrence after therapy and in prophylaxis and preemptive strategies. There are now several assays to measure CMV-specific CMI, some of which are commercially available. These assays measure gamma-interferon or other cytokine markers in response to CMV-specific peptides.[23,55] A recent study demonstrated the feasibility of using CMV-specific CMI (QuantiFERON-CMV, Qiagen, Hilden, Germany) to guide the use of antiviral secondary prophylaxis in 27 SOT recipients completing treatment of CMV viremia and disease.[56] Those with evidence of CMV CMI at the end of treatment had antivirals successfully stopped without significant viremia on follow-up. Additional validated studies to determine the optimal use of these assays is required but will, it is hoped, help limit prophylaxis and CMV DNA monitoring only to those who benefit the most.

There is no way to restore CMV-specific immunity other than delicate reduction of immunosuppression as able. Adoptive immunotherapy (stimulating donor T lymphocytes in vitro with CMV peptides and infusing into patients) has been used successfully in hematopoietic stem cell transplantation recipients but is not available for widespread use and has not been performed in SOT recipients.[57]

ANTIVIRAL RESISTANCE

Resistance mutations in CMV UL97 protein kinase and UL54 DNA polymerase genes confer varied degrees of resistance to ganciclovir, foscarnet, and cidofovir. **Table 3** highlights the common mutations associated with antiviral resistance. Genotypic testing is currently the method of choice for determining antiviral resistance. Phenotypic resistance testing has been available but can take weeks to result and may be affected by fitness characteristics of drug-resistant viral strains.[58]

CMV resistance should be suspected when CMV viremia or disease persist or worsen despite appropriate therapeutic doses of ganciclovir or valganciclovir for greater than 2 weeks. One should expect at least a 0.5 to 1.0 log reduction from baseline of CMV DNA viral load in 2 weeks. However, of those with suspected drug resistance, only one-quarter have genotypic resistance.[59] Therefore, concern should prompt an evaluation of drug dosing in the context of renal function and drug absorption. Oral valganciclovir can be changed to intravenous ganciclovir, and higher dosing could be considered (up to 10 mg/kg every 12 hours) or combining ganciclovir and

Table 3
Cytomegalovirus resistance mutations

	Ganciclovir High-Level Resistance >5× EC50	Ganciclovir Low-Level Resistance <5× EC50	Foscarnet	Cidofovir	Letermovir[a]
UL97 Frequent	M460VI H520Q A594V L595S C603W	C592G	—	—	—
UL97 Infrequent	M460T A594G 595del L595FW E596Y K599T Del601–3 C603R C607Y	L405P V466G A594ET E596G L600del C603S C607F I610T A613V	—	—	—

(continued on next page)

Table 3
(continued)

	Ganciclovir High-Level Resistance >5× EC50	Ganciclovir Low-Level Resistance <5× EC50	Foscarnet	Cidofovir	Letermovir[a]
UL54	V526L	D301N, N408DKS, N410K, F412CV, D413EAN, L501I, T503I, A505V, K513ENR, L516R, I521T, P522AS, C524del, V526L, C539G, D542E, L545S, Q578L, D588N, I726TV, E756K, L773V, L776M, V781I, Del981-2, L987G	N495K, V526L, Q578L, D588EN, T700A, V715 AM, E756DKQ, L773V, L776M, V781I, V787L, L802M, A809V, V812L, T813S, T821I, A834P, T838A, G841AS, Del981-2	D301N, N408DKS, N410K, F412CV, D413EAN, L501I, T503I, A505V, K513ENR, L516R, I521T, P522AS, C524del, V526L, C539G, D542E, L545S, I726TV, L773V, K805Q, V812L, T813S, A834P, G841A, Del981-2, L987G	—
UL56	—	—	—	—	Codons 231–369, V236M, E237D, C325F/R

Abbreviation: EC50, 50% effective concentration.
[a] More data required to identify clinically significant resistance mutations.
Data from Refs.[63–66]

foscarnet while awaiting genotypic drug resistance testing.[60,61] Persisting CMV infection should also prompt a review of immunosuppressive therapy with reductions as able. Consideration to switching to an mTOR inhibitor-based regimen can be given.[13]

Risk factors for CMV drug resistance include D+/R− serostatus, high peak viral load (>10^5 IU/mL), increased duration of antiviral exposure (including >6 months CMV prophylaxis), and suboptimal antiviral drug concentrations. Lung, intestinal, and kidney/pancreas transplant recipients seem to be at higher risk for antiviral drug resistance.[15,62] Most patients with ganciclovir resistance have mutations in UL97 that confer high- or low-grade resistance. Mutations in the UL54 polymerase gene can increase the degree of ganciclovir resistance and confer coincident cidofovir or foscarnet resistance, even without prior exposure to cidofovir or foscarnet.

Treatment of low-level ganciclovir-resistant virus (<5-fold increase in 50% effective concentration [EC50]) includes increasing the dose of ganciclovir to 7.5 to 10.0 mg/kg every 12 hours or combined ganciclovir/foscarnet.[60,61] Treatment of high-level ganciclovir-resistant virus (>5-fold increase in EC50) includes foscarnet or cidofovir, assuming no cross-resistance. There have traditionally been no available drugs for multidrug-resistant CMV infection, but letermovir may successfully change that.

SUMMARY

Prevention and management of CMV infection and disease has been a major advance in SOT. Given the goals of immunosuppressive therapies, it is unlikely that organ transplantation will soon be free of CMV disease risk. Optimizing prevention and treatment strategies remains the responsibility of each transplant center. Newer monitoring assays and available antivirals may help reduce the toxicities of existing therapies and create more opportunities for patients to adapt to lifelong CMV latency.

REFERENCES

1. Britt W. Manifestations of human cytomegalovirus infection: proposed mechanisms of acute and chronic disease. In: Shenk T, Stinski MF, editors. Human cytomegalovirus: 325. Current topics in microbiology and immunology. Springer Berlin Heidelberg; 2008.
2. Zhang LJ, Hanpf P, Rutherford C, et al. Detection of cytomegalovirus, DNA, RNA and antibody in normal blood donor blood. J Infect Dis 1995;171:1002–6.
3. Rubin R. Summary of a workshop on cytomegalovirus infections in organ transplantation. J Infect Dis 1979;139:728–34.
4. Crough T, Khanna R. Immunobiology of human cytomegalovirus: from bench to bedside. Clin Microbiol Rev 2009;22:76.
5. Gandhi MK, Khanna R. Human cytomegalovirus: clinical aspects, immune regulation, and emerging treatments. Lancet Infect Dis 2004;4:725.
6. Beersma MF, Bijlmakers MJ, Ploegh HL. Human cytomegalovirus down-regulates HLA class I expression by reducing the stability of class I H chains. J Immunol 1993;151:4455–64.
7. Sylwester AW, Mitchell BL, Edgar JB, et al. Broadly targeted human cytomegalovirus-specific CD4 and CD8 T cells dominate the memory compartments of exposed subjects. J Exp Med 2005;202:673.
8. Gerna G, Sarasina A, Patrone M, et al. Human cytomegalovirus serum neutralizing antibodies block virus infection of endothelial/epithelial cells, but not fibroblasts, early during primary infection. J Gen Virol 2008;89(4):853–65.
9. LaRosa C, Diamond DJ. The immune response to human CMV. Future Virol 2012; 7(3):279–93.

10. Sester M, Gartner BC, Sester U, et al. Is the cytomegalovirus serologic status always accurate? A comparative analysis of humoral and cellular immunity. Transplantation 2003;76:1229.

11. Brennan DC, Legendre C, Patel D, et al. Cytomegalovirus incidence between everolimus versus mycophenolate in de novo renal transplants: pooled analysis of three clinical trials. Am J Transplant 2011;11(11):2453–62.

12. Vigano M, Dengler T, Mattei MF, et al. Lower incidence of cytomegalovirus with everolimus versus mycophoenolate mofetil in de novo cardiac transplant recipients: a randomized, multicenter study. Transpl Infect Dis 2010;12:23–30.

13. Torre-Cisneros J, Aguado JM, Caston JJ, et al. Management of cytomegalovirus infection in solid organ transplant recipients: SET/GESITRA-SEIMC/REIPI recommendations. Transplant Rev (Orlando) 2016;30:119–43.

14. Timpone JG, Girlanda R, Rudolph L, et al. Infections in intestinal and multivisceral transplant recipients. Infect Dis Clin North Am 2013;27(2):359–77.

15. Timpone JG, Yimen M, Cox S, et al. Resistant cytomegalovirus in intestinal and multivisceral transplant recipients. Transpl Infect Dis 2016;18:202–9.

16. Florescu DF, Langnas AN, Grant W, et al. Incidence, risk factors, and outcomes associated with cytomegalovirus disease in small bowel transplant recipients. Pediatr Transplant 2012;16:294–301.

17. Balthesen M, Messerle M, Reddehase MJ. Lungs are a major organ site of cytomegalovirus latency and recurrence. J Virol 1993;67:5360–6.

18. Rubin RH. The indirect effects of cytomegalovirus infection on the outcome of organ transplantation. JAMA 1989;261:3607–9.

19. Hodson EM, Jones CA, Webster AC, et al. Antiviral medications to prevent cytomegalovirus disease and early death in recipients of solid organ transplants: a systematic review of randomized controlled trials. Lancet 2005;365:2105–15.

20. Humar A, Limaye AP, Blumberg EA, et al. Extended valganciclovir prophylaxis in D+/R- kidney transplant recipients is associated with long term reduction in cytomegalovirus disease: two year results of the IMPACT study. Transplantation 2010; 90:1427–31.

21. Tamm M, Aboyoun CL, Chhajed PN, et al. Treated cytomegalovirus pneumonia is not associated with bronchiolitis obliterans syndrome. Am J Respir Crit Care Med 2004;170:1120–3.

22. Kotton CN, Kumar D, Caliendo AM, et al. Updated international consensus guidelines on the management of cytomegalovirus in solid-organ transplantation. Transplantation 2010;96:333–60.

23. Nagai S, Mangus RS, Anderson E, et al. Cytomegalovirus infection after intestinal/multivisceral transplantation: a single-center experience with 210 cases. Transplantation 2016;100:451–60.

24. Hirsch HH, Lautenschlager I, Pinsky BA, et al. An international multicenter performance analysis of cytomegalovirus load tests. Clin Infect Dis 2013;56:367–73.

25. Bodro M, Sabe N, Llado L, et al. Prophylaxis versus preemptive therapy for cytomegalovirus disease in high-risk liver transplant recipients. Liver Transpl 2012; 18(9):1093–9.

26. Hodson EM, Ladhani M, Webster AC, et al. Antiviral medications for preventing cytomegalovirus disease in solid organ transplant recipients. Cochrane Database Syst Rev 2013;(2):CD003774.

27. Palmer SM, Limaye A, Banks M, et al. Extended valganciclovir prophylaxis to prevent cytomegalovirus after lung transplantation; a randomized controlled trial. Ann Intern Med 2010;152:761–9.

28. Finlen Copeland CA, Davis WA, Snyder LD, et al. Long-term efficacy and safety of 12 months of valganciclovir prophylaxis compared with 3 months after lung transplantation: a single-center, long-term follow-up analysis from a randomized controlled cytomegalovirus prevention trial. J Heart Lung Transplant 2011;30: 990–6.
29. Paya C, Humar A, Dominguez E, et al. Efficacy and safety of valganciclovir vs. oral ganciclovir for prevention of cytomegalovirus disease in solid organ transplant recipients. Am J Transplant 2004;4:611.
30. Limaye AP, Bakthavatsalam R, Kim HW, et al. Impact of cytomegalovirus in organ transplant recipients in the era of antiviral prophylaxis. Transplantation 2006;81: 1645–52.
31. Owers DS, Webster AC, Strippoli GFM, et al. Pre-emptive treatment for cytomegalovirus viremia to prevent cytomegalovirus disease in solid organ transplant recipients. Cochrane Database Syst Rev 2013;(2):CD005133.
32. Asberg A, Humar A, Rollag H, et al. Oral valganciclovir is noninferior to intravenous ganciclovir for the treatment of cytomegalovirus disease in solid organ transplant recipients. Am J Transplant 2007;7:2106–13.
33. Kotton CN. CMV: prevention, diagnosis and therapy. Am J Transplant 2013;13: 24–40.
34. Asberg A, Humar A, Jardine AG, et al. Long-term outcomes of CMV disease treatment with valganciclovir versus IV ganciclovir in solid organ transplant recipients. Am J Transplant 2006;2009(9):1205–13.
35. Avery RK, Arav-Boger R, Marr KA, et al. Outcomes in transplant recipients treated with foscarnet for ganciclovir-resistant or refractory cytomegalovirus infection. Transplantation 2016;100(10):e74–80.
36. Bonatti H, Sifri CD, Larcher C, et al. Use of cidofovir for cytomegalovirus disease refractory to ganciclovir in solid organ recipients. Surg Infect (Larchmt) 2017; 18(2):128–36.
37. Wilkens H, Sester M. Treatment of cytomegalovirus infection with cidofovir and CMV immune globulin in a lung transplant recipient. Case Rep Transplant 2016. https://doi.org/10.1155/2016/4560745.
38. Goldner T, Hewlett G, Ettischer N, et al. The novel anticytomegalovirus compound AIC246 (letermovir) inhibits human cytomegalovirus replication through a specific antiviral mechanism that involves the viral terminase. J Virol 2011;85(20): 10884–93.
39. Lischka P, Hewlett G, Wunberg T, et al. In vitro and in vivo activities of the novel anticytomegalovirus compound AIC246. Antimicrob Agents Chemother 2010; 54(3):1290–7.
40. Marty FM, Ljungman P, Chemaly RF, et al. Letermovir prophylaxis for cytomegalovirus in hematopoietic cell transplantation. N Engl J Med 2017;377(25): 2433–44.
41. Chemaly RF, Ullmann AJ, Stoelben S, et al. Letermovir for cytomegalovirus prophylaxis in hematopoietic cell transplantation. N Engl J Med 2014;370(19):1781–9.
42. US FDA. PREVYMISTM (letermovir) tablet and injection: NDA approval letter. 2017. Available at: https://www.fda.gov. Accessed March 15, 2018.
43. Stoelben S, Arns W, Renders L, et al. Preemptive treatment of cytomegalovirus infection in kidney transplant recipients with letermovir; results of a phase 2a study. Transpl Int 2014;27(1):77–86.
44. Kaul DR, Stoelben S, Cober E, et al. First report of successful treatment of multidrug-resistant cytomegalovirus disease with the novel anti-CMV compound AIC246. Am J Transplant 2011;11:1079–84.

45. Kropeit D, von Richter O, Stobernack HP, et al. Pharmacokinetics and safety of letermovir coadministered with cyclosporine A or tacrolimus in healthy subjects. Clin Pharmacol Drug Dev 2018;7(1):9–21.
46. Bonaros N, Mayer B, Schachner T, et al. CMV hyperimmune globulin for preventing cytomegalovirus infection and disease in solid organ transplant recipients: a meta-analysis. Clin Transpl 2008;22:89–97.
47. Rea F, Potena L, Yonan N, et al. Cytomegalovirus hyper immunoglobulin for CMV prophylaxis in thoracic transplantation. Transplantation 2016;100(3S):S19–26.
48. Verdonck LF, de Gast GC, Dekker AW, et al. Treatment of cytomegalovirus pneumonia after bone marrow transplantation with cytomegalovirus immunoglobulin combined with ganciclovir. Bone Marrow Transplant 1989;4(2):187–9.
49. Emanuel D, Cunningham I, Jules-Elysee K, et al. Cytomegalovirus pneumonia after bone marrow transplantation successfully treated with the combination of ganciclovir and high dose intravenous immune globulin. Ann Int Med 1988;15: 777–82.
50. Yamani MH, Avery R, Mawhorter WD, et al. The impact of CytoGam on cardiac transplant recipients with moderate hypogammaglobulinemia: a randomized single-center study. J Heart Lung Transplant 2005;24:1766–9.
51. Chon WJ, Kadambi PV, Xu C, et al. Use of leflunomide in renal transplant recipients with ganciclovir-resistant/refractory cytomegalovirus infection: a case series from the university of Chicago. Case Rep Nephrol Dial 2015;5:96–105.
52. Battiwalla M, Paplham P, Almyroudis NG, et al. Leflunomide failure to control recurrent cytomegalovirus infection in the setting of renal failure after allogeneic stem cell transplantation. Transpl Infect Dis 2007;9(1):28–31.
53. Shapira MY, Resnick IB, Chou S, et al. Artesunate as a potent antiviral agent in a patient with late drug-resistant cytomegalovirus infection after hematopoietic stem cell transplantation. Clin Infect Dis 2008;46:1455–7.
54. Lau PKH, Woods ML, Rantanjee SK, et al. Artesunate is ineffective in controlling valganciclovir-resistant cytomegalovirus infection. Clin Infect Dis 2011; 52(2):279.
55. Egli A, Humar A, Kumar D. State of the art monitoring of cytomegalovirus-specific immunity for the prediction of cytomegalovirus disease after organ transplant: a primer for the clinician. Clin Infect Dis 2012;55:1678–89.
56. Kumar D, Mian M, Singer L, et al. An interventional study using cell-mediated immunity to personalize therapy for cytomegalovirus infection after transplantation. Am J Transplant 2017;17(9):2468–73.
57. Neuenhahn M, Albrecht J, Odendahl M, et al. Transfer of minimally manipulated CMV-specific T cells from stem cell or third-party donors to treat CMV infection after allo-HSCT. Leukemia 2017;31(10):2161–71.
58. Emery VC, Griffiths PD. Prediction of cytomegalovirus load and resistance patterns after antiviral chemotherapy. Proc Natl Acad Sci U S A 2000;97:8039.
59. Lopez-Aladid R, Guiu A, Sanclemente G, et al. Detection of cytomegalovirus drug resistance mutations in solid organ transplant recipients with suspected resistance. J Clin Virol 2017;90:57–63.
60. Gracia-Ahufinger I, Gutierrez-Aroca J, Corderoa E, et al. Use of high-dose ganciclovir for the treatment of cytomegalovirus replication in solid organ transplant patients with ganciclovir resistance inducing mutations. Transplantation 2013; 95:1015–20.
61. Mylonakis E, Kallas WM, Fishman JA. Combination antiviral therapy for ganciclovir-resistant cytomegalovirus infection in solid-organ transplant recipients. Clin Infect Dis 2002;34:1337.

62. LePage AK, Jager MM, Iwasenk JM. Clinical aspects of cytomegalovirus antiviral resistance in solid organ transplant recipients. Clin Infect Dis 2013;56(7): 1018–29.

63. Chou S. Approach to drug-resistant cytomegalovirus in transplant recipients. Curr Opin Infect Dis 2015;28:293–9.

64. Lurain NS, Chou S. Antiviral drug resistance of human cytomegalovirus. Clin Microbiol Rev 2010;23(4):689–712.

65. Gohring K, Hamprecht K, Jahn G. Antiviral drug and multidrug resistance in cytomegalovirus infected SCT patients. Comput Struct Biotechnol J 2015;13:153–9.

66. Hakki M, Chou S. The biology of cytomegalovirus drug resistance. Curr Opin Infect Dis 2011;24:605–11.

Management of BK Polyomavirus Infection in Kidney and Kidney-Pancreas Transplant Recipients

A Review Article

Nissreen Elfadawy, MS, MD[a],*, Masaaki Yamada, MD[b],
Nagaraju Sarabu, MD[a]

KEYWORDS

- Kidney transplantation • BK virus • BKV-associated nephropathy (BKVAN)
- Polyomavirus

KEY POINTS

- BK virus (BKV) infection is common in kidney transplant recipients.
- BKV-associated nephropathy can cause premature graft loss in severe cases.
- Preventive strategy with active surveillance has improved outcomes of BKV infection but optimal management and specific therapy remain unclear and variable.
- Judicious immunosuppression adjustment is warranted in case of significant BK viremia and nephropathy.
- Currently, there is a limited role of use of antiviral agents either as prophylaxis or active treatment.

HISTORY AND BACKGROUND

BK virus (BKV) belongs to a large family called Polyomaviruses. Polyma in the Greek language means many (-poly) tumors (-oma). There are 77 recognized species in this family. Of these, 13 species, which are ubiquitous and usually asymptomatic, are known to infect humans.[1] However, 4 species of polyomaviruses are associated

Disclosure of Interest: None.
[a] Department of Nephrology and Hypertension, University Hospitals, Cleveland Medical Center, 11100 Euclid Avenue, Cleveland, OH 44106, USA; [b] Division of Nephrology, University of Cincinnati College of Medicine, 231 Albert Sabin Way, Suite 6213, Cincinnati, OH 45267-0585, USA
* Corresponding author.
E-mail address: Nissreen.elfadawy@uhhospitals.org

Infect Dis Clin N Am 32 (2018) 599–613
https://doi.org/10.1016/j.idc.2018.04.009
0891-5520/18/© 2018 Elsevier Inc. All rights reserved.

id.theclinics.com

with human diseases: BKV[2]; JC virus (JCV)[3]; Merkel cell virus[4]; and, most recently, New Jersey polyomavirus.[5]

JCV and BKV are 70% related in their genome sequence. JCV was first discovered in 1959[6] but it was not until 1971 that it was isolated from a brain of a patient with Hodgkin disease diagnosed with progressive multifocal leukoencephalopathy.[7] The same year and in the same issue of the Lancet, BKV was first described.[8]

BK Virus is named after a Sudanese patient who suffered from endstage renal disease secondary to chronic pyelonephritis and underwent a living-related kidney transplant. Postoperative course was complicated with 2 mild rejections. Five months after transplant, the patient was admitted with graft dysfunction and ureteric obstruction. Tissue culture from the donor's ureter revealed a virus with unique cytopathic effect that distinguished the newly discovered virus from the rest of the polyoma viruses.[8]

EPIDEMIOLOGY AND ROUTE OF TRANSMISSION

There have been 4 genotypes identified for BKV (I to IV). BKV type I has the higher prevalence in the 4 groups. Baksh and colleagues[9] described 19 cases of renal allograft viral interstitial nephritis due to BKV. Eleven out of the 19 grafts (58%) corresponded to genotype I. Interestingly, in addition to BKV, JCV was seen in 7 interstitial nephritis grafts (37%), suggesting that both JCV and BKV can be isolated from renal tissue. This is consistent with some case reports linking JCV with a milder form of nephropathy seen in renal transplant patients.[10–12]

BKV is ubiquitous, with a worldwide seroprevalence in adults of 75% (range 46%–94%)[13] and of 30% to 90%.in the United States and Europe.[14,15] In several anecdotal reports, 60% to 100% of children are seropositive to BKV by the age of 10 years, indicating that infection occurs early in life and is usually asymptomatic.[16] The antibodies then decline to around 70% as age advances[17]; this observation suggests the role of maternal fetal antibodies transmission, which is supported by the identification of BKV IgM in newborns[18] and BKV genome in aborted fetuses.[19] However, there is no evidence in the literature suggesting teratogenicity or adverse fetal events secondary to BKV prenatal transmission. Following primary infection, the virus remains latent in the renal epithelium (tubular, transitional, and parietal epithelium) due to its tropism to the urinary tract.

The route of BKV transmission is believed to be human-to-human with no animal reservoir identified. To date, there is no specific route of transmission that has been identified. Some reports have identified BKV in stool[20,21] and sewage,[22] suggesting a possible fecal-oral route. Other studies detected BKV in tonsillar tissues,[23] which suggests either an oral or a respiratory route of transmission might be possible, with the latter the most important.

CLINICAL SIGNIFICANCE AND PREVALENCE AFTER KIDNEY AND KIDNEY-PANCREAS TRANSPLANTATION
BK Virus in Immunocompetent Population

As previously mentioned, BKV is highly seroprevalent in the healthy immunocompetent population, mostly presenting as asymptomatic low-grade viruria with no data suggesting clinical significance. Coleman and colleagues[24] showed evidence of high incidence of asymptomatic BKV viruria among 1235 pregnant women, which was attributed to impaired cell-mediated immunity, with no evidence of subsequent complications or fetal transmission.

BK Virus in Immunocompromised Population

BKV is reported to be pathogenic in the immunocompromised population mainly among patients with transplants. Interestingly, among kidney and kidney-pancreas transplantation patients, BKV reactivation primarily causes tubulointerstitial nephritides known as BKV-associated nephropathy (BKVAN) and ureteral stenosis.[25] On the other hand, BKV reactivation in allogeneic hematopoietic cell transplantation primarily causes hemorrhagic cystitis, which is rarely observed in the kidney transplant population.[26] BKVAN in native kidneys after nonkidney organ transplantation is rarely reported, even in settings of the same degree of immunosuppression.[27] This observation suggests that factors associated with the process of kidney transplantation might play a role, such as ischemia-reperfusion injury, and tissue trauma that might activate the latent virus in the donated kidney; therefore, donor–recipient transmission can be supported. Bohl and colleagues[28] demonstrated the homology of the BKV capsid component viral protein 1 by performing polymerase chain reaction (PCR) of BKV in donor–recipient pairs to suggest that BKV is derived from the donor.

Course of BK Virus Reactivation

Previous reports have described that the course of the BKV disease spectrum among the kidney and kidney-pancreas transplant population evolves from reactivation of the latent BKV in the urinary tract epithelium and manifests as BK viruria; to BK viremia; to BKVAN; to graft dysfunction, "which is the most common clinical presentation in this population"; to, eventually, graft failure.[29–31]

BK Virus and Graft Rejection

It is strongly believed that the main mechanism of graft dysfunction after BKV reactivation is related to the direct cytopathic injury caused by viral invasion. Another proposed mechanism is that decreased immunosuppressive medication after BKV reactivation might induce rejection.[32] Recently, Sawinski and colleagues[33] reported a novel association between BKV and the development of de novo donor-specific antibodies and subsequent graft rejection owing to an allosensitization effect induced by changing in the net immunosuppression state from over-immunosuppression to under-immunosuppression after reduction in immunosuppression medication.

BK Virus and Malignancy

As the name of the family, polyoma, or many tumors, implies (as suggested in the literature), there might be a link between BKV and malignancy, especially in prostate cancer and bladder cancer. Monini and colleagues[34] identified BKV particles in normal and neoplastic tissue samples of prostatic cancer by DNA PCR. Interestingly, the DNA load was significantly higher in neoplastic tissue compared with normal tissue, ruling out the possibility that detection of the virus from the malignant tissues was due to the ubiquitous presence of BKV. Conversely, Keller and colleagues[35] reported BKV seropositive status was associated with better prognosis in 226 subjects with prostate cancer, owing to beneficial immune response. Similar controversy is reported regarding the possible association of BKV and bladder cancer.[36,37] There is no definitive association between BKV and malignancy in humans.[38]

Risk Factors for BK Virus Reactivation and BK Virus–Associated Nephropathy

The literature is inconsistent concerning the risk factors for BKV. **Table 1** summarizes the reported risk factors of BKV reactivation and BKVAN.[25,30–33]

Table 1
Risk factors of BK virus reactivation and BK virus–associated nephropathy

Risk Factors of BKV Reactivation After Transplantation		
Recipient-Related	**Donor-Related**	**Transplant-Related**
• Older age	• Female gender	• High immunosuppression drug levels
• Male gender	• African American	• Use of tacrolimus
• Steroid exposure	• Deceased donors	• Thymoglobulin induction
• Antirejection treatment	• BKV seropositive	• Ureteral stents
• Diabetes mellitus	status	• HLA mismatch
• Negative BKV serostatus		• A,B, OR O blood groups incompatibility
		• Ischemia or reperfusion injury
		• Long ischemia time

In a prospective study that included 240 kidney-only transplant recipients, Sood and colleagues[39] reported African American recipients to be protected against BKV reactivation. A recent retrospective study, which included 573 kidney and kidney-pancreas transplant cases, identified vitamin D insufficiency (25-hydroxvitmain D <30 ng/mL) to be an independent risk factor for infections, including BKV reactivation, after adjusting for the degree of immunosuppression in a logistic regression model.[40]

We previously reported that cytomegalovirus (CMV) reactivation after kidney transplantation might be protective against BKV reactivation, possibly due to decreased immunosuppression after CMV infection is identified.[41]

The key element for the risk and pathogenesis of BKV reactivation is believed to be the imbalance between the BKV replication and BKV- specific immunity.[2] As previously mentioned, risk factors of BKV are inconsistent among various studies. However, it is clear that the degree of immunosuppression is the strongest risk factor for BKV reactivation. This fact caused some investigators to consider that BKV reactivation may be a marker for over-immunosuppression.[42] Brennan and colleagues[43] evaluated the incidence of BKV reactivation with 4 different immunosuppressive regimens in a prospective study that included 200 subjects after kidney transplantation. The subjects were randomly assigned to receive tacrolimus (n = 134) or cyclosporine (n = 66). As a second immunosuppression agent, azathioprine (n = 112) was used. Mycophenolate mofetil (MMF) (n = 88) was used instead of azathioprine under certain circumstances (eg, second transplant, panel reactive antibody >20%) and all subjects received prednisone tapered by month 3 to 5 to 7.5 mg daily. By year 1, their study revealed no difference in the rate of BK viruria or viremia among those receiving tacrolimus compared with cyclosporine. In addition, no differences were found with azathioprine compared with MMF. Although there is no definitive single immunosuppressive medication or specific combination that has been confirmed to be associated with BKV reactivation, Hirsch and colleagues[44] recently reported that the mammalian target of rapamycin (mTOR) inhibitor sirolimus can inhibit BKV replication during early gene expression, supporting the notion that BKV replication depends on mTOR activity. Calcineurin inhibitor (CNI) cyclosporine A also inhibited BKV replication. On the other hand, tacrolimus was reported as an enhancer to BKV replication; moreover, it reversed the sirolimus inhibition effect. These findings definitely open new horizons for clinical trials aiming to find a specific anti-BKV drug and provide guidance for modifying immunosuppressive medications in patients with BK viremia.

Low Versus High BK Viremia

In agreement with other studies, the authors previously reported that BK viral loads less than 10,000 copies/mL were not associated with graft adverse effects at 3, 6, or 12 months posttransplant, increased graft rejection rate, or increased risk of BKVAN when compared with BKV-negative transplant recipients.[45–49] Moreover, spontaneous clearance rate in the low viremia population was reported to be as high as 95% without intervention or change in the immunosuppression protocol, suggesting that close observation might be a reasonable option for those patients.[45] On the other hand, BK viral loads greater than 10,000 copies/mL were reported to be the cutoff for significant BK viremia and subsequent negative outcomes, including graft dysfunction, graft rejection, and development of BKVAN, which mandates immediate intervention.[46–48] Indeed, recent reports support that a plasma PCR viral load greater than 10,000 copies/mL for greater than 3 weeks is a surrogate marker for presumptive BKVAN.[47–49]

DIAGNOSIS

The prevalence of BK viremia among the kidney and kidney-pancreas transplant population has been reported to range from 7% to 27%,[46–48] with most cases observed during the first year particularly, as early as 2 to 6 months posttransplant.[49] The incidence of BKVAN in several reports ranged between 1% to 27%, depending on the surveillance protocol, and possible early detection and intervention of BKV reactivation before graft injury occurs.[44–49] Owing to better awareness of the BKV and its adverse effect on renal graft outcome, the incidence of graft loss due to BKVAN has significantly declined over the past 20 years.[25,50]

BKV infection is almost always asymptomatic and only manifests as a functional impairment of kidney transplant. Active replication of BKV in the urinary tract occurs before renal function impairment; hence transplant centers now routinely use screening methods for early detection.

Screening Protocols

Screening can be performed by 1 of 3 ways:

1. Decoy cells: First described by Coleman and colleagues,[51] these are urothelial cells with characteristic large basophilic nuclear inclusions that can be identified by urine cytology. Presence of these in urine is suggestive of BK viral replication.[52]
2. BK viruria: Genomic detection and quantification in urine, by PCR technique.
3. BK viremia: Genomic detection and quantification in blood, again, by PCR technique.

In North America, quantitative plasma BKV PCR measurement is the preferred screening method. Urine cytology (decoy cells) and urine BKV PCR are not commonly used. As previously mentioned, the initial process of BKV infection in renal transplant recipients is BK viruria; however, two-thirds of patients with BK viruria do not develop either viremia or BKVAN. This reflects the low positive predictive value of BK viruria. In summary, plasma BKV PCR is the preferred method.

Nevertheless, the quantification of BK viral load should be interpreted with caution because of interassay variation. To standardize quantitative BK viral load testing, the World Health Organization (WHO) proposed an international standard for BKV PCR.[53] This initiative is expected to enhance clinical research focusing on BKV management.

Utility of these screening methods has been extensively investigated. **Table 2** summarizes sensitivities and specificities, and advantages and disadvantages of each screening method.

Table 2
Utility of BK virus screening methods

Method	Utility	Sensitivity[a]	Specificity[a]	PPV[a]	NPV[a]	Disadvantage	Advantage
1. Urine							
Decoy Cells	++	100%	45%	Low	High	• Decoy cells identification needs experience • Not to monitor decline in viral load after decrease immuno-suppression due to delayed response	• Less cost • Precedes BK viremia by 6–12 wk and flags patients who require intervention and intensive screening by plasma PCR
Qualitative PCR	+						
Quantitative PCR	+++						
2. Plasma							
Qualitative PCR	+	100%	66%[b]	High	Low	• Expensive • May progress to BKVAN quickly, with a window period of only 2 wk	• High PPV • Immediate response to reduction in immunosuppression
Quantitative PCR	++++						

+ Scale 1 to 4: + not commonly used, ++++ very commonly used.
Abbreviations: NPV, negative predictive value; PPV, positive predictive value.
[a] For detecting BKV reactivation.
[b] Specificity increases to 90% if viral load is greater than 10,000 copies/mL of blood.

Frequency of surveillance varies from center to center but most commonly, including in University Hospitals, is done during months 1, 3, 6, 9, and 12 of the first year posttransplant, then for cause when unexplained graft dysfunction is noticed. Because this frequency might occasionally miss early stages of BK viremia, some centers screen monthly for the first 6 months, then every other month until 1 year, quarterly for the second year, then as clinically indicated afterward.[54] According to the Kidney Disease: Improving Global Outcomes (KDIGO) guidelines and the American Society of Transplantation recommendations, options include (1) monthly screening with quantitative plasma BKV PCR test for the first 3 to 6 months, followed by every 3 months until 24 months after transplant; or (2) biweekly urine tests (BKV PCR or cytology), followed by a quantitative plasma PCR test, if positive, for the first 3 months, then monthly until month 6, and then every 3 months until 24 months after transplant.[55]

Kidney Biopsy

Although the diagnosis of presumptive BKVAN can be made based on a quantitative plasma BK viral load greater than 10,000 copies/mL,[56] kidney biopsy remains the gold standard to diagnose definitive BKVAN.[2] However, early BKV infection can be limited to focal areas and easily missed. Indeed, discordance of histologic findings was observed in up to 37% of simultaneously obtained biopsy tissue cores.[57] Virus-infected atypical tubular cells can be prominent but additional virus staining should be sought to safely differentiate BKVAN from acute rejection, which resembles it morphologically (**Fig. 1**). Simian virus 40 is widely used and in situ hybridization of BKV can be applied if necessary.[58]

TREATMENT

Reduction of immunosuppression is the mainstay of treatment of persistent BK viremia and/or biopsy-proven BKVAN. Reduction is done carefully in a stepwise manner while closely monitoring quantitative plasma BKV PCR and serum creatinine, generally every 2 weeks. Opinions regarding which immunosuppressive drug to be withdrawn first are variable. One strategy is to first reduce CNI (tacrolimus or cyclosporine) dosing in a stepwise manner until discontinuation. Another strategy is to first

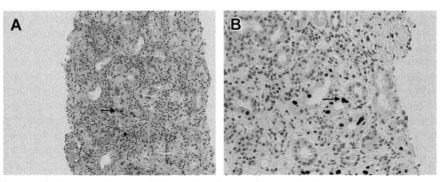

Fig. 1. (A) Hematoxylin-eosin (H&E) stain of renal biopsy showing positive tubular cells viral inclusions and interstitial inflammation. Tubular epithelial cells with cytopathic changes due to BK inclusions (black arrow). Interstitial inflammation (black star). (B) Immunohistochemical stain of renal biopsy showing positive staining for the BK T antigen. Tubular epithelial cells showing viral inclusions that are positive for simian virus 40 antigen by immunohistochemistry (arrow).

reduce the antiproliferative drugs (mycophenolate, azathioprine, sirolimus) in a stepwise manner of 50% each step, until discontinuation. Sometimes, if BK viremia persists at a high level of greater than 10, 000 copies/mL even after discontinuation of 1 drug, reduction of another drug is needed. Due to the lack of an objective testing that can measure an individual's immunity level against the development of BKVAN, and because different individuals have different immunosuppression responses, reduction in immunosuppression is done arbitrarily while monitoring BK viral load. At our center, we occasionally withdrew both CNI and antiproliferative drugs until downtrend in BK viremia was achieved (**Fig. 2**). In such circumstances, when rejection becomes of concern due to under-immunosuppression, other options might be sought. Alternatively, switching from tacrolimus to cyclosporine is embraced at some institutions.[59]

Alternative to the standard CNI regimen, belatacept was approved by the US Food Drug Administration in June 2011. There are limited data regarding BKV infection with belatacept use. The maintenance dose of belatacept is administered parentally. In contrast to CNI, dose adjustment is not typically required. In cases of BKV reactivation with belatacept regimen, reduction or withdrawal of antiproliferative drugs is the first step to manage BKV infection; however, the proper measure to adjust maintenance belatacept dose has not been studied. The frequency of belatacept is typically extended to every 6 weeks instead of the routine 4 weeks if further reduction of immunosuppression medication is warranted, although this lacks evidence.[60]

Leflunomide

Leflunomide is a prodrug whose active metabolite, teriflunomide A77 1726, inhibits dihydroorotate dehydrogenase, a key enzyme in the pyrimidine synthesis pathway of BKV replication, and tyrosine kinase. The inhibition of these enzymes leads to reduction in BK large T antigen expression and DNA replication.[61] In vitro studies have shown antipolyomavirus activity and clearance of BK viremia[62,63] but recent reports that studied the correlation between leflunomide usage and A77 1726 levels with BKV clearance has shown no significant benefit of its use in clearing BK viremia.[64] This drug has fallen out of favor, at least at the United States, due to limited efficacy and side effects, mainly neuropathy, lethargy, gastrointestinal intolerance, and loss of taste without any correlation to plasma concentration. Because leflunomide has some immunosuppressive activity, its use might be considered in conjunction with reduced does of immunosuppressive regiments. When used, the loading dose of leflunomide is 100 mg daily for 3 to 5 days, followed by maintenance at 20 to 60 mg daily, aiming for target leflunomide trough levels of 40 to 80 mg/dL. Without a loading dose, leflunomide might take up to 2 months to reach its target levels; hence, it is not expected to cause a rapid effect on viral clearance.[65] Pregnancy is a contraindication for receiving leflunomide owing to its reported teratogenicity, and elimination of the drug from the circulation might take up to several months owing to long half-life.[66] If major toxicity or unplanned pregnancy occurs, a washout procedure is undertaken with oral cholestyramine (typically 8 g 3 times daily for 11 days) or activated charcoal. Teriflunomide cannot be removed by dialysis; therefore, hemodialysis is not a treatment approach for patients who are experiencing major toxicity or who have taken an overdose of leflunomide.

Cidofovir and Brincidofovir

Cidofovir has modest in vitro activity against polyomaviruses by an unclear mechanism.[59] Several case reports have claimed its efficacy as an adjunctive treatment of

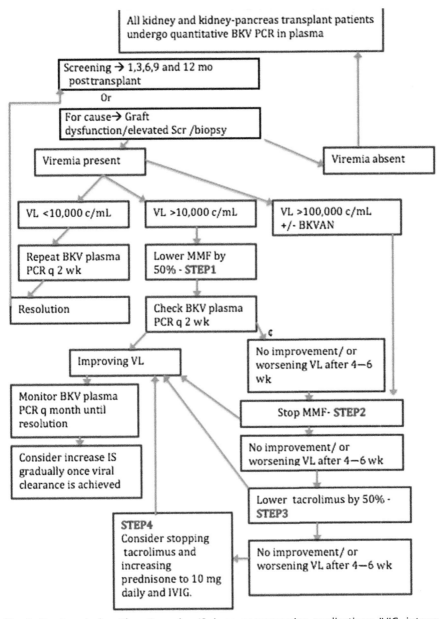

Fig. 2. Treatment algorithm. C, copies; IS, immunosuppression medications; IVIG, intravenous immunoglobulin; q, every; Scr, serum creatinine; VL, viral load. (*Courtesy of* Kidney and Kidney-Pancreas program at University Hospitals, Cleveland Medical Center, Cleveland, OH; with permission.)

BK viremia or BKVAN. A retrospective review by Kuten and colleagues,[67] including 75 kidney and kidney-pancreas recipients ascribed preservation of graft function to cidofovir usage in conjunction with reduced immunosuppression. This favorable result was not appreciated in older recipients with higher BK viral loads. Cidofovir dosage is

1 mg/kg induction and 0.5 mg/kg maintenance every 2 weeks. Major side effects include nephrotoxicity and acute uveitis. Many centers do not use cidofovir at all.

Brincidofovir is the prodrug and lipid-ester formulation of cidofovir (ie, CMX001). Some case reports suggested its use in pediatric renal transplant population, which seems well-tolerated except for diarrhea; however, it lacks randomized controlled trial (RCT) data and further scientific data are warranted.[68] Trials in hematopoietic stem cell transplantation have been halted owing to high graft-versus-host disease–related mortality; and no research is currently ongoing.

Intravenous Immunoglobulin

Similar to other conditions that respond to intravenous immunoglobulin (IVIG), the exact mechanism of action in BKV management remains unclear; however, a detection of BKV-neutralizing antibodies in IVIG preparation was reported.[69] Vu and colleagues[70] reported the efficacy of IVIG administered to 30 kidney transplant recipients after reduction in immunosuppression and leflunomide failed to decrease BK viremia after 8 weeks. Following IVIG administration, 90% of subjects had a decrease in viremia. Although IVIG is not routinely used at university hospitals, the safety and ease of administration of IVIG is encouraging. Occasionally use IVIG in cases of persistent BK viremia after reduction of immunosuppression, and when BK viremia occurred with or after an episode of antibody-mediated rejection. Several limitations apply when interpreting the literature claiming the efficacy of IVIG in clearing BK viremia or BKVAN. RCTs are warranted to prove the efficacy of this intervention. When used, the dose of IVIG is 1 to 2 g/kg divided over 2 to 5 days.

Fluoroquinolones Use as Prophylaxis and Adjunctive Therapy

Fluoroquinolones (FQs) are broad-spectrum antimicrobial agents that inhibit bacterial topoisomerase II and IV, and are widely used in clinical practice. In vitro, FQs interfere with helicase activity of BKV large T antigen protein, which is essential for viral replication.[71] One retrospective study showed a potential benefit of prophylactic ciprofloxacin use in reduction of early BKV infection.[72] Currently, an RCT is ongoing to prove efficacy of prophylactic ciprofloxacin use in BKV infection in renal transplant recipients (ClinicalTrials.gov identifier: NCT01789203). Nonetheless, 3-month levofloxacin use did not reduce the incidence of BK viruria (levofloxacin group 29% vs placebo group 33%, $P > .05$) in a prospective study that was stopped early owing to lack of funding.[73] Furthermore, there was a significantly higher rate of levofloxacin-resistant bacterial organisms isolated (relative risk 1.75, 95% CI 1.01–2.98), which substantially affects the outpatient treatment strategy for common urinary tract infections caused by Enterobacteriaceae and *Pseudomonas aeruginosa*. Levofloxacin at 500 mg daily was tested as adjunctive therapy for BK viremia in a different RCT.[74] There was no statistical difference in plasma BK viral load during the study period, up to 6 months. A recent report studied effect of 3 months of ciprofloxacin in a group of 29 kidney transplant recipients compared with matched 43 control subjects. Ciprofloxacin prophylaxis showed no difference in the incidence of BK infection.[75] In conclusion, there is no current recommendation regarding the usage of FQs as a prophylactic or adjunctive treatment of BKV reactivation after kidney transplantation.

Retransplantation after BK Virus–Associated Nephropathy Graft Loss

As previously mentioned, graft loss due to BKVAN has been significantly declining over the last 2 decades owing to understanding of the disease process and improvement in its management; however, retransplantation after graft loss from BKVAN remains a challenge for transplant physicians. A history of BKVAN does not preclude another transplant candidacy. An analyses of United Network for Organ Sharing and Organ Procurement Transplant Network database reported a general acceptance and favorable results of retransplantation after BKVAN graft loss, although it requires special considerations.[76] Retransplantation is recommended after BK viremia clearance to decrease risk of BKVAN in the retransplanted kidney.[77] Nephrectomy of prior failed allograft if BK viremia persists despite minimization of immunosuppression remains controversial with no supporting evidence. The key to successful retransplantation is balance of overall immunosuppression, risk of BKV replication, and risk of rejection.

SUMMARY

BKV is the most common opportunistic viral infection encountered in kidney allografts and high viral load can lead to graft failure. Fortunately, due to effective preemptive monitoring and early reduction of immunosuppressive medication, graft failure due to BKVAN has decreased considerably. Owing to the unproven efficacy of antiviral drugs against BK, reduction in immunosuppression is the only effective measure in the treatment of this complication; however, protocols of reduction in immunosuppression vary among institutions and can be very challenging due to the risk of subsequent rejection.

ACKNOWLEDGMENTS

The authors greatly appreciate the assistance of Dr Parmjeet Randhawa, MD, Department of Pathology, UPMC-Montefiore, with article review and editing.

REFERENCES

1. Polyomaviridae Study Group of the International Committee on Taxonomy of, Viruses, Calvignac-Spencer S, Feltkamp MC, Daugherty MD, et al. A taxonomy update for the family Polyomaviridae. Arch Virol 2016;161:1739–50.

2. Hirsch HH, Randhawa P. AST Infectious Diseases Community of Practice. BK polyomavirus in solid organ transplantation. Am J Transplant 2013;4:179–88.

3. Tan CS, Koralnik IJ. Progressive multifocal leukoencephalopathy and other disorders caused by JC virus: clinical features and pathogenesis. Lancet Neurol 2010; 9:425–32.

4. Santos-Juanes J, Fernández-Vega I, Fuentes N, et al. Merkel cell carcinoma and Merkel cell polyomavirus: a systematic review and meta-analysis. Br J Dermatol 2015;173:42–50.

5. Mishra N, Pereira M, Rhodes RH, et al. Identification of a novel polyomavirus in a pancreatic transplant recipient with retinal blindness and vasculitic myopathy. J Infect Dis 2014;210(10):1595–9.

6. Stewart SE, Eddy BE. Tumor induction by SE polyoma virus and the inhibition of tumors by specific neutralizing antibodies. Am J Public Health 1959;49:1493–9.

7. Padgett BL, Walker DL, ZuRhein GM, et al. Cultivation of papova-like virus from human brain with progressive multifocal leucoencephalopathy. Lancet 1971; 1(7712):1257–64.

8. Gardner SD, Field AM, Coleman DV, et al. New human papovavirus (B.K.) isolated from urine after renal transplantation. Lancet 1971;1(7712):1253–60.

9. Baksh FK, Finkelstein SD, Swalsky PA, et al. Molecular genotyping of BK and JC viruses in human polyomavirus-associated interstitial nephritis after renal transplantation. Am J Kidney Dis 2001;38(2):354–62.

10. Drachenberg CB, Hirsch HH, Papadimitriou JC, et al. Polyomavirus BK versus JC replication and nephropathy in renal transplant recipients: a prospective evaluation. Transplantation 2007;84(3):323–9.

11. Kazory A, Ducloux D, Chalopin JM, et al. The first case of JC virus allograft nephropathy. Transplantation 2003;76(11):1653–61.

12. Costa C, Bergallo M, Sidoti F, et al. Polyomaviruses BK- And JC-DNA quantitation in kidney allograft biopsies. J Clin Virol 2009;44(1):20–8.

13. Knowles W. The epidemiology of BK virus and the occurrence of antigenic and genomic subtypes. In: Khalili K, GS, editors. Human polyomaviruses: molecular and clinical perspectives. New York: Wiley-Liss; 2001. p. 527–60.

14. Egli A, Infanti L, Dumoulin A, et al. Prevalence of polyomavirus BK and JC infection and replication in 400 healthy blood donors. J Infect Dis 2009;199(6):837–44.

15. Kean JM, Rao S, Wang M, et al. Seroepidemiology of human polyomaviruses. PLoS Pathog 2009;5(3):e1000363.

16. Knowles WA, Pipkin P, Andrews N, et al. Population-based study of antibody to the human polyomaviruses BKV and JCV and the simian polyomavirus SV40. J Med Virol 2003;(1):115–23.

17. Schmidt T, Adam C, Hirsch HH, et al. BK polyomavirus-specific cellular immune responses are age-dependent and strongly correlate with phases of virus replication. Am J Transplant 2014;14(6):1334–45.

18. Gibson PE, Field AM, Gardner SD, et al. Occurrence of IgM antibodies against BK and JC polyomaviruses during pregnancy. J Clin Pathol 1981;34(6):674–82.

19. Boldorini R, Allegrini S, Miglio U, et al. BK virus sequences in specimens from aborted fetuses. J Med Virol 2010;82(12):2127–32.

20. Wong AS, Cheng VC, Yuen KY, et al. High frequency of polyoma BK virus shedding in the gastrointestinal tract after hematopoietic stem cell transplantation: a prospective and quantitative analysis. Bone Marrow Transplant 2009;43(1):43–7.

21. Vanchiere JA, Abudayyeh S, Copeland CM, et al. Polyomavirus shedding in the stool of healthy adults. J Clin Microbiol 2009;47(8):2388–97.

22. Bofill-Mas S, Pina S, Girones R. Documenting the epidemiologic patterns of polyomaviruses in human populations by studying their presence in urban sewage. Appl Environ Microbiol 2000;66(1):238–47.

23. Goudsmit J, Wertheim-van Dillen P, van Strien A, et al. The role of BK virus in acute respiratory tract disease and the presence of BKV DNA in tonsils. J Med Virol 1982;10(2):91–9.

24. Coleman DV, Wolfendale MR, Daniel RA, et al. A prospective study of human polyomavirus infection in pregnancy. J Infect Dis 1980;142(1):91–9.

25. Randhawa PS, Finkelstein S, Scantlebury V, et al. Human polyoma virus-associated interstitial nephritis in the allograft kidney. Transplantation 1999;67(1):103–9.

26. Peinemann F, de Villiers EM, Dörries K, et al. Clinical course and treatment of haemorrhagic cystitis associated with BK type of human polyomavirus in nine paediatric recipients of allogeneic bone marrow transplants. Eur J Pediatr 2000;159(3):182–96.

27. Vigil D, Konstantinov NK, Barry M, et al. BK nephropathy in native kidneys of patients with organ transplants: clinical spectrum of BK infection. World J Transplant 2016;6(3):472–504.

28. Bohl DL, Storchb GA, Ryschkewitschc C, et al. Donor origin of BK virus in renal transplantation and role of HLA C7 in susceptibility to sustained BK viremia. Am J Transplant 2005;5(9):2213–21.

29. Hirsch HH, Brennan DC, Drachenberg CB, et al. Polyomavirus- associated nephropathy in renal transplantation: interdisciplinary analyses and recommendations. Transplantation 2005;79:1277–86.
30. Hardinger KL, Koch MJ, Bohl DJ, et al. BK- virus and the impact of pre-emptive immunosuppression reduction: 5-year results. Am J Transplant 2010;10:407–15.
31. Babel N, Fendt J, Karaivanov S, et al. Sustained BK viruria as an early marker for the development of BKV-associated nephropathy: analysis of 4128 urine and serum samples. Transplantation 2009;88:89–95.
32. Alméras C, Vetromile F, Garrigue V, et al. Monthly screening for BK viremia is an effective strategy to prevent BK virus nephropathy in renal transplant recipients. Transpl Infect Dis 2011;13:101–8.
33. Sawinski D, Forde KA, Trofe-Clark J, et al. Persistent BK viremia does not increase intermediate- term graft loss but is associated with de novo donor-specific antibodies. J Am Soc Nephrol 2015;26:966–75.
34. Monini P, Rotola A, Di Luca D, et al. DNA rearrangements impairing BK virus productive infection in urinary tract tumors. Virology 1995;214(1):273–9.
35. Keller XE, Acevedo C, Sais G, et al. Antibody response to BK polyomavirus as a prognostic biomarker and potential therapeutic target in prostate cancer. Oncotarget 2015;6(8):6459–69.
36. Weinreb DB, Desman GT, Amolat-Apiado MJ, et al. Polyoma virus infection is a prominent risk factor for bladder carcinoma in immunocompetent individuals. Diagn Cytopathol 2006;34(3):201–3.
37. Rollison DE, Sexton WJ, Rodriguez AR, et al. Lack of BK virus DNA sequences in most transitional-cell carcinomas of the bladder. Int J Cancer 2007;120(6):1248–51.
38. Dalianis T, Hirsch HH. Human polyomaviruses in disease and cancer. Virology 2013;437(2):63–72.
39. Sood P, Senanayake S, Sujeet K, et al. Lower prevalence of BK virus infection in African American renal transplant recipients: a prospective study. Transplantation 2012;93(3):291–6.
40. Kalluri HV, Sacha LM, Ingemi AI, et al. Low vitamin D exposure is associated with higher risk of infection in renal transplant recipients. Clin Transplant 2017;31:e12955.
41. Elfadawy N, Flechner SM, liu X, et al. CMV Viremia is associated with a decreased incidence of BKV reactivation after kidney and kidney-pancreas transplantation. Transplantation 2013;96(12):1097–103.
42. Budde K, Matz M, Durr M, et al. Biomarkers of over-immunosuppression. Clin Pharmacol Ther 2011;90:316–22.
43. Brennan DC, Agha I, Bohl DL, et al. Incidence of BK with tacrolimus versus cyclosporine and impact of preemptive immunosuppression reduction. Am J Transplant 2005;5:582–94.
44. Hirsch HH, Yakhontova K, Lu M, et al. BK polyomavirus replication in renal tubular epithelial cells is inhibited by sirolimus, but activated by tacrolimus through a pathway involving FKBP-12. Am J Transplant 2016;16(3):821–32.
45. Sood P, Senanayake S, Sujeet K, et al. Management and out- come of BK viremia in renal transplant recipients: a prospective single-center study. Transplantation 2012;94:814–9.
46. Hirsch HH, Knowles W, Dickenmann M, et al. Prospective study of polyomavirus type BK replication and nephropathy in renal-transplant recipients. N Engl J Med 2002;347:488–93.

47. Nickeleit V, Klimkait T, Binet IF, et al. Testing for polyoma- virus type BK DNA in plasma to identify renal-allograft recipients with viral nephropathy. N Engl J Med 2000;342:1309–14.
48. Chung BH, Hong YA, Kim HG, et al. Clinical usefulness of BK virus plasma quantitative PCR to prevent BK virus associated nephropathy. Transpl Int 2012;25: 687–95.
49. Elfadawy N, Flechner S, Liu X, et al. The impact of surveillance and rapid reduction in immunosuppression to control BK virus-related graft injury in kidney transplantation. Transpl Int 2013;26:822–35.
50. Knight R, Gaber L, Patel S, et al. Screening for BK viremia reduces but does not eliminate the risk of BK nephropathy: a single-center retrospective analysis. Transplantation 2013;95:949–58.
51. Coleman DV, Field AM, Gardner SD, et al. Virus-induced obstruction of ureteric and cystic duct in allograft recipients. Transplant Proc 1973;5(1):95–8.
52. Nickeleit V, Hirsch HH, Binet IF, et al. Polyomavirus infection of renal allograft recipients: from latent infection to manifest disease. J Am Soc Nephrol 1999;10(5): 1080–9.
53. Collaborative study to establish the 1st WHO International Standard for BKV DNA for nucleic acid amplification technique (NAT)-based assays. Expert committee on biological standardization. Geneva, 12–16 2015.
54. Elfadawy N, Flechner AM, Schold JD, et al. Transient versus persistent BK viremia and long term outcomes after kidney and kidney-pancreas transplantation. Clin J Am Soc Nephrol 2014;9(3):553–61.
55. Kidney Disease. Improving Global Outcomes (KDIGO) Transplant Work Group. KDIGO clinical practice guideline for the care of kidney transplant recipients. Am J Transplant 2009;9(3):5–6.
56. Pollara CP, Corbellini S, Chiappini S, et al. Quantitative viral load measurement for BKV infection in renal transplant recipients as a predictive tool for BKVAN. New Microbiol 2011;34:165–71.
57. Drachenberg CB, Papadimitriou JC, Hirsch HH, et al. Histological patterns of polyomavirus nephropathy: correlation with graft outcome and viral load. Am J Transplant 2004;4(12):2082–92.
58. Nickeleit V, Singh HK, Randhawa P, et al. The Banff working group classification of definitive polyomavirus nephropathy: morphologic definitions and clinical correlations. J Am Soc Nephrol 2018;29(2):680–93.
59. Hirsch HH, Vincenti F, Friman S, et al. Polyomavirus BK replication in de novo kidney transplant patients receiving tacrolimus or cyclosporine: a prospective, randomized, multicenter study. Am J Transplant 2013;13(1):136–45.
60. Bassil N, Rostaing L, Mengelle C, et al. Prospective monitoring of cytomegalovirus, Epstein-Barr virus, BK virus, and JC virus infections on belatacept therapy after a kidney transplant. Exp Clin Transplant 2014;12(3):212–9.
61. Liacini A, Seamone ME, Muruve DA, et al. Anti-BK virus mechanisms of sirolimus and leflunomide alone and in combination: toward a new therapy for BK virus infection. Transplantation 2010;90(12):1450–7.
62. Farasati NA, Shapiro R, Vats A, et al. Effect of leflunomide and cidofovir on replication of BK virus in an in vitro culture system. Transplantation 2005;79(1):116–8.
63. Williams JW, Javaid B, Kadambi PV, et al. Leflunomide for polyomavirus type BK nephropathy. N Engl J Med 2005;352(11):1157–8.
64. Faguer S, Hirsch HH, Kamar N, et al. Leflunomide treatment for polyomavirus BK associated nephropathy after kidney transplantation. Transpl Int 2007;20(11): 962–9.

65. Rozman B. Clinical pharmacokinetics of leflunomide. Clin Pharmacokinet 2002; 41:421–3.

66. Brent RL. Teratogen updates: reproductive risks of leflunomide (Arava); a pyrimidine synthesis inhibitor: counseling women taking leflunomide before or during pregnancy and men taking leflunomide who are contemplating fathering a child. Teratology 2001;63:106–12.

67. Kuten SA, Patel SJ, Knight RJ, et al. Observations on the use of cidofovir for BK virus infection in renal transplantation. Transpl Infect Dis 2014;16(6):975–83.

68. Reisman L, Habib S, McClure GB, et al. Treatment of BK virus associated nephropathy with CMX001 after kidney transplantation in a young child. Pediatr Transplant 2014;18(7):231–9.

69. Randhawa PS, Schonder K, Shapiro R, et al. Polyomavirus BK neutralizing activity in human immunoglobulin preparations. Transplantation 2010;89(12):1462–5.

70. Vu D, Shah T, Ansari J, et al. Efficacy of intravenous immunoglobulin in the treatment of persistent BK viremia and BK virus nephropathy in renal transplant recipients. Transplant Proc 2015;47(2):394–8.

71. Portolani M, Pietrosemoli P, Cermelli C, et al. Suppression of BK virus replication and cytopathic effect by inhibitors of prokaryotic DNA gyrase. Antiviral Res 1988; 9(3):205–18.

72. Wojciechowski D, Chanda R, Chandran S, et al. Ciprofloxacin prophylaxis in kidney transplant recipients reduces BK virus infection at 3 months but not at 1 year. Transplantation 2012;94(11):1117–23.

73. Knoll GA, Humar A, Fergusson D, et al. Levofloxacin for BK virus prophylaxis following kidney transplantation: a randomized clinical trial. JAMA 2014; 312(20):2106–14.

74. Lee BT, Gabardi S, Grafals M, et al. Efficacy of levofloxacin in the treatment of BK viremia: a multicenter, double-blinded, randomized, placebo-controlled trial. Clin J Am Soc Nephrol 2014;9(3):583–9.

75. Lebreton M, Esposito L, Mengelle C, et al. A 3-month course of ciprofloxacin does not prevent BK virus replication in heavily immunosuppressed kidney-transplant patients. J Clin Virol 2016;79:61–7.

76. Dharnidharka VR, Cherikh WS, Neff R, et al. Retransplantation after BK virus nephropathy in prior kidney transplant: an OPTN database analysis. Am J Transplant 2010;10(5):1312–5.

77. Geetha D, Sozio SM, Ghanta M, et al. Results of repeat renal transplantation after graft loss from BK virus nephropathy. Transplantation 2011;92(7):781–6.

Human Immunodeficiency Virus Organ Transplantation

Alan J. Taege, MD

KEYWORDS

- HIV • Organ transplantation • Hepatitis C virus • Organ rejection
- HIV positive to positive organ transplantation

KEY POINTS

- HIV is a chronic disease associated with potential organ failure.
- Organ transplantation is a proven option for HIV patients with organ failure.
- Organ rejection rates remain high.
- Hepatitis C virus remains a challenge in HIV organ transplantation.
- HIV-positive donor to HIV-positive recipient transplantation offers potential future options.

INTRODUCTION

The human immunodeficiency virus (HIV) epidemic remains a serious worldwide health problem with more than 35 million people infected. The last four decades have produced tremendous advances in the understanding of HIV and the development of highly active antiretroviral therapy (cART). The success of cART has made HIV a manageable chronic disease and allowed those afflicted to have a near normal lifespan. As a result, aging HIV patients face many of the same chronic health conditions and organ failure as the general population. Liver failure occurs at an accelerated rate for HIV patients because of HIV and hepatitis C. Consequently, chronic conditions outnumber opportunistic infections (OI) as a cause of death for HIV patients.

Organ transplantation is an accepted modality of therapy for organ failure in the general population and more recently in HIV patients. Unfortunately, donor organs are in short supply, whereas the list of those needing organs continues to expand. Currently there are more than 115,000 people listed on the United Network for Organ Sharing waiting list who need donor organs, but only approximately 10,000 transplants are performed annually from available donors, making the supply of organs a critical need.[1] It is unclear how many of the listed individuals are HIV positive because they are not specifically identified.

Dr A.J. Taege: Gilead Community Speaker's bureau. Speaker Clinical Care Options (supported by Viiv grant).
Department of Infectious Disease, Cleveland Clinic, 9500 Euclid Avenue, Cleveland, OH 44195, USA
E-mail address: taegea@ccf.org

This article provides an overview of the transplantation needs in the HIV population focusing on kidney and liver transplants with a brief history of HIV organ transplantation, critical information learned from early experience, and the developing (controversial) approach of transplanting HIV-positive organs into HIV-positive patients.

The pretreatment and early treatment era of the HIV epidemic were marked by death in a few short years from the time of diagnosis, most commonly from OI. With the advent of cART, OI were replaced by chronic conditions of aging and organ failure as leading causes of death. The most common organs failing are the kidney and liver. Renal failure in HIV is most commonly caused by HIV-associated nephropathy (HIVAN), immune complex disease, and thrombotic microangiopathy.[2,3] Diabetes mellitus and hypertension are becoming additional etiologies, similar to the general population. Liver failure is usually the result of hepatitis C virus (HCV); hepatitis B virus (HBV); and secondary hepatocellular carcinoma (HCC), alcohol abuse, and adverse effects of medications. The direct-acting agents (DAA) for HCV have replaced interferon and ribavirin with unprecedented success ushering in a new era for HCV-infected patients.

EARLY YEARS

Organ transplantation was viewed unfavorably in the early years of the epidemic. HIV patients were excluded from consideration because of concerns of hastening disease progression by use of immune suppression, wasting scarce organs in patients with a terminal incurable disease and concerns about exposure of health care workers to the virus while working with HIV patients.[4–6]

Early attempts with organ transplantation in HIV patients, intentional and accidental, in the pre-cART era had poor results.[7–12] Interestingly, HIV did not affect the outcome of the transplanted organ.[13]

The cART era produced marked improvements in survival and life expectancy, quality of life, and decreases in OI.[14,15] Subsequently interest and efforts continued in HIV organ transplantation. Ethical concerns persisted along with reluctance by some to perform the necessary care culminating in the Sounding Board article published in the *New England Journal of Medicine* in 2002, which provided support for solid organ transplantation in HIV patients.[16]

KIDNEY TRANSPLANTATION

HIV patients have an ongoing, increased risk of end-stage renal disease (ESRD) that is 2- to 20-fold higher than the general population even after the benefits of cART.[17] Today HIV patients comprise 1% to 1.5% of the US dialysis population resulting in a rate that is 3.2 times higher than the general population (4.5 for black patients) and will likely continue to rise.[18] ESRD is six-fold higher in black HIV patients than white HIV patients. The racial disparity of HIVAN and ESRD in black HIV patients has a genetic association with the Apo lipoprotein L 1 gene.[17] In addition to HIVAN, the cause of this racial disparity for ESRD in the black HIV population comes from the higher rates of diabetes mellitus and hypertension in the black population.[19] Once placed on dialysis, HIV patients have a significantly worse outcome with survival rates approximately one-third less than HIV-negative dialysis patients.[20,21] The cART era has fortunately resulted in a decreased occurrence of HIVAN[22] but excess ESRD persists in HIV patients.

A survival benefit of kidney transplantation over continuous dialysis was demonstrated for HIV-negative patients.[23–26] This has now been demonstrated in HIV kidney transplantation recipients.[27] Mortality was 79% lower at 5 years after kidney transplant compared with dialysis in HIV monoinfected recipients. The mortality benefit for HIV/HCV coinfected patients was 91% lower at 5 years, although it required a longer post-transplant period to demonstrate this benefit.

HIV transplant candidates are only listed approximately 20% of the time.[28] Contributing factors to this listing disparity include a history of substance abuse, black race, low CD4 count (<200 cells/mm³), or a lack of CD4 documentation. Once listed it is difficult to determine mortality for HIV candidates on the waiting list because HIV status is not indicated. Cross-referencing of the Scientific Registry of Transplant Recipients and Integrated Management System Pharmacy databases revealed 25% of kidney transplant candidates died before achieving transplantation.[27] This equals an 8.7% annual death rate compared with a 4.9% annual death rate for the HIV-negative waiting list group. Mortality was even higher for older individuals and those with HCV/HIV coinfection.

Outcomes in HIV renal transplantation have been very good in the cART era. The National Institutes of Health (NIH)-sponsored HIV-TR study with 150 HIV patients demonstrated patient and graft survival rates between that of the total transplant population and older recipients (>65 years).[29] This cohort was predominantly black (69%) and included 19% with HIV/HCV confection. Delayed graft function (DGF) was common, occurring in 46%. Acute rejection (AR) occurred at high rates, with 1- and 3-year rates of 31% (vs ~12% in HIV-negative recipients) and 41%, respectively, and higher resulting graft failure. Infections occurred in 38% of the cohort, most occurring in the first 6 months involving the respiratory and genitourinary tracts. Similar results have been demonstrated from European transplant centers, although with a lower rate of AR (15%).[30] Contrary to initial concerns, HIV remained controlled and no increase in malignancies was noted, although increases in high-grade intraepithelial anal squamous cell lesions were found.

Several reasons for higher rejection and graft failure rates were considered.[29] HIV-TR did not have a uniform induction or maintenance immunosuppressive regimen stated in the protocol. Each center made their own determinations for induction and maintenance immunosuppression regimens. Concern existed over drug-drug interactions (DDI) involving cART and immunosuppressive medications, particularly protease inhibitors (PI) and nonnucleoside reverse transcription inhibitors (NNRTI), causing inconsistent drug levels and inadequate immune suppression.

A larger comparative analysis of HIV-positive and HIV-negative kidney transplant recipients from the Scientific Registry of Transplant Recipients reviewed 510 HIV-positive kidney recipients.[31] HIV patients had a significantly lower 5- and 10-year graft survival, 69.2% versus 75.3% and 49.8% versus 54.4%. However, if HIV/HCV coinfected patients were removed from the analysis, leaving only HIV monoinfected recipients to be compared with HIV-negative recipients, graft and patient survival were similar. Significant differences exist between these populations (**Boxes 1** and **2**). A living donor and using calcineurin inhibitor (CNI) maintenance immune suppression were associated with better graft outcomes. Higher weight, living donor, and use of lymphocyte-depleting induction immune suppression resulted in lower death rates. Risk factors for kidney graft loss and patient death are listed in **Boxes 3** and **4**. An additional study has shown superior outcomes in HIV monoinfected patients compared with HIV-negative/HCV-positive or HIV/HCV coinfected patients.[32]

A different approach to data capture confirmed several of the previously mentioned factors but also noted HIV-positive transplant candidates spent more time on dialysis, a marker for less favorable outcome, and were less likely to remain on the waiting list.[33] Mortality was similar between HIV-positive and HIV-negative waiting list patients

Box 1
Demographics of HIV-positive and HIV-negative groups

	HIV-Positive (%)	HIV-Negative (%)
<50 y	61.4	41.2
Body mass index >30	18.1	33.3
Male	79.6	61
African American	71.0	26.5
HCV-positive	24.2	5.5
Maintenance steroids	75.1	66.1
Living donor	27.7	38.4
Antithymocyte globulin induction	27.8	42.6
Acute rejection	17.8	8.8

Data from Locke JE, Mehta S, Reed RD, et al. A national study of outcomes among HIV-infected kidney transplant recipients. J Am Soc Nephrol 2015;265:2222–9.

but the likelihood of receiving a transplant was lower for HIV-positive patients with the lowest rates occurring in minorities.

As experience accrued, outcomes have improved in more recent years, even outside of large sponsored trials.[34] Hepatitis C and AR continue to impact outcomes. Efforts to engage, successfully list HIV patients, and keep them listed must be enhanced. Thus, carefully selected patients and donors can lead to excellent outcomes for HIV-positive kidney transplantation candidates.

LIVER TRANSPLANTATION

Liver disease in HIV patients is related to HCV and HBV, substance abuse, predominantly alcohol and adverse drug events. HIV increases the rate of progression of liver disease to cirrhosis particularly in combination with HCV.[35] Presentation occurs at a younger age with significantly reduced survival after the first episode of decompensation.

Liver Transplantation in Human Immunodeficiency Virus/Hepatitis C Virus Coinfected Patients

Liver transplantation had encouraging results in the early cART era.[36] A small US series reported 94% 1-year survival but six episodes of AR (38%) and almost universal

Box 2
Graft and patient survival HIV with matched control subjects

	HIV Monoinfected (%)	HIV-Negative/HCV-Negative (%)
Male	79.1	63.5
Maintenance steroids	77.2	67.0
Acute rejection	17.4	10.3
Body mass index >30	17.1	37.5
Antithymocyte globulin induction	29.5	47.1
1-y graft/patient survival	93.3/96.1	95.3/96.9
3-y graft/patient survival	89.2/92.0	89.4/93.8
5-y graft/patient survival	85.1/88.7	84.9/89.1
10-y graft/patient survival	81.4/63.5	73.6/77.6

Data from Locke JE, Mehta S, Reed RD, et al. A national study of outcomes among HIV-infected kidney transplant recipients. J Am Soc Nephrol 2015;265:2222–9.

Box 3
Risk factors for kidney graft loss

Delayed graft function

HCV

Plasma reactive antibody >80

Acute rejection

Cold ischemia time >10 hours

Data from Locke JE, Mehta S, Reed RD, et al. A national study of outcomes among HIV-infected kidney transplant recipients. J Am Soc Nephrol 2015;265:2222–9.

---

recurrence of HCV after transplantation in HIV/HCV coinfected patients. A European cohort reported similar results with a numerically lower 1-year survival.[37]

The largest HIV liver transplant trial was the HIV-TR cohort with 125 HIV recipients including 89 HIV/HCV coinfected subjects.[38,39] Graft and survival rates were lower for HIV/HCV coinfected patients than HCV monoinfected patients. HIV/HCV coinfected patients had higher rates of rejection (1.6 times). Predictors of graft loss were HIV infection, older donor age, lower body mass index less than 21 kg/m^2, combined kidney-liver transplant, and an anti-HCV-positive donor. HIV infection was identified as the major factor in reduced graft and patient survival. However, excluding those with body mass index less than 21 kg/m^2, anti-HCV-positive donor and combined kidney-liver transplant, the resulting patient and graft survival were similar to those of the overall US liver transplant recipients. It was concluded that HIV/HCV coinfection was not a contraindication to transplantation but exclusion of several identified key factors in patient and donor selection could maximize outcomes.

A meta-analysis of European and US HIV liver transplantation in the cART era was performed to evaluate outcomes.[40] Survival at 1 and 5 years was 84.5% and 63.8% for HIV patients. HBV coinfected patients did well with optimal outcomes but HCV coinfected patients did less well. Near universal recurrence of HCV was noted again and HCV was a predictor of worse outcome. Survival was noted be to better for those with an undetectable HIV viral load at the time of transplantation.

A prospective Spanish study enrolled 84 HIV/HCV coinfected patients matched 1:3 to HCV monoinfected liver recipients. Five-year survival rates were 54% and 71%, respectively.[41] AR was high, 38% versus 20%. HIV was found to be an independent predictor of mortality. HCV recurrence resulted in 21% mortality at 1 year in HCV/HIV recipients compared with 12% mortality in HCV monoinfected patients. This

---

Box 4
Risk factors for death

HCV

Age >50 years

Diabetes mellitus

Hypertension

Data from Locke JE, Mehta S, Reed RD, et al. A national study of outcomes among HIV-infected kidney transplant recipients. J Am Soc Nephrol 2015;265:2222–9.

reinforces the finding of a more aggressive post-transplant course for HCV in HIV/HCV coinfected patients. HCV genotype 1 and higher donor risk index (DRI) were associated with increased mortality. Negative HCV RNA, before or after transplant, predicted better outcomes and lower mortality. Pretransplant variables of HCV genotype 1, pretransplant Model for End-State Liver Disease score of 15, and lower center experience were associated with negative outcome but when removed from analysis, the 5-year prognosis was similar to HCV monoinfected patients.

Risk factors for adverse outcomes in HIV/HCV liver transplantation have emerged from several major studies[38,41–43] and are compiled in **Box 5**.

HIV/HCV coinfected patients receive a low rate of early referral for transplant evaluation despite published guidelines and recommendations. A UK study revealed only 16.3% of appropriate patients were referred for transplant evaluation.[44] The reasons for low referral rates were not clear.

Human Immunodeficiency Virus/Hepatitis B Virus Coinfection

Results of HIV/HBV coinfected transplants have been excellent and comparable with HIV-negative patients.[45] Patient and graft survival were similar to HIV-uninfected recipients, although rejection rates were higher (22% vs 10%). HBV remained well controlled throughout follow-up but required ongoing antiviral medications for HBV and hepatitis B immunoglobulin to prevent relapse.

HEPATOCELLULAR CARCINOMA

HCC is an increasing cause of morbidity and mortality in HIV patients. They have a four-fold higher risk of developing HCC than the general population with a more aggressive course.[46–48] A multicenter cohort study revealed HIV/HCV coinfected patients with HCC were older, had more HBV infection, lower current CD4 counts, and cirrhosis, all potential markers for the condition.[49]

Medical treatments are available for HCC, but scant data exist for HIV patients. Liver transplantation is an option. A prospective Spanish study of matched 74 HIV and 222 non-HIV patients with HCC who received liver transplantation identified HCV and nodule diameter greater than 3 cm at explant as risk factors for mortality in both

Box 5
Risk factors decreased outcomes HIV/HCV liver transplantation
HIV
HCV genotype 1
Post-transplant recurrent HCV
Low body mass index <21 kg/m²
Combined kidney-liver transplant
Low-volume transplant center
Donor age >50 years
High donor risk index
HCV-positive donor
Donor diabetes mellitus
Pretransplant Model for End-Stage Liver Disease

groups.[50] Recurrence rates were similar, 16% and 14%, respectively, with only micro-vascular invasion seen on pathologic examination as a risk factor for recurrence. Survival at 1, 3, and 5 years was similar. HIV was not a risk factor for recurrence or mortality, thus transplantation should be considered for HIV patients with HCC.

Once a patient has been referred and evaluated, time is of the essence. Studies have demonstrated that survival is shorter for HIV patients on the waiting list.[51,52] HIV accelerates the course of HCV with more rapid progression of fibrotic cholestatic hepatitis to cirrhosis. A Spanish study reaffirms these data, particularly in the first year of listing, despite including a small number of HIV/HCV coinfected patients.[53,54] The 1-, 3-, 6-, and 12-month survival by intention-to-treat analysis for HCV monoinfected patients and HIV/HCV coinfected patients are shown in **Table 1**. Independent negative predictors for survival were HIV/HCV coinfection, United Network for Organ Sharing status 1, Model for End-Stage Liver Disease score of 15, and donor age greater than 70 years. Shorter time on the wait list was protective.

RETRANSPLANTATION

Retransplantation is a consideration for liver allograft failure. The most common reasons for it are vascular complications, primary graft nonfunction, or AR. A small early study demonstrated poor results of retransplantation in HIV patients leading some to not recommend it.[53] A recent international multicenter evaluation supports retransplantation but noted HCV replication at the time of retransplantation predicted a much worse outcome.[55] Thus retransplantation seems to be a reasonable option for those with HBV, undetectable HCV, or other causes but not someone with active HCV replication.

Multiple factors should be considered during referral, evaluation, and liver transplantation for HIV patients especially HIV/HCV coinfected patients. **Box 6** includes several considerations or recommendations based on a recent review[56] and additional information. This could be considered a checklist. The standard eligibility criteria are list in **Box 7**. Some items will be revised as more is learned about this population and the use of DAA to treat HCV.

Supply cannot meet demand for organ transplantation. The gap continues to widen for patients on the waiting list and suitable organs available while patients die as they lie in wait. Waiting lists often last 3 to 5 years or longer for transplantation.

Each year many organs have been discarded because of real or suspected HCV or HIV infection. To better use available donor organs, the University of Pennsylvania performed a pilot study transplanting HCV-positive kidneys into 10 HCV-negative

Table 1		
HIV wait list survival		
Months	**HIV-Negative/HCV-Positive Survival (%)**	**HIV/HCV Coinfected Survival (%)**
1	96	76
3	91	70
6	87	64
12	75	52

Data from Araiz JJ, Serrano MT, Garcia-Gil FA, et al. Intention-to-treat survival analysis of hepatitis C virus/human immunodeficiency virus coinfected liver transplant: is it the waiting list? Liver Transpl 2016;22:1186–96.

Box 6
Considerations for HIV liver transplantation in HIV/HCV coinfection

Refer at first episode of hepatic decompensation

Follow standard eligibility criteria

Avoid deceased donors >50 years of age

HCV donors should be avoided

Avoid candidates with body mass index <21 kg/m^2

Avoid combined liver-kidney transplant

Avoid low-volume transplant centers

Avoid transplant centers without organized multidisciplinary team

Monitor HCV recurrence closely with biopsy and elastography

Treat recurrent HCV early (moderate or severe hepatitis, progressive fibrosis)

Use direct-acting agents (and ribavirin)

Avoid interferon-based regimens

When possible treat existing HCV pretransplant

Avoid protease inhibitor–containing cART regimens if possible

Base cART regimen on patient needs favoring integrase inhibitor and NRTI-based therapy

Consider HCC patients based on Milan Criteria; consider Model for End-Stage Liver Disease exceptions

Retransplantation can be considered

---

recipients followed by treatment with DAA for HCV.[57] The results were excellent. All developed HCV viremia, and were treated and cured of HCV. Graft function was also excellent. This could provide a new avenue to better use donated organs while helping more patients, shortening the waiting list, and decreasing mortality while on the waiting list. Transplanting HCV-positive organs into HIV patients is problematic as already noted, resulting in worse outcomes. The new DAA could mitigate those issues.

Box 7
Eligibility criteria for HIV liver and kidney transplant candidates

CD4 >200 cells/mm^3 (kidney)

CD4 >100 cell/mm^3 (liver)

Undetectable HIV RNA (or perceived ability to control)

Stable cART regimen

No current opportunistic infection or malignancy

No history of chronic cryptosporidiosis, primary central nervous system lymphoma, or progressive multifocal leukoencephalopathy

No HCV-positive donor

BMI >21 kg/m^2

No need for combined liver and kidney transplant

HUMAN IMMUNODEFICIENCY VIRUS–POSITIVE DONOR TO HUMAN IMMUNODEFICIENCY VIRUS–POSITIVE RECIPIENT TRANSPLANTATION

A different approach was born out of necessity in South Africa, a resource poor area with limited access to dialysis for renal failure patients, particularly those with HIV. Dr. Elmi Muller boldly pioneered the first four HIV-positive to HIV-positive kidney transplants in 2008.[58] Outcomes for the initial cohort and a subsequent total cohort of 27 patients have been good. The 1-, 3-, and 5-year patient and graft survival and rejection rates are shown in **Table 2**. Antithymocyte globulin induction was used. Because of her efforts, HIV patients became eligible for dialysis and kidney transplantation from HIV-positive or HIV-negative donors.

This was not the first time HIV-positive to HIV-positive transplantation had been considered or proposed. In 2004, the state of Illinois passed a law allowing use of HIV-positive organs for transplantation. However, this state law was never enacted because of the supremacy of the 1984 Federal National Organ Transplant Act stating HIV-positive organs could not be used. In 2007, Switzerland amended the Swiss Federal Act on Transplantation allowing HIV-positive to HIV-positive transplantation. Thus far only one liver transplant was performed under this amendment, occurring in 2015.[59]

After the South African experience was announced, feasibility of HIV-positive to HIV-positive transplantation was researched in the United States. However, there were significant differences between the HIV-positive population of South Africa and the US HIV population to be considered. HIV drug resistance is low in South Africa, the donors were generally younger with a median age of 30, only one donor had been exposed to cART, and most were trauma victims. The recipient's median age was 41, they had not been on dialysis, 74% had HIVAN, and HIV was well controlled. In the United States, baseline cART HIV drug resistance is much higher, 15% to 19% depending on geographic location.[60] Many US patients have been exposed to more than one cART regimen and therefore have a greater risk to harbor or develop further drug resistance. Donors and recipients may have archived resistance resulting in loss of HIV control in the recipient. Furthermore, the size of the potential donor pool was unknown in the United States.

HUMAN IMMUNODEFICIENCY VIRUS–POSITIVE DONORS

A 2011 study provided insight and a crude conservative estimate of 500 to 600 potential HIV deceased donors annually.[61] These donors could provide greater than 1000 organs for transplantation. This would provide a direct benefit to HIV-positive patients and an indirect benefit to HIV-negative patients. This study lacked many demographic details on the donors.

Table 2
Patient and graft survival and rejection rates

	1 Year (%)	3 Years (%)	5 Years (%)
Patient survival	84	84	74
Graft survival	93	84	74
Rejection rates	8	22	Not available

Data from Muller E, Bardat Z, Mendelson M, et al. HIV-positive –to-HIV-positive kidney transplantation: results at 3 to 5 years. N Engl J Med 2015;372:613–20.

A single site study retrospectively reviewed six deceased HIV patients in detail as potential organ donors.[62] The information was used to extrapolate estimates of the potential US HIV-positive donor pool. Their analysis suggested lower numbers than the original estimate[61] with 356 HIV deceased donors yielding 192 kidneys and 247 livers per year. They also noted some DRIs that raised additional questions about the quality of donated kidneys.

To this pool of donors could be added a small number who have false-positive HIV tests at the time of screening evaluation for donation. These organs are traditionally discarded but could be used for HIV-positive patients. The estimate of false-positive testing is 0.1% to 0.85%.

The HIV Organ Policy Equity (HOPE) Act was introduced in 2013 to amend the 1984 National Organ Transplant Act. It proposed to allow kidney and liver transplants between HIV-positive donors and HIV-positive recipients as a clinical research protocol. It was signed into law November 2013 by President Barack Obama.[63]

ETHICS

Many issues and questions surfaced. Ethical considerations were debated over the primary concepts of beneficence (benefit, alleviate suffering, and potential cost involved) and nonmaleficence (use caution; cause no harm), efficacy, urgency, and equity.

HIV is a form of suffering that can lead to an increase in organ failure and subsequently results in disparity between need and access to relief through organ transplantation mostly because of the small donor pool. Allowing positive to positive transplantation would be an additional attempt to alleviate suffering, beyond standard HIV-negative to HIV-positive organ transplants. This could benefit the HIV-positive and HIV-negative populations and improve equity while improving the ongoing urgent need for donors.

Caution must be exercised in positive to positive transplants because of limited data sets available to offer guidance. This should be carefully explained to potential recipients with detailed informed consent. The HOPE Act[63] mandates the use of an independent recipient advocate to avoid intentional or unintentional improper influence in obtaining consent. This will ensure full disclosure and voluntary consent. The risks of immune suppression, organ rejection and graft failure, superinfection, and the psychological implications to the patient and partner should be included. The medical team should understand the risk of acquiring HIV through exposure during care of donors and recipients. Additional care needs to be taken to avoid inadvertent transplantation of an HIV-positive organ into an HIV-negative recipient. The privacy of the deceased donor should be carefully guarded and not violated but equity must be exercised by allowing these individuals the right to exercise their ability to be donors. This would provide opportunity to exercise personal autonomy, potentially reducing stigma and allowing more acceptance of those with HIV.[64,65]

Attitudes of HIV-positive patients toward donating or receiving an HIV-positive organ were evaluated in the United Kingdom.[66] The demographics of the study subjects were atypical of most Western European or North American HIV populations. Most were heterosexual (83%), black African (70%), and women (54%). Sixty-two percent offered to donate specific organs and 55% would accept HIV-positive organs. Thus, most favored the concept. Interestingly, the longer an individual was HIV infected, the less likely they would accept an HIV-positive organ. One possible explanation might be fear of acquiring a resistant virus.

SUPERINFECTION

HIV superinfection has been hypothesized for decades. The donated organ could contain a resistant strain of HIV because of existing baseline resistance of 15% to 19% in the United States. A CXCR4 tropic virus could be transplanted with the donor organ. This strain is typically associated with advanced disease that progresses more rapidly. If the donor had adequate detectable virus in the blood, a genotype could be performed to ascertain resistance mutations; however, it may require more time than is available for the deceased donor and harvest process. Thus far superinfection has not occurred; transmitted drug resistance has stabilized or declined in the United States; and resistance to integrase strand inhibitors, a newer and favored therapy, is low. Therefore, efficacy seems to be preserved.

PRIMARY DISEASE RECURRENCE

The possibility the original process could recur has been considered. This could lead to organ failure in the transplanted organ. Changes were noted in three renal biopsy specimens from the South African cohort with pathologic findings that could be interpreted as rejection or recurrent HIVAN.[67] A French group studied 19 HIV-positive kidney transplant patients (all received HIV-negative kidneys) and demonstrated HIV infection of podocytes or tubular epithelial cells in 68% of biopsy specimens even though all had undetectable viral loads in their blood.[68] The grafts with podocyte infection had nephrotic range proteinuria and more rapid declines in allograft function leading to the conclusion that HIV infection of the allograft leads to loss of kidney function. It was further postulated that HIV infection of cells within the allograft may stimulate an immune response that could be involved in higher rejection rates seen in this population. Other researchers suggested HIV inflammatory infiltrate may be misinterpreted as rejection.[69] The French group then developed a novel HIV DNA assay for urine samples that correlates with allograft infection. Thus, the kidney allograft may be a reservoir for HIV infection, although the mechanism by which these cells are infected is unclear because they lack the usual receptors for HIV infection.[70]

In addition to HIVAN possibly recurring in the kidney allograft[67,68,71] other HIV-associated renal disease could recur in a transplanted kidney. A case of immune complex glomerulonephritis has been reported.[72]

DRUG-DRUG INTERACTIONS

Combining cART treatment of HIV, its complications and immunosuppressive medications to prevent rejection in organ transplantation significantly increases the likelihood of DDI. The need to concurrently treat HCV may add an additional level of complexity depending on the regimens involved. PIs, some NNRTI, and the boosting agent cobicistat, used with several HIV medications, may be particularly troublesome. Most transplant teams include a pharmacist to review regimens and assist in managing the complex DDI. Integrase strand inhibitors in general lack interactions and have become the preferred agents in organ transplantation. In addition, they have a high barrier to drug resistance and have a low level of existing baseline drug resistance in the US HIV population.

Unresolved Questions in Human Immunodeficiency Virus–Positive to Human Immunodeficiency Virus–Positive Organ Transplantation

The quality of the donated organ is affected by donor age, underlying diseases, active or latent infections, cause of death, and ischemic time. All impact the ultimate outcome. The use of HIV-positive donors may result in higher risk organs that could lead to a less favorable outcomes. HIV patients are known to have higher rates of hypertension and chronic kidney and liver disease. They have higher rates of HCV and HBV. Antivirals used to treat HIV are associated with adverse effects on kidney and liver function. Sample DRI calculations[73] predictive of transplant outcomes, suggest HIV patients could be higher risk donors. Others believe the DRI is not fully applicable to the HIV population because of differences between HIV patients and the population on which the index was established. Similar concerns have been voiced on cardiac and bone risk calculators. Should these organs be considered increased risk?

Should a minimum CD4 count be required for donors? Would this lessen the risk of transmitted infections or malignancies? The risk of acquiring infections, particularly OI, and cancer has an inverse relationship with CD4 count. Should all cART-experienced donors be required to have an undetectable viral load to minimize the risk of transmitted drug resistance? If a patient has a detectable viral load while on therapy, the risk of drug resistance increases. Thoughtful review of current and past cART regimens and resistance tests of donor and recipient must occur to allow construction of the best regimen to treat HIV in the recipient.

In reality how will HIV-positive organ donation be received by potential HIV-positive recipients? A previously mentioned survey demonstrated reasonable acceptance but a subtotal embrace of the concept.[66] The additional levels of risk above standard transplantation require careful thought and counseling.

How should organ allocation occur to insure equity? Will standard listing and assignment apply? Will it be necessary to consider previous cART exposure in donor and recipient? How does one ensure access to complete donor information promptly to allow proper evaluation before accepting an organ?

Should HIV-positive patients provide living donations? The quality and risk of accepting the donated organ and the long-term safety of the donor must be considered. As noted, HIV patients are more likely to have hypertension, chronic kidney and liver disease, HBV, or HCV. Additional risks result from medications used, especially cART. Thus, a kidney donor could have a higher risk of kidney failure and eventual need for dialysis or kidney transplantation themselves. Opposition has been voiced to living donation with suggestions to use caution until more study can occur.

Routine insurance coverage for HIV organ transplantation did not occur until 2010. Will HIV-positive to HIV-positive transplantation be covered outside the research setting? Organ transplantation is a significant financial burden that cannot be borne by the providing centers without reimbursement.

FUTURE STUDY

Multiple areas of future study are listed in **Box 8**. Several are discussed next.

Rejection

AR has a multifactorial cause that includes HLA tissue matching, race, induction and maintenance immune suppression, type of immune suppression, viral infections, and consistency of immune suppression.

Early efforts in HIV organ transplantation were plagued by high levels of rejection. Induction immune suppression was often omitted because of concern of "excessive" immune suppression and an increased risk of infection to the recipient. This contributed to higher rates of rejection and DGF. A small multicenter study in Spain pointed to HIV itself as an additional cause for increased rates of DGF.[74] More recent studies support induction with antithymocyte globulin or interleuin-2 receptor blockers, which

Box 8
Areas for research
Optimal induction regimen
Best maintenance immunosuppression regimen
Ideal cART regimen
Improved understanding of HIV immune dysregulation and HIV-induced immune suppression
Approaches to decrease acute organ rejection
Study recurrent disease of allograft; mechanism and impact
Study HIV infection of allograft; mechanism, impact on graft
Impact of DAA on HCV; outcome for HIV allografts
Evaluate survival benefit of HIV-positive to HIV-positive organ transplantation
Study transplant complications in HIV: hypertension, diabetes mellitus, hyperlipidemia, cardiovascular disease, bone mineral density, malignancy, human papilloma virus, obesity
Impact of immunosuppressive medications on HIV reservoir

demonstrated lower rates of AR and DGF with less graft loss and no increased risk of infections.[75,76]

HIV stimulates immune activation and resultant immune dysregulation, which could play a role in AR. Even with prolonged HIV suppression and control, immune activation markers remain elevated, although significantly lower. A US group hypothesized that longer duration of HIV control could lead to lower rates of rejection in HIV transplantation.[77] Data supporting their view correlating lower rejection rates with longer duration of HIV suppression were demonstrated but higher overall rates of rejection were noted. They did not study activation markers or the HIV reservoir. Could a smaller HIV reservoir result in less activation thus explaining their result? Contrary to other studies, a UK study suggested HIV was not associated with graft rejection after adjusting for ethnicity and HLA mismatch.[78] Additional studies may resolve these questions.

Immunosuppressive Medications

Several immunosuppressive medications used in transplant care possess HIV antiretroviral and other properties. Sirolimus, mycophenylate mofetil, and cyclosporine have some degree of antiretroviral activity and could play a role as disease-modifying agents. Sirolimus has antiproliferative properties and salutary effects on Kaposi sarcoma, an HIV-associated malignancy and an uncommon malignancy in transplantation.[79] Sirolimus may provide a protective or therapeutic benefit.

The optimal maintenance immunosuppressive regimen has not been developed at this time. Tacrolimus has gained widespread use; however, it does not provide any direct antiviral activity similar to sirolimus, cyclosporine, or mycophenylate. Tacrolimus has been shown to have better outcomes based on lower rejection rates,[29,75] whereas sirolimus had a 2.2-fold increased risk of rejection.

Drug-Drug Interactions and Highly Active Antiretroviral Therapy

CNIs (tacrolimus and cyclosporine) are metabolized through the CYP3A4 hepatic enzyme system and interact with several antiretroviral medications. PI with ritonavir or cobicistat have a profound inhibitory effect on CYP3A4 and p-glycoprotein transporters. NNRTI are inducers of hepatic metabolism. Although early concerns existed about DDI causing inconsistent levels of CNI by interacting with PI causing elevated rates of rejection, this has not been demonstrated. PI have been linked to reduced graft and patient survival, not related to AR or serious non-OI but by other unclear mechanisms.[80,81] Integrase strand inhibitors (dolutegravir and raltegravir) seem to be better choices for cART regimens because of a lack of CYP3A4 interaction and are preferred by many centers. They can be dosed once daily and are well tolerated by patients. P-glycoprotein may be involved with raltegravir transport and metabolism and may interact with CNI, thus influencing drug levels of raltegravir.[82] Therapeutic drug monitoring evaluation may need to be considered to avoid toxic or subtherapeutic levels.

The NRTI class has evolved to the use of tenofovir, tenofovir alfenamide, emtricitibine or lamivudine, and abacavir. Tenofovir is known for its potency and durability but has adverse renal and bone effects, whereas the new formulation, alfenamide, seems to have significantly less effect on kidneys and bone mineral density.[83] Both are associated with high barriers to HIV drug resistance. Abacavir has a known genetic association with a hypersensitivity reaction[84] that is predicted by testing for the HLA-B5701 marker.[85] Abacavir has also been linked to adverse cardiac events in some studies but not others.[86] Emtricitibine and lamivudine are generally well tolerated. All NRTIs require some degree of renal dose adjusting except abacavir.[87] Maraviroc, a CCR5 receptor inhibitor, is occasionally used if the patient harbors a CCR5 tropic virus. CCR5 blockade may also be beneficial in preventing organ rejection.[88]

Malignancies

All transplant patients are at increased risk of developing several malignancies. HIV transplantation patients have an additional risk because of their underlying disease with chronic immune dysregulation.[89] Viral-associated malignancies caused by Epstein-Barr virus, human herpesvirus 8, and possibly human papilloma virus are of particular concern. Some transplant-associated cancers are mitigated by reduction of immune suppression. Similar declines are noted in HIV patients as their CD4 counts rise during successful cART therapy. This does not seem to apply to human papilloma virus–associated cancer where the risk does not decline significantly after discontinuation of immune suppression or improvement in CD4 counts. Human papilloma virus is not routinely evaluated or aggressively pursued in transplant patients. This may be an area of future clinical focus and study. Late transplant non-Hodgkin lymphoma is more likely to be Epstein-Barr virus–related and extranodal, often occurring at the site of transplantation.[90] Will transplanting HIV-positive organs into HIV-positive patients increase this risk?

The pretransplant and post-transplant evaluation and care of HIV patients is the same as non-HIV patients.[91] OI prophylaxis should be used liberally. The difficult decision may be to determine when it is safe to stop prophylaxis.

Human Immunodeficiency Virus–Positive to Positive Transplant Research

After passage of the HOPE Act, the NIH and the Department of Health and Human Services published specific criteria and guidance to be followed for HIV-positive to HIV-positive organ transplants.[92] The general inclusion and exclusion criteria are similar to what has been previously followed for HIV-negative organ transplantation into HIV-positive recipients. Living organ donation is not specifically addressed and remains a topic of ongoing debate. Independent advocates will be used for each transplant candidate to ensure understanding of risks and benefits while obtaining impartial consent.

The Organ Procurement and Transplantation Network was directed to revise standards for the acquisition and transportation of HIV-positive organs. Particular attention was directed to avoid inadvertent transplantation of HIV-positive organs into HIV-negative recipients. These standards were completed and published in November of 2015.[93]

A pilot protocol was developed, opened in January 2016 and administrated through Johns Hopkins University.[94] The intent of the pilot is to demonstrate the feasibility and safety of this approach leading to the opening of a much larger trial. The first HIV-to-HIV kidney and liver transplants were performed at Johns Hopkins in March 2016 under an ongoing multicenter pilot trial (ClinicalTrials.gov, NCT02602262).[95,96] An NIH-funded trial of HIV-to-HIV deceased donor kidney transplantation launched at 19 transplant centers in January 2018 and a trial of HIV-to-HIV deceased donor liver transplantation is expected in the near future.

SUMMARY

HIV has evolved through dramatic advancement and understanding from the early years of despair and death to hope and near normal lifespan. The early attempts at HIV organ transplantation produced poor results but now with more understanding of HIV, cART, and transplantation, results have dramatically improved. HCV and AR rates continue to be problematic confounders. HIV-positive to HIV-positive organ transplantation, although controversial, seems feasible in properly selected patients and requires ongoing research. It is an approach that may help alleviate widespread organ shortage. This is not an option for all and not likely to be accepted by all. Currently the benefits seem to outweigh the risks. Although this ground-breaking work has been clinically and intellectually exciting, many aspects are still poorly understood and in need of further careful thought and research.

REFERENCES

1. Available at: http://optn.transplant.hrsa.gov/. Accessed February 4, 2018.
2. Fine DM, Perazella MA, Lucas GM, et al. Renal disease in patient with HIV infection. Drugs 2008;68:963–80.
3. Kalayjian RC, Lau B, Mechekano RN, et al. Risk factors for chronic kidney disease in a large cohort of HIV-1 infected individuals initiating antiretroviral therapy in routine care. AIDS 2012;26:1907–15.
4. Rubin RH, Jenkins RL, Shaw BW, et al. The acquired immunodeficiency syndrome and transplantation. Transplantation 1987;44:1–4.
5. Rubin RH, Tokoff-Rubin NE. The problem of human immunodeficiency virus (HIV) infection and transplantation. Transpl Int 1988;1:36–42.
6. Boyd AS. Organ transplantation in HIV positive patients. N Engl J Med 1990; 323(21):1492–3.
7. Centers for Disease Control (CDC). Human immunodeficiency virus infection transmitted from an organ donor screened for HIV antibody-North Carolina. MMWR Morb Mortal Wkly Rep 1987;36:306–8.
8. Feduska NJ, Perkins HA, Melzer J, et al. Observations relating to the incidence of AIDS and other possibly associated conditions in a large population of renal transplant recipients. Transplant Proc 1987;19:2161–6.
9. Kumar P, Pearson JE, Martin DH, et al. Transmission of human immunodeficiency virus by transplantation of a renal allograft with development of the acquired immunodeficiency syndrome. Ann Intern Med 1987;106:244–5.

10. L'Age-Stehr J, Schwarz A, Offermann G, et al. HTLV-III infection in kidney transplant recipients. Lancet 1985;2:1361–2.
11. Margreiter R, Fuchs D, Hansen A, et al. HIV infection in renal allograft recipients. Lancet 1986;2:398.
12. Milgrom M, Esquenazi V, Fuller L, et al. Acquired immunodeficiency syndrome in a transplant patient. Transplant Proc 1985;17(Suppl 2):75–6.
13. Erice A, Rhame FS, Heussner RC, et al. Human immunodeficiency virus infection in patients with solid-organ transplants: report of five cases and review. Rev Infect Dis 1991;13:537–47.
14. Ahuja TS, Zingman B, Glicklich D. Long-term survival in an HIV-infected renal transplant recipient. Am J Nephrol 1997;17:480–2.
15. Antiretroviral therapy cohort collaboration. Life expectancy of individuals on combination antiretroviral therapy in high: income countries; a collaborative analysis of 14 cohort studies. Lancet 2008;372:293–9.
16. Halpern SC, Ubel PA, Caplan AL. Solid-organ transplantation in HIV infected patients. N Engl J Med 2002;347:284–7.
17. Abraham AG, Althoff KN, Yuezhou J, et al. End-stage renal disease among HIV-infected adults in North America. Clin Infect Dis 2015;60(6):941–9.
18. Wright AJ, Gill JS. Kidney transplantation in HIV-infected recipients: encouraging outcomes, but registry data are no longer enough. J Am Soc Nephrol 2015;26: 2070–1.
19. Lucas GM, Eustace JA, Socio S, et al. Highly active antiretroviral therapy and the incidence of HI-1-associated nephropathy: a 12-year cohort study. AIDS 2004;18: 541–6.
20. Trullos J, Cofan F, Barril G, et al. Outcome and prognostic factors in HIV-1-infected patients on dialysis in the cART era: a GESIDA/SEN cohort study. J Acquir Immune Defic Syndr 2011;57:276–83.
21. Bickel M, Marben W, Betz C, et al. ESRD and dialysis in HIV-positive patients: observations from a long-term cohort study with a follow up of 22 years. HIV Med 2013;14:127–35.
22. Wyatt CM. The kidney in HIV infection: beyond HIV-associated nephropathy. Top Antivir Med 2012;20:106–10.
23. Oniscu GC, Brown H, Forsythe JL. How great is the survival advantage of transplantation over dialysis in elderly patients? Nephrol Dial Transplant 2004;19: 945–51.
24. Reese PP, Shults J, Bloom RD, et al. Functional status, time to transplantation, and survival benefit of kidney transplantation among wait-listed candidates. Am J Kidney Dis 2015;66:837–45.
25. Lloveras J, Arcos E, Comas J, et al. A paired survival analysis comparing hemodialysis and kidney transplantation from deceased elderly donors older than 65 years. Transplantation 2015;99:991–6.
26. Wolfe RA, Ashby VB, Milford EL, et al. Comparison of mortality in all patients on dialysis, patients on dialysis awaiting transplantation, and recipients of a first cadaveric transplant. N Engl J Med 1999;341:1725–30.
27. Locke JE, Gustafson MD, Mehta S, et al. Survival benefit of kidney transplantation in HIV-infected patients. Ann Surg 2017;265(3):604–8.
28. Sawinski D, Wyatt CM, Casagrande L, et al. Factors associated with failure to list HIV positive kidney transplant candidates. Am J Transplant 2009;9:1467–71.
29. Stock PG, Barin B, Murphy B, et al. Outcomes of kidney transplantation in HIV infected recipients. N Engl J Med 2010;363:2004–14.

30. Touzot M, Pillebout E, Matignon M, et al. Renal transplantation in HIV-infected patients: the Paris experience. Am J Transplant 2010;10:2263–9.
31. Locke JE, Mehta S, Reed RD, et al. A national study of outcomes among HIV-infected kidney transplant recipients. J Am Soc Nephrol 2015;265:2222–9.
32. Sawinski D, Forde KA, Eddinger K, et al. Superior outcomes in HIV-positive kidney transplant patients compared with HCV-infected or HIV/HCV-coinfected recipients. Kidney Int 2015;88:341–9.
33. Locke JE, Mehta S, Sawinski D, et al. Access to kidney transplantation among HIV-infected waitlist candidates. Clin J Am Soc Nephrol 2017;12:467–75.
34. Locke JE, Reed RD, Mehta SG, et al. Center-level experience and kidney transplant outcomes in HIV-infected recipients. Am J Transplant 2015;15:2096–104.
35. Hernandez MD, Sherman KE. HIV/hepatitis C coinfection natural history and disease progression. Curr Opin HIV AIDS 2011;6:478–82.
36. Neff GW, Bonham A, Tzakis AG, et al. Orthotopic liver transplantation in patients with human immunodeficiency virus and end-stage liver disease. Liver Transpl 2003;9:239–47.
37. Norris S, Taylor C, Muiesan P, et al. Outcome of liver transplantation in HIV-infected individuals: the impact of HCV and HBV infection. Liver Transpl 2004; 10:1271–8.
38. Terrault NA, Roland ME, Schiano T, et al. Outcomes of liver transplant recipients with hepatitis C and HIV coinfection. Liver Transpl 2012;18:716–26.
39. Roland ME, Barin B, Huprikar S, et al. Survival in HIV-positive transplant recipients compared with transplant candidates and with HIV-negative controls. AIDS 2016;30:435–44.
40. Cooper C, Kanters S, Klein M, et al. Liver transplant outcomes in HIV-infected patients: a systemic review and meta-analysis with synthetic cohort. AIDS 2011;25: 777–86.
41. Miro JM, Montegjo M, Castells L, et al. Outcome of HCV/HIV-coinfected liver transplant recipients: a prospective and multicenter study. Am J Transplant 2012;12:1866–76.
42. Duclos-Valle JC, Feray C, Sevagh M, et al. Survival and recurrence of hepatitis C after liver transplantation in patients coinfected with human immunodeficiency virus and hepatitis C virus. Hepatology 2008;47:407–17.
43. Campos-Varela I, Dodge JL, Stock PG, et al. Key donor factors associated with graft loss among liver transplant recipients with human immunodeficiency virus. Clin Transplant 2016;30:1140–5.
44. Warren-Gash C, Childs K, Thornton A, et al. Cirrhosis and liver transplantation in patients co-infected with HIV and hepatitis B or C: an observational cohort study. Infection 2017;45:215–20.
45. Coffin CS, Stock PG, Dove LM, et al. Virologic and clinical outcomes of hepatitis B virus infection in HIV-HBV coinfected transplant recipients. Am J Transplant 2010; 10:1268–75.
46. Merchane N, Marino E, Lopez-Aldeguer J, et al. Increase incidence of hepatocellular carcinoma in HIV-infected patients in Spain. Clin Infect Dis 2013;56:143–50.
47. Sahasrabudde VU, Shiels MS, McGlynn KA, et al. The risk of hepatocellular carcinoma among individuals with acquired immunodeficiency syndrome in the US. Cancer 2012;118:6226–33.
48. Puoti M, Rossotti R, Garlaschelli A, et al. Hepatocellular carcinoma in HIV hepatitis C virus. Curr Opin HIV AIDS 2011;6:534–8.
49. Gjarerde LI, Sheperd L, Jablonowska E, et al. Trends in incidence and risk factors for hepatocellular carcinoma and other liver events in HIV and hepatitis C virus

coinfected individuals from 2001 to 2014: a multi cohort study. Clin Infect Dis 2016;63:821–9.

50. Aguero F, Forner A, Manzardo C, et al. Human immunodeficiency virus infection does not worsen prognosis of liver transplantation for hepatocellular carcinoma. Hepatology 2016;63:488–98.

51. Ragni MV, Eghtesad B, Schlesinger KW, et al. Pretransplant survival is shorter in HIV-positive than HIV-negative subjects with end-stage liver disease. Liver Transpl 2005;11:1425–30.

52. Pineda JA, Romero-Gomez M, Diaz-Garcia F, et al. HIV coinfection shortens the survival of patients with hepatitis C virus-related decompensated cirrhosis. Hepatology 2005;41:779–89.

53. Araiz JJ, Serrano MT, Garcia-Gil FA, et al. Intention-to-treat survival analysis of hepatitis C virus/human immunodeficiency virus coinfected liver transplant: is it the waiting list? Liver Transpl 2016;22:1186–96.

54. Gastaca M, Valdivieso A, Montejo M, et al. Is antithrombotic prophylaxis required after liver transplantation in HIV-infected recipients? Am J Transplant 2012;12:2258.

55. Aguero F, Rimola A, Stock P, et al. Liver retransplantation in patients with HIV-1 infection: an international multicenter cohort study. Am J Transplant 2016;16:679–87.

56. Miro JM, Stock P, Teicher E, et al. Outcome and management of HCV/HIV coinfection pre- and post-liver transplantation. A 2015 update. J Hepatol 2015;62:701–11.

57. Goldberg DS, At PL, Blumberg EA, et al. Trial of transplantation of HCV-infected kidneys in uninfected recipients. N Engl J Med 2017;376:2394–5.

58. Muller E, Bardat Z, Mendelson M, et al. HIV-positive –to-HIV-positive kidney transplantation: results at 3 to 5 years. N Engl J Med 2015;372:613–20.

59. Calmy A, van Delden C, Giostra E, et al. HIV-positive –to-positive liver transplantation. Am J Transplant 2016;16:2473–8.

60. Kim K, Ziebell R, Saduvala N. Trend in transmitted HIV-1 drug resistance-associated mutation: 10 HIV surveillance areas, US, 2007-2010. 20th Conference on Retroviruses and Opportunistic Infections (CROI). Atlanta, GA, March 3–6, 2013. [abstract: 149].

61. Boyarsk BJ, Hall EC, Singer AL, et al. Establishing the pool of HIV-infected deceased donors in the US. Am J Transplant 2011;11:1209–17.

62. Richterman A, Sawinski D, Reese PP, et al. An assessment of HIV-infected patients dying in care for deceased organ donation in a United States urban center. Am J Transplant 2015;15:2105–16.

63. Health Resources and Services Administration (HRSA), Department of Health and Human Services (HHS). Organ procurement and transplantation: implementation of the HIV Organ Policy Equity Act. Final rule. Fed Regist 2015;80(89):26464. February 4, 2018.

64. Mgbako O, Glazier A, Blumberg E, et al. Allowing HIV-positive organ donation: ethical, legal and operational considerations. Am J Transplant 2013;13:1636–42.

65. Durand CM, Segev D, Sugarman J, et al. The ethics of organ transplantation from HIV infected donors. Ann Intern Med 2016;165(2):138–42.

66. Taha H, Newby K, Das A, et al. Attitude of patients with HIV infection towards organ transplant between HIV patients. A cross-sectional questionnaire survey. Int J STD AIDS 2016;27(1):13–8.

67. Canaud G, Avettand-Fenoel V, Legendre C. HIV-positive-to-HIV-positive kidney transplantation. N Engl J Med 2015;372:21.

68. Canaud G, Dejucq-Rainsford N, Avettand-Fenoel V, et al. The kidney as a reservoir for HIV-1 after renal transplantation. J Am Soc Nephrol 2014;25:407–19.

69. Stock PG. Kidney infection with HIV-1 following kidney transplantation. J Am Soc Nephrol 2014;25:212–5.

70. Avettand-Fenoel V, Rouzioux C, Legendre C, et al. Infection in the native and allograph kidney: implications for management, diagnosis and transplantation. Transplantation 2017;101:2003–8.

71. Anil Kumar MS, Sierka DR, Damask AM, et al. Safety and success of kidney transplantation and concomitant immunosuppression in HIV-positive patients. Kidney Int 2005;67:1622–9.

72. Chandran S, Jen K, Laszik ZG. Recurrent HIV-associated immune complex glomerulonephritis with lupus-like features after kidney transplantation. Am J Kidney Dis 2013;62(2):335–8.

73. Feng S, Goodrich NP, Bragg-Gresham JL, et al. Characteristics associated with liver graft failure: the concept of a donor risk index. Am J Transplant 2006;6:783–90.

74. Mazuecos A, Fernandez A, Zarraga S, et al. High incidence of delayed graft function in HIV-infected kidney transplant recipients. Transpl Int 2013;26:893–902.

75. Locke JE, James NT, Mannon RB, et al. Immunosuppression regimen and the risk of acute rejection in HIV-infected kidney transplant recipients. Transplantation 2014;97(4):446–50.

76. Kucirka LM, Durand CM, Bae S, et al. Induction immunosuppression and clinical outcomes in kidney transplant recipients infected with human immunodeficiency virus. Am J Transplant 2016;16:2368–76.

77. Husson J, Stafford K, Bromberg J, et al. Association between duration of human immunodeficiency virus (HIV)-1 suppression prior to renal transplantation and acute cellular rejection. Am J Transplant 2017;17:551–6.

78. Gathogo EN, Shah S, Post FA. Kidney transplant outcomes in HIV serodiscordant recipient pairs. AIDS 2017;31(8):1199–201.

79. Stock PG, Barin B, Hatano H, et al. Reduction of HIV persistence following transplantation in HIV-infected kidney transplant recipients. Am J Transplant 2014;14:1136–41.

80. Rosa R, Suarez JF, Lorio MA, et al. Impact of antiretroviral therapy on clinical outcomes in HIV+ kidney transplant recipients: review of 58 cases. F1000 Res 2016;5:2893.

81. Sawinski D, Shelton BA, Mehta S, et al. Impact of protease inhibitor-based antiretroviral therapy on outcomes for HIV+ kidney transplant recipients. Am J Transplant 2017;17:3114–22.

82. Cottaneo D, Puoti M, Sollima S, et al. Reduced raltegravir clearance in HIV-infected liver transplant recipients: an unexpected interaction with immunosuppressive therapy? J Antimicrob Chemother 2016;71:1341–5.

83. Cohen SD, Kopp JB, Kimmel JL. Kidney diseases associated with human immunodeficiency virus infection. N Engl J Med 2017;377:2363–74.

84. Symonds W, Cutrell A, Edwards M, et al. Risk factor analysis of hypersensitivity reactions to abacavir. Clin Ther 2002;24(2):565–73.

85. Martin AM, Nolan D, Gaudieri S, et al. Predisposition to abacavir hypersensitivity conferred by HLA-B*5701 and a haplotypic Hsp70-Hom variant. Proc Natl Acad Sci U S A 2004;101(12):4180–5.

86. Nadel J, Holloway CJ. Screening and risk assessment for coronary artery disease in HIV infection: an unmet need. HIV Med 2017;18:292–9.

87. Available at: https://aidsinfo.nih.gov/guidelines/html/1/adult-and-adolescent-arv-guidelines/44/arv-dosing-for-renal-or-hepatic-insufficiency. Accessed February 4, 2018.

88. Fishereder M, Luckow B, Hocher B, et al. CC chemokine receptor 5 and renal-transplant survival. Lancet 2001;357:1758–61.

89. Grulich AE, Vajdic CM. The epidemiology of cancers in human immunodeficiency virus infection and after organ transplantation. Semin Oncol 2015;42(2):247–57.

90. Gibson TM, Engels EA, Clarke CA, et al. Risk of diffuse large B-cell lymphoma after solid organ transplantation in the United States. Am J Hematol 2014; 89(7):714–20.

91. Miro JM, Aguero F, Duclos-Vallee JC, et al. Infections in solid organ transplant HIV-infected patients. Clin Microbiol Infect 2014;20(suppl7):119–30.

92. Final Human Immunodeficiency Virus (HIV) Organ Policy Equity (HOPE) Act Safeguards and Research Criteria for Transplantation of Organs Infected With HIV. Fed Regist 2015;80(227):73785–96. February 4, 2018.

93. Available at: https://www.federalregister.gov/documents/2015/05/08/2015-11048/organ-procurement-and-transplantation-implementation-of-the-hiv-organ-policy-equity-act. Accessed February 4, 2018.

94. Pilot Protocol HIV + organ transplantation into HIV positive recipients. Clinicaltrials.govNCT02602262. Available at: https://clinicaltrials.gov/ct2/results?cond=&term=NCT02602262&cntry=&state=&city=&dist=. Accessed February 4, 2018.

95. Malani P. HIV and transplantation: new reasons for HOPE. JAMA 2016;316(2): 136–8.

96. Available at: https://www.hopkinsmedicine.org/transplant/news_events/hiv-positive-to-hiv-positive-transplants.html. Accessed February 4, 2018.

Management of Viral Hepatitis in Solid Organ Transplant Recipients

Elizabeth Buganza-Torio, MD[a],
Karen Elizabeth Doucette, MD, MSc[b],*

KEYWORDS

- Hepatitis B virus • Hepatitis C virus • Hepatitis E virus • Liver transplantation
- Kidney transplantation • Thoracic transplantation

KEY POINTS

- Hepatitis B virus (HBV) has declined as an indication for liver transplant in North America, but remains a common indication in Asia. Outcomes following transplant are now excellent in liver and nonliver recipients with chronic HBV infection with modern management strategies including potent antiviral therapy with or without hepatitis B immunoglobulin tailored to patient risk.
- Hepatitis C virus (HCV) remains a leading indication for liver transplant globally. However, direct-acting antiviral therapy can now cure virtually all liver and nonliver transplant candidates and recipients with excellent short-term results, although the optimal timing of therapy remains controversial.
- The use of organs from donors who are either hepatitis B surface antigen or HCV RNA positive has been increasingly described in case series and with modern antiviral therapy seems to be safe in selected cases, although the optimal use of such donors remains to be evaluated.
- Chronic hepatitis E virus infection is an emerging cause of chronic hepatitis and cirrhosis in immunocompromised hosts in the developed world. A high clinical suspicion is needed to make this diagnosis because signs and symptoms may be minimal and serology negative in up to 20%.

Disclosures: E. Buganza-Torio has nothing to disclose. K.E. Doucette has received research support and educational grants from Gilead Sciences, Merck Canada, AbbVie Canada, Astellas, and GSK in addition to speaking honoraria from Gilead and Merck Canada.
[a] Division of Gastroenterology, University of Alberta, 11350 83 Avenue, Edmonton, Alberta T6G2G3, Canada; [b] Division of Infectious Diseases, University of Alberta, 11350 83 Avenue, Edmonton, Alberta T6G2G3, Canada
* Corresponding author. Division of Infectious Diseases, Department of Medicine, University of Alberta, 11350 83 Avenue, Clinical Sciences Building 1-139, Edmonton, Alberta T6G 2G3, Canada.
E-mail address: karen.doucette@ualberta.ca

Infect Dis Clin N Am 32 (2018) 635–650
https://doi.org/10.1016/j.idc.2018.04.010
0891-5520/18/© 2018 Elsevier Inc. All rights reserved.

id.theclinics.com

INTRODUCTION

In recent years, strategies for the prevention and treatment of hepatitis B virus (HBV) and hepatitis C virus (HCV) in organ transplant candidates and recipients have evolved rapidly. Although these viral infections no longer threaten transplant outcomes, in either hepatic or nonhepatic transplantation, they continue to be a focus of research. Strategies are needed to optimize cost-effective management that improve survival and quality of life because viral hepatitis remains a leading cause of death globally from liver failure and hepatocellular carcinoma (HCC). Remaining controversies include the ideal timing of HCV antiviral therapy and the use of HCV viremic donors in hepatic and nonhepatic transplantation. Hepatitis E virus (HEV) is an emerging pathogen in organ transplantation, now recognized to be a cause of chronic hepatitis post-transplantation with a significant risk of progression to cirrhosis. This article reviews the current management of HBV, HCV, and HEV in organ transplantation, highlighting remaining priorities for research.

HEPATITIS B VIRUS
Liver Transplant

In 2015, an estimated 257 million people were living with chronic hepatitis B infection globally.[1] Despite a highly effective vaccine and potent antiviral medications for treatment, the global attributable mortality because of HBV increased between 1990 and 2013[2] with most deaths attributable to HCC, followed by liver failure. In the United States, and other Western countries, however, HBV-related liver disease has become an uncommon indication for liver transplant (LT), although it remains a common indication in Asian countries.[3,4] Before the introduction of hepatitis B immunoglobulin (HBIg) and the development of potent nucleos(t)ide analogues (NA) used to prevent HBV recurrence in the graft, early graft loss and mortality were common, but outcomes now for this indication are among the best.[5] Although early data with the use of lamivudine or adefovir in combination with HBIg demonstrated improved early outcomes and lower risk of HBV recurrence, potent NAs with a high barrier to resistance (entecavir [ETV], tenofovir disoproxil fumarate [TDF], or tenofovir alafenamide fumarate [TAF]) are now preferred.

The risk of recurrent HBV after LT is related to the HBV DNA load at the time of transplantation[6] and thus all patients on the LT waiting list with HBV-related liver disease should be treated with a potent NA and a goal of achieving an undetectable HBV DNA. After LT, all patients should receive the combination of HBIg and a potent NA, which reduces the risk of HBV recurrence to less than 5%.[7,8] The NA therapy should continue indefinitely in all; however, in those at low risk for recurrence, HBIg discontinuation is considered, generally after a minimum of 1 to 3 months, although in select patients, potent NA therapy alone, without HBIg has been shown to effectively prevent recurrence.[9,10] Conversely, in those with risk factors for recurrent HBV, including those with detectable HBV DNA at the time of transplant, those with HCC, and those with coinfection with human immunodeficiency virus or hepatitis delta virus, combination HBIg and potent NA therapy should continue indefinitely.

In addition to the potency of NAs, renal function and prior antiviral exposure should be considered in choosing the preferred agent. In those with renal dysfunction, ETV or TAF is preferred. In those with prior lamivudine exposure, TDF or TAF are preferred.[11] Although the risk of recurrence is low with prophylaxis, monitoring is recommended to pick up recurrent disease early and limit the impact on long-term outcomes. HBV recurrence is defined as the reappearance of hepatitis B surface antigen (HBsAg) after LT and quantifiable levels of DNA, although patients on antiviral prophylaxis may develop HBsAg positivity without detectable DNA, or abnormal biochemistry and histology.[7] The monitoring protocol for HBV recurrence varies among centers, but HBsAg and HBV DNA every 3 months for the first year and every 6 months thereafter is suggested.[12]

The use of liver donors with prior HBV infection, as demonstrated by a negative HBsAg but positive anti–hepatitis B core antibody (anti-HBc), with or without anti–hepatitis B surface antibody (anti-HBs), has been shown to be safe with appropriate prophylaxis in the recipient and is generally accepted as a way to increase the donor pool without compromising outcomes.[7,13] Despite this, there continues to be significant center-to-center variability in the use of anti-HBc-positive liver donors.[14] Recipients of a liver from a donor with past HBV infection (anti-HBc-positive) should receive NA therapy to prevent HBV recurrence, which otherwise occurs in 50% to 80% of cases. Data support the use of lamivudine monotherapy in this setting with a low risk of recurrence of less than 3% and no additional benefit of HBIg.[13,15] Some centers, however, prefer to use potent NA therapy. Most centers also continue NA therapy indefinitely, although in low-risk recipients with prior HBV infection themselves and natural immunity (positive anti-HBc and anti-HBs) NA discontinuation is considered.[13]

There are less data regarding the use of HBsAg-positive donors; however, several case series suggest this is a safe option to expand the donor pool.[13,16] If being considered, donor liver biopsy is required to exclude significant hepatic fibrosis. In most cases, HBsAg-positive liver grafts have been used preferentially for HBsAg-positive recipients and under prophylaxis with HBIg and NA therapy.[16,17] Although recurrence or persistence of HBsAg is common in these cases, reported graft function and survival is excellent. The exception is in hepatitis delta virus coinfected recipients where the use of HBsAg-positive liver grafts should be avoided because of early hepatitis delta virus reinfection and severe liver disease.[18,19]

Nonliver Transplant

The prevalence of HBV in patients with end-stage renal, heart, and lung disease is generally similar to that of the general population of the region. Although response rates are poor, approximating 50%, all nonimmune transplant candidates should be vaccinated against hepatitis B using a high-dose preparation.[20]

Historically, HBsAg-positive kidney transplant recipients had markedly reduced graft and overall survival primarily because of accelerated progression of liver disease.[21] However, with NA therapy, particularly potent agents, such as ETV and TDF,[22,23] outcomes have improved dramatically with survival rates similar to HBsAg-negative recipients.[24,25] As a result, the use of HBIg has been abandoned in this population in most programs.[12,26]

Pretransplant assessment of patients with HBV should be done by a specialist to determine the staging of hepatic fibrosis and need for therapy. In the past staging was done using liver biopsy; however, several noninvasive methods are now validated, including transient elastography, magnetic resonance elastography, shear-wave elastography, and serologic panels. Each one has advantages and disadvantages, although all give comparable classification to liver biopsy, particularly to exclude cirrhosis.[27] Any patients meeting standard criteria for HBV therapy in the general population should be initiated on treatment.[11] HCC surveillance should also be undertaken as recommended in the general population.

Post-transplant treatment in patients with HBV should be started as soon as the immunosuppressive therapy is commenced. The ideal duration of antiviral therapy has not been studied; however, because the risk of reactivation persists lifelong while on immunosuppressive therapy, potent NA therapy is recommended to continue indefinitely.[12] Although ETV and TDF have both been used successfully to treat HBV post–kidney transplant, many programs prefer to use ETV because of the low, but established risk of renal tubular toxicity with TDF and safety of ETV in renal dysfunction. In those with prior lamivudine exposure, however, TDF is preferred. To date there is no published experience with the use of TAF in kidney transplantation, but this could be considered as an alternative in those with renal dysfunction.

The use of kidneys from donors who are anti-HBc-positive has been shown to be safe, without prophylaxis, in recipients who are immune to HBV (anti-HBs titer >10 IU/mL).[28]

Limited data exist regarding use of HBsAg-positive donors. In a recent study by Chancharoenthana and colleagues,[29] they compare outcomes of kidney HBsAg-negative transplant recipients with anti HBs titer greater than 100 IU/mL from HBsAg-positive donors and HBsAg-negative donors. With a median follow-up of 58.2 months, no significant differences in graft and patient survival were found. In heart transplant, where most available data are from Taiwan and Korea,[30–32] protocols including pretransplant vaccination and post-transplant antiviral therapy with or without HBIg prophylaxis has been shown to be effective in the prevention of HBV transmission from HBsAg-positive donor hearts. In North America, where the prevalence of HBV in donors is also low, organs from HBsAg-positive donors continue to be used selectively weighing the risks and benefits in individual recipients and following strict informed consent (**Table 1**).[13]

HEPATITIS C VIRUS

HCV is estimated to infect 2% to 3% of the global population, corresponding to 150 to 190 million people worldwide.[33] HCV-related end-stage liver disease and HCC remain the leading indications for LT worldwide. Before effective direct-acting antiviral (DAA) therapy, hepatic and nonhepatic transplant recipients with HCV had significantly reduced graft and overall survival compared with HCV-uninfected patients.[21,34] There are now several DAA therapies that are well tolerated and highly effective and can cure more than 90% of those infected, including those post-transplant. As a result, HCV no longer limits access to or outcomes of transplantation and there is growing interest and data to consider HCV viremic organs in HCV-negative recipients.

Liver Transplant

The DAAs currently used for the treatment of chronic HCV infection are effective in patients with advanced cirrhosis and post-LT. The combinations of sofosbuvir and ribavirin, sofosbuvir and ledipasvir, with or without ribavirin, sofosbuvir and daclatasvir,

Table 1 HBV summary		
	Treatment of Liver Recipient	Treatment of Nonliver Recipient
Recipient with HBV infection (HBsAg positive)	NA ± HBIg	NA
Donor anti-HBc + ve	NA	Preferred anti-HBs >10 IU/mL If anti-HBs <10 IU/mL, assess donor HBV DNA ± NA
Donor HBsAg + ve	Only HBsAg + ve NA + HBIg	Preferred anti-HBs >100 IU/mL NA ± HBIg

with or without ribavirin, sofosbuvir/velpatasvir and daclatasvir/sofosbuvir have all been shown to improve clinical and biochemical outcomes in those with decompensated liver disease.[35–38] However, whether DAA therapy should be administered in patients awaiting transplantation, or deferred to post-transplant remains controversial.

Data continue to demonstrate that sustained virologic response (SVR) significantly reduces the risk of progressive liver disease, hepatic decompensation, HCC, liver-related mortality, and all-cause mortality.[39] Achieving SVR in patients with cirrhosis may improve the model for end-stage liver disease (MELD) score. Stabilization or improvement in hepatic function may occur in 60% of the patients, whereas about a quarter experience declining liver function and the remainder are unchanged.[40–42] For some, this may result in a lower priority for LT allocation, without improving the poor quality of life associated with complications of end-stage liver disease. This situation has been termed "MELD limbo" or "MELD purgatory."[43,44] In addition, the cure rate in those with decompensated liver disease is significantly lower than those with compensated cirrhosis or post-LT. A recent analysis by Foster and colleagues[45] included 467 patients with Child-Turcotte-Pugh class B/C that received treatment of all HCV genotypes (GTs). Treatment was chosen by clinician and included sofosbuvir with ledipasvir or daclatasvir, and with or without ribavirin. The overall SVR was only 83.5%. Primarily for these reasons, when to treat HCV-infected patients awaiting LT remains controversial. Treatment before LT in this cohort of patients might also limit the donor pool if a listed patient cured of HCV would then no longer be considered for an HCV-viremic donor.[41]

In a recent modeling study by Chhatwal and colleagues[40] long-term outcomes of pre-LT versus post-LT HCV treatment with DAAs for patients with MELD scores between 10 and 40 were simulated using integrated data from United Network for Organ Sharing and the SOLAR 1 and 2 trials. Their findings suggest that at the US national level, treating HCV before LT increased life expectancy if MELD score was less than or equal to 27 but could decrease life expectancy at higher MELD scores. The International Liver Transplantation Society also recently released a consensus statement on HCV management in LT candidates.[42] This suggests that patients awaiting LT with HCV-related cirrhosis who are Child-Turcotte-Pugh B and/or have MELD score less than 20 and who are without refractory portal hypertension be treated with antiviral therapy, whereas those with Child-Turcotte-Pugh C and/or MELD score more than 30 should not undergo antiviral therapy. There are several additional factors that must be considered from an LT program and patient perspective. These include the anticipated wait times in the region, availability of HCV viremic donors, availability of a living donor, and access to DAA therapy.

In patients with HCV-related HCC awaiting LT, decisions regarding the timing of HCV therapy are also complex. Prenner and colleagues[46] studied a total of 421 patients with HCV cirrhosis where 33% had active or a history of HCC. The SVR rate was only 79% in patients with HCC compared with 88% in patients without HCC ($P = .009$). Of the 29 patients with HCC who did not achieve SVR, 93% of these had an active tumor at the time of treatment. DAA therapy in patients with inactive tumor or after removal (resection/LT) had better SVR rates ($P<.001$). These findings suggest that a primary predictor of DAA failure is the presence of active HCC at the time of treatment (odds ratio, 8.5; 95% confidence interval, 3.90–18.49). Presently, The International Liver Transplantation Society consensus statement on HCV management in LT candidates[44] suggests that HCV-infected patients with HCC and either compensated cirrhosis or those with decompensated cirrhosis who are not expected to undergo LT within 3 to 6 months be treated with antiviral therapy. Only in those with HCV-related HCC and decompensated disease who are expected to receive an LT within 3 to 6 months is deferral of DAA therapy suggested. **Table 2** summarizes the advantages and disadvantages of treating patients with DAAs for HCV-related liver diseases before LT.[43,47,48]

Following LT, cure of HCV results in a significant decrease in morbidity and mortality.[49] Several DAA regimens have been studied in the post-LT population in those with GT1, GT4, GT5, or GT6. The SOLAR-1 study included 223 LT patients with a broad spectrum of fibrosis, including six with fibrosing cholestatic hepatitis, who received sofosbuvir/ledipasvir/ribavirin for 12 or 24 weeks. The overall SVR was 96% to 98% (12 weeks and 24 weeks, respectively) and all with fibrosing cholestatic hepatitis achieved SVR.[50] SOLAR-2 included 168 LT recipients who similarly received sofosbuvir/ledipasvir/ribavirin for 12 or 24 weeks and SVR was comparable in patients without cirrhosis at 94% to 100% (12 weeks and 24 weeks, respectively).[35] The MAGELLAN-2 study included 80 LT recipients and demonstrated glecaprevir/pibrentasvir for 12 weeks to be well tolerated with an SVR of 98%.[51] Real-world cohorts have also demonstrated a high SVR rate with or without the inclusion of ribavirin in combination with ledipasvir/sofosbuvir.[52,53] However, because factors leading clinicians to include ribavirin in the regimen in the observational studies cannot be determined, the addition of ribavirin is still recommended, particularly for patients with unfavorable baseline characteristics, such as cirrhosis or prior treatment experience, by many experts. In those with post-transplant HCV recurrence and GT2 or GT3 infection glecaprevir/pibrentasvir and daclatasvir/sofosbuvir/ribavirin for 12 weeks have been shown to be effective.[51,54,55] There have been no studies published evaluating sofosbuvir/velpatasvir therapy in LT recipients and further data are awaited. Given the limited options for therapy, however, particularly in patients with decompensated cirrhosis, this may be used, based on expert opinion, with or without the addition of ribavirin.

In summary, those with decompensated HCV-cirrhosis where LT is contraindicated or not accessible should receive HCV treatment with the expectation of improved hepatic function in about 60% of cases and resultant longer survival. To optimize outcomes in those who are LT candidates, however, one must consider primarily the severity of the liver disease as measured by MELD and the presence and stage of HCC. In addition, the anticipated wait time at the center, patient treatment history and access to DAA therapy, and availability and local philosophy of HCV viremic donor use (only in HCV viremic recipient or any recipient) remain important factors in the timing of HCV therapy.

Table 2
Advantages and disadvantages of treating patients with decompensated cirrhosis caused by HCV infection before LT

Advantages	Disadvantages
SVR is achieved in >80% of patients	May eliminate the opportunity to have a curative treatment (LT) of liver disease; and place the patient into the "MELD purgatory" situation where quality of life is still poor
Liver function often improves	
May obviate LT (up to 30% of patients)	
Improved liver function may increase options for local regional treatment of HCC and reduce HCC recurrence	
	Still at risk of progressive liver disease and HCC
Prevent post-LT HCV recurrence	
Fewer drug-drug interactions (compared with treating LT recipients)	May preclude the use of HCV viremic organs
	Treatment after LT is associated with higher SVR rates compared with treatment in decompensated cirrhosis before LT
	In those who fail therapy, exposure to NS5A inhibitors decreases options when retreating after LT

Nonliver Transplant

The prevalence of hepatitis C in patients with end-stage renal disease (ESRD) varies worldwide, but is higher in those on hemodialysis compared with peritoneal dialysis and in those on dialysis longer. In the United States and Western Europe, it stands at 5% to 10%.[56] Most new infections in ESRD are now caused by the usual risk factors for community acquisition, most notably infection drug use; however, there continue to be cases of health-care acquired HCV in dialysis centers worldwide.[57] With the screening of blood products and the use of erythropoiesis-stimulating agents, the risk of transfusion-related HCV infection in dialysis patients has dramatically declined.

Historically, chronic HCV infection has been associated with a significant decrease in patient and graft survival at 10 years following transplantation.[21] However, even in the era before DAA therapy, there was a clear survival advantage to transplantation versus remaining on dialysis in those with chronic HCV infection. In a recent systematic review and meta-analysis performed by Ingsathit and colleagues,[58] they concluded that patients with chronic HCV who remain on dialysis are at higher risk of death when compared with those who received kidney transplantation (relative risk, 2.19; 95% confidence interval, 1.50–3.20; $P = .004$), comparable with previous meta-analyses.[59,60]

There are now several DAA regimens that have been studied in both ESRD and post–kidney transplant that are safe and effective. In ESRD, elbasvir/grazoprevir for 12 weeks was studied in GT1 HCV-infected patients in the C-SURFER trial and resulted in an SVR of 99%.[61] The pangenotypic combination of glecaprevir/pibrentasvir for 12 weeks, studied in the EXPEDITION-4 trial, demonstrated excellent safety and efficacy in those with ESRD, including those on dialysis resulting in a 100% SVR in 104 patients.[62] As a result, these are the primary recommended treatment options in this population. Published clinical trials to date of sofosbuvir-based regimens have excluded those with estimated glomerular filtration rate less than 30 mL/min and use of these regimens in those with advanced renal disease is not currently recommended. There are, however, accumulating real-world data that suggest sofosbuvir-based regimens are safe and effective[63–65] and clinical trials are ongoing.

Ruling out cirrhosis before HCV therapy and transplantation is important to risk stratify those who would need HCC surveillance and/or endoscopic assessment for varices, and to identify the few that may be better served by combined liver-kidney transplant. The Kidney Disease: Improving Global Outcomes (KDIGO) group, in their most recent guidelines, recommend that patients with chronic kidney disease be assessed for liver fibrosis with noninvasive tests, such as transient elastography or serum markers.[66]

In the post–kidney transplant setting clinical trials in addition to multiple real-world studies have demonstrated excellent efficacy and safety using several DAA regimens. In a phase 2 open label study of 114 kidney transplant recipients with either GT1 or GT4 HCV infection randomized to receive ledipasvir/sofosbuvir for 12 or 24 weeks all patients achieved SVR and treatment was well tolerated.[67] In a Spanish cohort of 103 kidney transplant recipients treated with DAA post-transplant an SVR of 98% was achieved. The most commonly used combinations were sofosbuvir/ledipasvir (n = 59; 57%) and sofosbuvir/daclatasvir (n = 18; 17%), with ribavirin being added in 41%.[68] The combination of glecaprevir/pibrentasvir for 12 weeks in 20 kidney transplant recipients was well tolerated with an SVR of 98%. Several additional cohort studies have reported excellent outcomes following DAA therapy in renal transplant recipients, with SVR comparable with the nontransplant population.[52,69–71]

In thoracic organ transplant candidates, the prevalence of HCV infection has not been studied. The impact of HCV on outcomes of thoracic organ transplant in the pre-DAA is limited in interpretation by the study design. Most are database analysis with a paucity of clinical information and ability to control for confounding factors, and many classify patients' HCV status based solely on serology without data on HCV RNA status.[72-74] Only short-term outcomes following DAA therapy are available to date in case reports and small case series in thoracic transplantation; however, these are encouraging. Three patients post–lung transplant all achieved SVR with sofosbuvir-based regimens, with excellent drug tolerability and no major adverse reactions or immunosuppressive dose adjustment requirements.[75] Similar outcomes were observed in a cohort of 12 chronically HCV-infected heart transplant recipients treated with sofosbuvir combined with either ledipasvir or daclatasvir.[76] In one patient treated post–lung transplant with sofosbuvir/daclatasvir for rapidly progressive fibrosis, cure was also achieved.[77] Although data are limited to date, cure rates with DAA therapy in thoracic organ transplant recipients are anticipated to be excellent and similar to the general population and that observed in liver and kidney transplant recipients.

As in LT, an important unresolved question is the optimal timing of HCV therapy in renal and other nonhepatic transplant candidates. One of the strongest arguments to defer therapy until after transplant is to expand the donor pool for the recipients who would be eligible to receive an allograft from an HCV-viremic donor. However, there are several additional factors that must be considered because HCV viremic patients on dialysis also have an increased risk of death not only compared with transplantation, but also compared with those who are HCV-negative on dialysis. The severity of liver disease and anticipated wait times for transplant are key considerations, and access to DAA therapy. **Table 3** outlines the considerations of HCV therapy before or after kidney transplant. In a medical decision analysis published in abstract form, delayed HCV treatment seemed most cost effective; however, the robustness of this finding is limited by unknown net treatment benefit with DAA on mortality.[78]

For any recipient undergoing DAA therapy post-transplant, drug interactions and the risk of rejection must be considered. Overall there are few significant drug interactions between immunosuppressants and DAAs.[79] Sofosbuvir in combination with daclatasvir, ledipasvir, or velpatasvir is used safely with calcineurin inhibitors and sirolimus. Cyclosporine is contraindicated in combination with HCV protease inhibitors including grazoprevir, simeprevir, and voxilaprevir because of marked elevations in exposure to the protease inhibitor. Coadministration of glecaprevir/pibrentasvir with cyclosporine requires close monitoring because concentrations of glecaprevir/pibrentasvir may increase and this protease inhibitor should be avoided in those requiring a daily dose of cyclosporine of more than 100 mg.

Table 3
Considerations in timing of DAA therapy for HCV viremic kidney transplant candidates

Treat Before Transplant	Defer Treatment Until After Transplant

• Advanced liver disease
• Expected long wait for transplant
  ○ No living donor
  ○ Highly sensitized
  ○ Center average for blood group
• Unwilling to consider HCV viremic donor or not expected to be available rapidly
	• Mild/moderate liver disease (stage F2 or less)
	• Willing to accept HCV viremic kidney
	• Expect possibility of receiving HCV viremic kidney rapidly

Several case reports of acute rejection in patients cured with DAA therapy have emerged. Proposed potential mechanisms for this include improved liver function post-treatment with increased clearance of immunosuppressant agents, reduced calcineurin inhibitor levels attributed to HCV protease inhibitor use, and potential loss of the HCV-immunosuppressive effects that follow HCV cure. Although there is no proof of causation and rejection rates are low,[52] patients should be monitored for rejection during and after therapy.

Hepatitis C Virus Viremic Donors

Three primary factors have led to the international transplant community considering the use of HCV viremic organs for HCV negative recipients: (1) the advancements in HCV DAA therapy and the ability to cure nearly all those infected; (2) the organ shortage and possibility to expand the donor pool; and (3) in North America in particular, the growing number of often young, otherwise excellent, donors with HCV as a consequence of the opioid epidemic.[80] A recently published American Society of Transplantation Consensus suggests that transplantation from HCV viremic donors to negative recipients only be considered in the setting of clinical research at this time.[81] However, emerging data suggest the benefits of accepting an HCV viremic donor likely outweigh this risk of HCV infection in the era of DAA therapy.

In a pilot trial, 10 kidneys from GT1 HCV viremic donors were transplanted into HCV-negative recipients. After documentation of viremia in the recipients, all received elbasvir/grazoprevir for 12 weeks, achieving SVR in 100%.[82] Excellent short-term outcomes have also been seen in liver, lung, and heart recipients, including in cases of unintentional and intentional transplantation of organs from HCV-infected donors.[83–86] Mathematical modeling by Chhatwal and colleagues[87] simulating a trial of HCV-negative patients awaiting LT compared long-term outcomes in those willing to accept HCV-positive livers versus those willing only to accept HCV-negative livers. Patients receiving HCV-positive livers were treated with DAA therapy for 12 weeks. They demonstrated that willingness to accept HCV-negative or viremic livers resulted in an increase in patients' life expectancy when the MELD score was more than 20. Similar modeling in renal transplantation suggests HCV-negative recipients willing to accept HCV viremic kidneys would result in improved survival and be cost effective and under some conditions cost saving.[88]

Although there are practical and financial considerations, most notably ensuring access to DAA therapy for post-transplant treatment, and the need to obtain strict informed consent, the use of HCV viremic donors for HCV-negative recipients is a promising additional advance in expanding the donor pool (**Table 4**).

HEPATITIS E VIRUS

Approximately 3.7 million people worldwide are affected by HEV infection and associated mortality is 70,000 per year.[1] HEV GT1 and GT2 are waterborne and are the cause of infection in developing countries and associated with acute hepatitis and a characteristic high mortality of up to 30% in pregnant women. GT3 and GT4, however, are prevalent in developed countries and are zoonoses with animal reservoirs including pigs, wild boar, and rabbits. HEV infection occurs through drinking contaminated water or consumption of meat from infected animals. Transfusion-transmitted infection plays a minor role as source of infection in the risk group of solid-organ recipients with primary risk factors identified to be consumption of pork or game meat.[89,90] Prevention relies on avoiding raw or undercooked meat. Unlike HEV infection in immunocompetent hosts where infections are self-limited, organ transplant

Table 4
HCV summary

	Treatment of Liver Recipient	Treatment of Nonliver Recipient
Recipient with HCV infection	Timing of DAA (before or after transplant) depends on MELD, CTP class, *portal* HTN, regional anticipated wait list time, availability of living donor, availability of HCV viremic donor, access to DAA, and HCC.	Timing of DAA (before or after transplant) depends on severity of liver disease, regional anticipated wait list time, availability of living donor (kidney only), availability of HCV viremic donor, access to DAA.
Donor with HCV viremia	Previously HCV viremic recipients only. Currently HCV –ve acceptable with DAA after transplant.	

Abbreviations: CTP, Child-Turcotte-Pugh; HTN, hypertension.

recipients develop chronic infection in approximately 60% of cases and this leads to progressive fibrosis and cirrhosis in up to 10%.[91,92]

The diagnosis of HEV infection in immunosuppressed hosts is missed because of the absence of typical clinical signs and symptoms. Clinicians must have a high index of suspicion for infection and should consider HEV in transplant recipients with raised liver enzymes of any degree, although typically alanine aminotransferase levels are between 100 and 200 U/L.[93] The diagnose of HEV infection is by HEV RNA in serum or stool, because HEV antibodies may be absent in up to 20%, and the persistence of at least 6 months defines chronic disease.[89] Clearance of infection occurs spontaneously in more than 30% of cases. Where possible, a reduction in immunosuppression should be considered.

In transplant patients who develop persistent infection, ribavirin has been shown to be effective in the treatment of GT3 chronic HEV infection. A retrospective multicenter study demonstrated ribavirin monotherapy, given for a median of 3 months, to achieve a sustained virologic rate of ~90%.[94] Patients without detectable HEV RNA in the serum, but with persistent HEV RNA detected in the feces at the end of therapy, have a significantly higher risk of relapse,[95] whereas rapid decrease in serum HEV RNA within the first week of ribavirin therapy has been identified as a positive predictive factor for SVR.[96]

Up to 40% of transplant recipients with persistent HEV relapse after 3 months of treatment with ribavirin.[95,96] Most patients who relapse respond to a longer course of treatment with ribavirin, even in those harboring the G1634R mutation that is detected post-treatment.[97] The optimal duration and dose of ribavirin has not yet been determined. Retreating with a longer course of ribavirin in patients that relapse, however, should be considered and continued until two HEV RNA are negative in blood or stool with at least 1 month apart.[94]

REFERENCES

1. World Health Organization. Global hepatitis report 2017. Available at: http://www.who.int/hepatitis/publications/global-hepatitis-report2017/en/. Accessed January 14, 2018.
2. Stanaway JD, Flaxman AD, Naghavi M, et al. The global burden of viral hepatitis from 1990 to 2013: findings from the Global Burden of Disease Study 2013. Lancet 2016;388(10049):1081–8.

3. Stepanova M, Wai H, Saab S, et al. The portrait of an adult liver transplant recipient in the United States from 1987 to 2013. JAMA Intern Med 2014;174(8):1407–9.
4. Global Burden of Disease Liver Cancer Collaboration, Akinyemiju T, Abera S, Ahmed M, et al. The burden of primary liver cancer and underlying etiologies from 1990 to 2015 at the global, regional, and national level: results from the Global Burden of Disease Study 2015. JAMA Oncol 2017;3(12):1683–91.
5. Cholongitas E, Goulis J, Akriviadis E, et al. Hepatitis B immunoglobulin and/or nucleos(t)ide analogues for prophylaxis against hepatitis B virus recurrence after liver transplantation: a systematic review. Liver Transpl 2011;17(10):1176–90.
6. Marzano A, Gaia S, Ghisetti V, et al. Viral load at the time of liver transplantation and risk of hepatitis B virus recurrence. Liver Transpl 2005;11(4):402–9.
7. European Association for the Study of the Liver. EASL clinical practice guidelines: liver transplantation. J Hepatol 2016;64(2):433–85. Electronic address.
8. Lucey MR, Terrault N, Ojo L, et al. Long-term management of the successful adult liver transplant: 2012 practice guideline by the American Association for the Study of Liver Diseases and the American Society of Transplantation. Liver Transpl 2013;19(1):3–26.
9. Perrillo R, Buti M, Durand F, et al. Entecavir and hepatitis B immune globulin in patients undergoing liver transplantation for chronic hepatitis B. Liver Transpl 2013;19(8):887–95.
10. Fox AN, Terrault NA. The option of HBIG-free prophylaxis against recurrent HBV. J Hepatol 2012;56(5):1189–97.
11. European Association for the Study of the Liver. Electronic address: easloffice@easloffice.eu, European Association for the Study of the Liver. EASL 2017 clinical practice guidelines on the management of hepatitis B virus infection. J Hepatol 2017;67(2):370–98.
12. Levitsky J, Doucette K, AST Infectious Diseases Community of Practice. Viral hepatitis in solid organ transplantation. Am J Transplant 2013;13(Suppl 4): 147–68.
13. Huprikar S, Danziger-Isakov L, Ahn J, et al. Solid organ transplantation from hepatitis B virus-positive donors: consensus guidelines for recipient management. Am J Transplant 2015;15(5):1162–72.
14. Perrillo R. Hepatitis B virus prevention strategies for antibody to hepatitis B core antigen-positive liver donation: a survey of North American, European, and Asian-Pacific transplant programs. Liver Transpl 2009;15(2):223–32.
15. Cholongitas E, Papatheodoridis GV, Burroughs AK. Liver grafts from anti-hepatitis B core positive donors: a systematic review. J Hepatol 2010;52(2):272–9.
16. Loggi E, Conti F, Cucchetti A, et al. Liver grafts from hepatitis B surface antigen-positive donors: a review of the literature. World J Gastroenterol 2016;22(35): 8010–6.
17. Zanetto A, Ferrarese A, Bortoluzzi I, et al. New perspectives on treatment of hepatitis B before and after liver transplantation. Ann Transplant 2016;21:632–43.
18. Loggi E, Micco L, Ercolani G, et al. Liver transplantation from hepatitis B surface antigen positive donors: a safe way to expand the donor pool. J Hepatol 2012; 56(3):579–85.
19. Franchello A, Ghisetti V, Marzano A, et al. Transplantation of hepatitis B surface antigen-positive livers into hepatitis B virus-positive recipients and the role of hepatitis delta coinfection. Liver Transpl 2005;11(8):922–8.
20. Danziger-Isakov L, Kumar D, AST Infectious Diseases Community of Practice. Vaccination in solid organ transplantation. Am J Transplant 2013;13(Suppl 4): 311–7.

21. Mathurin P, Mouquet C, Poynard T, et al. Impact of hepatitis B and C virus on kidney transplantation outcome. Hepatology 1999;29(1):257–63.
22. Daude M, Rostaing L, Saune K, et al. Tenofovir therapy in hepatitis B virus-positive solid-organ transplant recipients. Transplantation 2011;91(8):916–20.
23. Kamar N, Milioto O, Alric L, et al. Entecavir therapy for adefovir-resistant hepatitis B virus infection in kidney and liver allograft recipients. Transplantation 2008; 86(4):611–4.
24. Harmanci O, Ilin S, Ocal S, et al. The effect of hepatitis B virus on graft and overall survival in kidney transplant patients. Exp Clin Transplant 2015;13(Suppl 3): 36–40.
25. Park KS, Han DJ, Park JB, et al. Long-term outcome of hepatitis B-positive renal allograft recipients after development of antiviral treatment. Clin Nephrol 2012; 78(5):391–8.
26. Halegoua-De Marzio D, Fenkel JM, Doria C. Hepatitis B in solid-organ transplant procedures other than liver. Exp Clin Transplant 2017;15(2):130–7.
27. Castera L. Non-invasive tests for liver fibrosis progression and regression. J Hepatol 2016;64(1):232–3.
28. Pilmore HL, Gane EJ. Hepatitis B-positive donors in renal transplantation: increasing the deceased donor pool. Transplantation 2012;94(3):205–10.
29. Chancharoenthana W, Townamchai N, Pongpirul K, et al. The outcomes of kidney transplantation in hepatitis B surface antigen (HBsAg)-negative recipients receiving graft from HBsAg-positive donors: a retrospective, propensity score-matched study. Am J Transplant 2014;14(12):2814–20.
30. Chen YC, Chuang MK, Chou NK, et al. Twenty-four year single-center experience of hepatitis B virus infection in heart transplantation. Transplant Proc 2012;44(4): 910–2.
31. Shin HS, Cho HJ, Jeon ES, et al. The impact of hepatitis B on heart transplantation: 19 years of national experience in Korea. Ann Transplant 2014;19: 182–7.
32. Wang SS, Chou NK, Ko WJ, et al. Heart transplantation using donors positive for hepatitis. Transplant Proc 2004;36(8):2371–3.
33. Petruzziello A, Marigliano S, Loquercio G, et al. Global epidemiology of hepatitis C virus infection: an up-date of the distribution and circulation of hepatitis C virus genotypes. World J Gastroenterol 2016;22(34):7824–40.
34. Forman LM, Lewis JD, Berlin JA, et al. The association between hepatitis C infection and survival after orthotopic liver transplantation. Gastroenterology 2002; 122(4):889–96.
35. Manns M, Samuel D, Gane EJ, et al. Ledipasvir and sofosbuvir plus ribavirin in patients with genotype 1 or 4 hepatitis C virus infection and advanced liver disease: a multicentre, open-label, randomised, phase 2 trial. Lancet Infect Dis 2016;16(6):685–97.
36. Welzel TM, Petersen J, Herzer K, et al. Daclatasvir plus sofosbuvir, with or without ribavirin, achieved high sustained virological response rates in patients with HCV infection and advanced liver disease in a real-world cohort. Gut 2016;65(11): 1861–70.
37. Curry MP, O'Leary JG, Bzowej N, et al. Sofosbuvir and velpatasvir for HCV in patients with decompensated cirrhosis. N Engl J Med 2015;373(27):2618–28.
38. Samuel D, Manns M, Forns X, et al. Ledipasvir/sofosbuvir with ribavirin is safe in >600 decompensated and post liver transplantation patients with HCV infection: an integrated safety analysis of the solar 1 and solar 2 trials. J Hepatol 2015;62:S620–1.

39. van der Meer AJ, Veldt BJ, Feld JJ, et al. Association between sustained virological response and all-cause mortality among patients with chronic hepatitis C and advanced hepatic fibrosis. JAMA 2012;308(24):2584–93.

40. Chhatwal J, Samur S, Kues B, et al. Optimal timing of hepatitis C treatment for patients on the liver transplant waiting list. Hepatology 2017;65(3):777–88.

41. Ofosu A, Durand CM, Saberi B, et al. Implications of treating hepatitis C virus infection among patients awaiting cadaveric liver transplant: a single-center experience. Exp Clin Transplant 2015;13(Suppl 3):7–10.

42. Terrault NA, McCaughan GW, Curry MP, et al. International liver transplantation society consensus statement on hepatitis C management in liver transplant candidates. Transplantation 2017;101(5):945–55.

43. Bunchorntavakul C, Reddy KR. Treat chronic hepatitis C virus infection in decompensated cirrhosis: pre- or post-liver transplantation? The ironic conundrum in the era of effective and well-tolerated therapy. J Viral Hepat 2016;23(6):408–18.

44. Carrion AF, Khaderi SA, Sussman NL. Model for end-stage liver disease limbo, model for end-stage liver disease purgatory, and the dilemma of treating hepatitis C in patients awaiting liver transplantation. Liver Transpl 2016;22(3):279–80.

45. Foster GR, Irving WL, Cheung MC, et al. Impact of direct acting antiviral therapy in patients with chronic hepatitis C and decompensated cirrhosis. J Hepatol 2016;64(6):1224–31.

46. Prenner SB, VanWagner LB, Flamm SL, et al. Hepatocellular carcinoma decreases the chance of successful hepatitis C virus therapy with direct-acting antivirals. J Hepatol 2017;66(6):1173–81.

47. Belli LS, Duvoux C, Berenguer M, et al. ELITA consensus statements on the use of DAAs in liver transplant candidates and recipients. J Hepatol 2017;67(3):585–602.

48. Coilly A, Roche B, Duclos-Vallee JC, et al. Optimum timing of treatment for hepatitis C infection relative to liver transplantation. Lancet Gastroenterol Hepatol 2016;1(2):165–72.

49. Picciotto FP, Tritto G, Lanza AG, et al. Sustained virological response to antiviral therapy reduces mortality in HCV reinfection after liver transplantation. J Hepatol 2007;46(3):459–65.

50. Charlton M, Everson GT, Flamm SL, et al. Ledipasvir and sofosbuvir plus ribavirin for treatment of HCV infection in patients with advanced liver disease. Gastroenterology 2015;149(3):649–59.

51. Reau N, Kwo PY, Rhee S, et al. Magellan-2: safety and efficacy of glecaprevir/pibrentasvir in liver or renal transplant adults with chronic hepatitis C genotype 1-6 infection. In: Program and abstracts of the International Liver Conference. Amsterdam, The Netherlands, April 13–22, 2017.

52. Saxena V, Khungar V, Verna EC, et al. Safety and efficacy of current direct-acting antiviral regimens in kidney and liver transplant recipients with hepatitis C: results from the HCV-TARGET study. Hepatology 2017;66(4):1090–101.

53. Kwok RM, Ahn J, Schiano TD, et al. Sofosbuvir plus ledispasvir for recurrent hepatitis C in liver transplant recipients. Liver Transpl 2016;22(11):1536–43.

54. Poordad F, Schiff ER, Vierling JM, et al. Daclatasvir with sofosbuvir and ribavirin for hepatitis C virus infection with advanced cirrhosis or post-liver transplantation recurrence. Hepatology 2016;63(5):1493–505.

55. Fontana RJ, Brown RS Jr, Moreno-Zamora A, et al. Daclatasvir combined with sofosbuvir or simeprevir in liver transplant recipients with severe recurrent hepatitis C infection. Liver Transpl 2016;22(4):446–58.

56. Marinaki S, Boletis JN, Sakellariou S, et al. Hepatitis C in hemodialysis patients. World J Hepatol 2015;7(3):548–58.

57. Pereira BJ, Levey AS. Hepatitis C virus infection in dialysis and renal transplantation. Kidney Int 1997;51(4):981–99.

58. Ingsathit A, Kamanamool N, Thakkinstian A, et al. Survival advantage of kidney transplantation over dialysis in patients with hepatitis C: a systematic review and meta-analysis. Transplantation 2013;95(7):943–8.

59. Pereira BJ, Natov SN, Bouthot BA, et al. Effects of hepatitis C infection and renal transplantation on survival in end-stage renal disease. The New England Organ Bank Hepatitis C Study Group. Kidney Int 1998;53(5):1374–81.

60. Fabrizi F, Takkouche B, Lunghi G, et al. The impact of hepatitis C virus infection on survival in dialysis patients: meta-analysis of observational studies. J Viral Hepat 2007;14(10):697–703.

61. Roth D, Nelson DR, Bruchfeld A, et al. Grazoprevir plus elbasvir in treatment-naive and treatment-experienced patients with hepatitis C virus genotype 1 infection and stage 4-5 chronic kidney disease (the C-SURFER study): a combination phase 3 study. Lancet 2015;386(10003):1537–45.

62. Gane E, Lawitz E, Pugatch D, et al. Glecaprevir and pibrentasvir in patients with HCV and severe renal impairment. N Engl J Med 2017;377(15): 1448–55.

63. Beinhardt S, Al Zoairy R, Ferenci P, et al. DAA-based antiviral treatment of patients with chronic hepatitis C in the pre- and postkidney transplantation setting. Transpl Int 2016;29(9):999–1007.

64. Desnoyer A, Pospai D, Le MP, et al. Pharmacokinetics, safety and efficacy of a full dose sofosbuvir-based regimen given daily in hemodialysis patients with chronic hepatitis C. J Hepatol 2016;65(1):40–7.

65. Dumortier J, Bailly F, Pageaux GP, et al. Sofosbuvir-based antiviral therapy in hepatitis C virus patients with severe renal failure. Nephrol Dial Transplant 2017; 32(12):2065–71.

66. Kidney Disease: Improving Global Outcomes (KDIGO). KDIGO clinical practice guidelines for the prevention, diagnosis, evaluation, and treatment of hepatitis C in chronic kidney disease. Kidney Int Suppl 2008;(109):S1–99.

67. Colombo M, Aghemo A, Liu H, et al. Treatment with ledipasvir-sofosbuvir for 12 or 24 weeks in kidney transplant recipients with chronic hepatitis C virus genotype 1 or 4 infection: a randomized trial. Ann Intern Med 2017;166(2):109–17.

68. Fernandez I, Munoz-Gomez R, Pascasio JM, et al. Efficacy and tolerability of interferon-free antiviral therapy in kidney transplant recipients with chronic hepatitis C. J Hepatol 2017;66(4):718–23.

69. Hussein NR, Saleem ZS. Successful treatment of hepatitis C virus genotype 4 in renal transplant recipients with direct-acting antiviral agents. Am J Transplant 2016;16(7):2237–8.

70. Kamar N, Marion O, Rostaing L, et al. Efficacy and safety of sofosbuvir-based antiviral therapy to treat hepatitis C virus infection after kidney transplantation. Am J Transplant 2016;16(5):1474–9.

71. Sawinski D, Kaur N, Ajeti A, et al. Successful treatment of hepatitis C in renal transplant recipients with direct-acting antiviral agents. Am J Transplant 2016; 16(5):1588–95.

72. Englum BR, Ganapathi AM, Speicher PJ, et al. Impact of donor and recipient hepatitis C status in lung transplantation. J Heart Lung Transplant 2016;35(2): 228–35.

73. Fong TL, Cho YW, Hou L, et al. Outcomes after lung transplantation and practices of lung transplant programs in the United States regarding hepatitis C seropositive recipients. Transplantation 2011;91(11):1293–6.

74. Stepanova M, Locklear T, Rafiq N, et al. Long-term outcomes of heart transplant recipients with hepatitis C positivity: the data from the U.S. transplant registry. Clin Transplant 2016;30(12):1570–7.

75. D'Ambrosio R, Aghemo A, Rossetti V, et al. Sofosbuvir-based regimens for the treatment of hepatitis C virus in patients who underwent lung transplant: case series and review of the literature. Liver Int 2016;36(11):1585–9.

76. Liu CH, Chen YS, Wang SS, et al. Sofosbuvir-based interferon-free direct acting antiviral regimens for heart transplant recipients with chronic hepatitis C virus infection. Clin Infect Dis 2017;66(2):289–92.

77. Doucette K, Sumner S, Weinkauf J. Treatment of hepatitis C in a lung transplant recipient with sofosbuvir and daclatasvir. J Heart Lung Transplant 2016;35(6): 840–1.

78. Kiberd B, Tennankore K, Doucette K. Treating hepatitis C+ patients before or after kidney transplantation: a medical decision analysis. Am J Transplant 2017; 17(S3):265.

79. HEP Drug Interaction Checker. Available at: https://www.hep-druginteractions. org/. Accessed January 5, 2018.

80. Goldberg DS, Blumberg E, McCauley M, et al. Improving organ utilization to help overcome the tragedies of the opioid epidemic. Am J Transplant 2016;16(10): 2836–41.

81. Levitsky J, Formica RN, Bloom RD, et al. The American Society of Transplantation Consensus Conference on the Use of Hepatitis C Viremic Donors in Solid Organ Transplantation. Am J Transplant 2017;17(11):2790–802.

82. Goldberg DS, Abt PL, Blumberg EA, et al. Trial of transplantation of HCV-infected kidneys into uninfected recipients. N Engl J Med 2017;376(24):2394–5.

83. Khan B, Singer LG, Lilly LB, et al. Successful lung transplantation from hepatitis C positive donor to seronegative recipient. Am J Transplant 2017;17(4):1129–31.

84. O'Dell H. Retrospective review of liver transplantation of UNOS-defined hepatitis C positive donors into hepatitis C naive recipients. Hepatology 2017;66(S1): 879A.

85. Saberi B, Hamilton JP, Durand CM, et al. Utilization of hepatitis C virus RNA-positive donor liver for transplant to hepatitis C virus RNA-negative recipient. Liver Transpl 2018;24(1):140–3.

86. Theodoropoulos N, Whitson BA, Martin SI, et al. Successful treatment of donor-derived hepatitis C infection in a lung transplant recipient. Transpl Infect Dis 2017;19:e12659.

87. Chhatwal J, Samur S, Bethea ED, et al. Transplanting HCV-positive livers into HCV-negative patients with preemptive antiviral treatment: a modeling study. Hepatology 2017. https://doi.org/10.1002/hep.29723.

88. Kiberd B, Doucette K, Tennankore K. Use of hepatitis C infected organs for kidney transplantation: a cost-effective analysis. Am J Transplant 2017;17(S3):807.

89. Fang SY, Han H. Hepatitis E viral infection in solid organ transplant patients. Curr Opin Organ Transplant 2017;22(4):351–5.

90. Lhomme S, Bardiaux L, Abravanel F, et al. Hepatitis E virus infection in solid organ transplant recipients, France. Emerg Infect Dis 2017;23(2):353–6.

91. Kamar N, Garrouste C, Haagsma EB, et al. Factors associated with chronic hepatitis in patients with hepatitis E virus infection who have received solid organ transplants. Gastroenterology 2011;140(5):1481–9.

92. Kamar N, Selves J, Mansuy JM, et al. Hepatitis E virus and chronic hepatitis in organ-transplant recipients. N Engl J Med 2008;358(8):811–7.

93. McPherson S, Elsharkawy AM, Ankcorn M, et al. Summary of the British Transplantation Society UK Guidelines for Hepatitis E and Solid Organ Transplantation. Transplantation 2018;102(1):15–20.

94. Kamar N, Izopet J, Tripon S, et al. Ribavirin for chronic hepatitis E virus infection in transplant recipients. N Engl J Med 2014;370(12):1111–20.

95. Abravanel F, Lhomme S, Rostaing L, et al. Protracted fecal shedding of HEV during ribavirin therapy predicts treatment relapse. Clin Infect Dis 2015;60(1):96–9.

96. Kamar N, Lhomme S, Abravanel F, et al. An early viral response predicts the virological response to ribavirin in hepatitis E virus organ transplant patients. Transplantation 2015;99(10):2124–31.

97. Lhomme S, Kamar N, Nicot F, et al. Mutation in the hepatitis E virus polymerase and outcome of ribavirin therapy. Antimicrob Agents Chemother 2015;60(3):1608–14.

Yeast Infections in Solid Organ Transplantation

Sarah Taimur, MD

KEYWORDS

- Yeast infections in organ transplants • Invasive candidiasis after organ transplant
- Cryptococcosis after organ transplant
- Emerging fungal pathogens in organ transplant

KEY POINTS

- Invasive candidiasis (IC) remains the most common invasive fungal infection following solid-organ transplant (SOT) but risk factors have evolved over the past several years. Current challenges include drug resistant non-albicans and emerging novel species such as Candida auris. Preventive antifungal use in SOT needs to be re-examined in light of these current challenges.
- Cryptococcus gattii is an emerging pathogen in SOT and should be considered in cases of cryptococcosis with history of travel or residence in the Pacific NW of USA and Canada. Infections due to C. gattii might be associated with reduced in-vitro susceptibility to antifungals.
- Diagnosis of cryptococcus associated IRIS remains a clinical entity. Reduction in calcineurin inhibitors is associated with significantly increased risk of IRIS in SOT recipients with cryptococcosis. Data on optimal treatment is lacking and guidance is based on expert opinion.

INTRODUCTION

Invasive fungal infections (IFIs) remain a major cause of morbidity and mortality among solid organ transplant (SOT) recipients. Over time, better understanding has been gained of the pathophysiology and risk factors for these infections and significant changes in epidemiology and management approach have been observed. Although IFIs have remained a commonly encountered challenge among SOT, information on epidemiology of these infections has been limited mostly to single-center and retrospective studies. Transplant-Associated Infection Surveillance Network (TRANSNET), a consortium of 23 United States transplant centers, provided the first prospective multicenter database on IFIs in SOT.[1] Based on 5-year surveillance data contributed by 15 transplant centers under the TRANSNET consortium, 1208 IFIs were identified among 1063 organ transplant recipients. The 1-year cumulative incidence of first IFI after SOT were 11.6%, 8.6%, 4.7%, 4.0%, 3.4%, and 1.3% for small bowel (SBT),

Division of Infectious Diseases, Icahn School of Medicine at Mount Sinai, One-Gustave L. Levy Place, New York, NY 10029, USA
E-mail address: sarah.taimur@mssm.edu

Infect Dis Clin N Am 32 (2018) 651–666
https://doi.org/10.1016/j.idc.2018.04.005
0891-5520/18/© 2018 Elsevier Inc. All rights reserved.

id.theclinics.com

lung (LTX), liver (LT), heart (HT), pancreas (PTX), and kidney transplant (KT) recipients. The most common IFIs were invasive candidiasis (IC) at 53%, invasive aspergillosis (IA) at 19%, cryptococcosis (8%), non-*Aspergillus* molds (8%), endemic fungi (5%), and zygomycosis (2%).[1] This is a review of IC and cryptococcosis in SOT focusing on key aspects with significant change in the recent past.

INFECTIONS DUE TO *CANDIDA* SPECIES IN SOLID ORGAN TRANSPLANTATION

Infections due to *Candida* species remain the most common type of IFI across all types of SOT, with the exception of LTX, where IA is more common.[1] In the TRANS-NET database, the 12-month cumulative incidence of IC was 1.9%—highest in SBT, followed by PTX, LT, KT, HT, and LTX.[1,2] A subsequent analysis of the TRANSNET database looked at IC specifically and included proved and probable cases, as defined by the European Organization for Research and Treatment of Cancer/Mycosis Study Group criteria.[3,4] The most common sites of IC were bloodstream and intra-abdominal; and the median time to onset was 80 days post-SOT (interquartile range 14–545 days). Consistent with clinical observation and prior studies, IC was seen most frequently in abdominal transplant recipients (LT: 41.1%, KT: 35.3%, kidney-pancreas: 9.1%, and LTX: 8.7%). The most commonly encountered species were *Candida* albicans (46.3%), *C glabrata* (24.4%), *C parapsilosis* (8.1%), *C tropicalis* (3.9%), and *C krusei* (3.1%).[3]

Risk Factors for Invasive Candidiasis in Solid Organ Transplant Recipients

Risk factors for IC after SOT have been best described in LT recipients.[5–10] These risk factors have evolved significantly over the past 2 decades, hence are worthy of discussion in this review. The initial risk factor analysis provided by Collins and colleagues[5] showed that operative variables, such as length of transplant operation, retransplantation, and abdominal and intrathoracic reoperations, were independent predictors of IFIs post-LT. The impact of these operative variables, however, seems reduced based on data from more recent studies.[6,8,10] One of the earlier studies that revealed this was by Husain and colleagues.[6] Contrary to previous data, variables, including operative time and blood transfusion, were not found independent predictors of the risk of IFIs. Rather, the investigators found that post-transplant variables, including antibiotic prophylaxis for spontaneous bacterial peritonitis (odds ratio [OR] 8.3; P = .002), post-transplant dialysis (OR 7.6; P = .0009), and retransplantation (OR 16.4; P = .0018), were independent predictors of IC.[6] This evolution of risk factors is believed to reflect the changes in transplantation practices over the years. This correlation was demonstrated in a study by Singh and colleagues,[10] where, over a 10-year time period, significant decrease in the operation time, intraoperative transfusion requirements, cold-ischemia time, and rate of biopsy-proved rejection was observed. Over the same period, the investigators observed a decrease in the incidence of IC without an increase in medical risk factors for IC, such as CMV infection, hence proving the relationship to operative variables.[10]

Evolution in risk factors for IFI and paucity of data on risk assessment in the current era lead to study of Model for End-stage Liver Disease Score (MELD) as a predictor for IFIs.[7–9] MELD is a practical validated measure of the severity of hepatic failure and it is well-known that patients with higher MELD scores are at higher risk of complications, including infections. This was seen in a study by Saliba and colleagues,[9] who showed that MELD score of 20 to 30 or greater than or equal to 30 was associated with a 2-fold to 4.3-fold increase in relative risk of IFIs. In the same study, similar to earlier studies, other independent predictors for IFIs were choledochojejunostomy anastomosis,[11] bacterial infection,[12] and CMV infection.[5,11,13] Another study by Raghuram and colleagues[8] identified MELD score of greater than 25 as a risk factor for IFI (OR 2.4; 95% CI, 1.2–4.9; P = .02) in univariate analysis; however, it was not identified as an independent predictor in multivariate analysis. In this study, the only independent risk factor for IFI in multivariate analysis was pretransplant fungal colonization (OR 7.8; 95% CI, 3.9–16.2; P<.001),[8] which is similar to findings from earlier studies where pretransplant and early post-transplant colonization were identified as a risk factor for post-LT IFIs.[5,11,13]

Risk factors for IC specific to nonliver SOT are less well understood. A brief overview is provided of risk factors for IC described for nonliver abdominal and thoracic transplants. In addition to LT, IC occurs most frequently in SBT, PTX, and multivisceral transplant (MVT) recipients.[1,3] Florescu and colleagues[14] provided an overview of IC in pediatric SBT recipients and reported that fungal infection occurred in 25% of the SBT recipients and C albicans was the most commonly seen infection. The investigators noted that patients who developed fungal infection (predominantly represented by IC) were older in age compared with those who did not develop fungal infections (mean age 61 months vs 29.8 months, difference +31.2; P = .04). Although this finding is not fully explained in this cohort, the investigators correctly postulate that it may be of significance because older recipients undergo a longer time on intestinal rehabilitation therapy in comparison to those who are transplanted at a younger age.[14] The other noteworthy finding in this study is that IC manifests more commonly as an intra-abdominal/surgical site infection earlier on after transplant whereas fungemia occurs later (>6 months post-transplant) in 80% of the patients. This description of timeline of IC by site of infection after SBT/MVT is a unique finding and informative of the continued risk for IC after SBT/MVT beyond the early postoperative period.[14] The continued risk of IC post-transplant is also described by van Hal and colleagues,[15] who lend the concept of late-onset candidemia based on findings from their multicenter cohort where 54% of IC was seen greater than 6 months post-transplant. They note that majority of late-onset IC episodes occurred in KT recipients with multiple risk factors for IC including prolonged inpatient stay, indwelling catheters and broad-spectrum antibiotic therapy. This finding highlights the significance of general risk factors for IC in the SOT population, in addition to those specific to transplantation.[15] Many groups have described risk factors for infection after PTX. The impact of the type of pancreatic drainage (bladder vs enteric) on risk of infection remains controversial and most studies have examined the risk of infection in general.[16–19] One study that looked at the impact of type of pancreatic drainage specifically on intra-abdominal fungal infections found that enteric drainage carried greater risk versus bladder drainage (21% vs 10%); however, the same finding has not been seen in other studies.[16] In a more recent publication by Herrero-Martinez and colleagues,[18] the investigators looked at a large retrospective cohort of pancreas-kidney transplant recipients. They found 40 episodes of fungal infection in 32 patients (mostly due to Candida species) and identified independent risk of IFI in recipients with pretransplant evidence of peripheral arterial disease, longer cold ischemia time, and high transfusion requirements. This study also highlighted the morbidity associated with these infections and found IFIs an independent risk factor for severe pancreatic dysfunction (OR 8.4; 95% CI, 1.9–37.0; P = .005).[18]

According to the TRANSNET data, IC is the most common IFI in following HT and second most common in LTX recipients.[1] Risk factors contributing to occurrence of IC after thoracic transplantation, however, remain poorly understood. In HT, most studies have examined the risk of IFI in general (IC, IA, and others) and have identified delayed chest closure,[20] induction with lymphocyte depleting agents,[20,21] renal replacement therapy,[21,22] and extracorporeal membrane oxygenation as risk factors.[22] Another study that looked at epidemiology and risk factors for nosocomial bloodstream infections in SOT found that HT recipients were more likely to have IC than other SOT and the source seemed to be central venous lines.[23] As for LTX and combined HT-LTX recipients, although epidemiology and infection trends have been described, information on risk factors for development of IC is lacking and most research in HT, has focused on IA. Although *Candida* species are widely considered nonpulmonary pathogens, in the LTX population, respiratory disease in the form of airway anastomotic site infection leading to dehiscence,[24,25] candida empyema,[26] and disruption of large vessel anastomosis in HT-LTX has been described.[27] The risk of airway anastomotic site candidiasis seems higher in patients with partial dehiscence, necrosis, and airway stents,[24,26] and infection has been attributed not only to recipient but also to donor tracheal colonization with candida.[26,27] Based on these clinical observations, it is common practice to give systemic and inhaled antifungal prophylaxis in the early post-LTX period aimed at targeting *Aspergillus* and *Candida* species,[28,29] and although recent data are supportive of the efficacy of universal antifungal prophylaxis after LTX for prevention to IA, data specific to IC prevention were not examined.[29]

Shift in Spectrum of Candida Infections and Emergence of Novel Species

Epidemiologic data have shown a shift in the spectrum of candida infections over the past 2 decades with an increase in the number of nonalbicans species.[30,31] This shift in spectrum seems to coincide with a general increase in the use of fluconazole.[32] In the realm of SOT, Husain and colleagues[6] published one of the earliest reports highlighting this issue. Since then, there have been several publications bringing attention to the emergence of nonalbicans species and challenges in the management of these infections due to antifungal resistance.[8,33] The clinical impact of this shift was clearly shown in the TRANSNET data with higher mortality among those who had IC due to nonalbicans species than those with *C albicans* infection (80/255: 31.4% vs 67/296: 22.6%; $P = .02$).[3]

Analysis of the TRANSNET data by Lockhart and colleagues[33] revealed that most cases of IC in SOT were still due to *C albicans* with *C glabrata* and *C parapsilosis* the second and third most common species, respectively. Overall, 16% of the isolates in the cohort were fluconazole resistant and this was mostly due to *C glabrata* and *C krusei*. Although *C albicans* and other candida species were mostly fluconazole susceptible, this study conclusively showed the impact of fluconazole prophylaxis on the geometric mean minimum inhibitory concentration (MIC), which was significantly higher in the fluconazole prophylaxis group for all species (4.8676 µg/mL vs 1.020 µg/mL; $P<.001$).[33] Furthermore, on multivariate analysis, the investigators identified fluconazole use in the past 3 months prior to IFI onset as an independent risk factor for fluconazole nonsusceptibility (adjusted OR 2.65; 95% CI, 1.17–5.99).[33] Another study that highlights the emergence of nonalbicans species as significant pathogens in the SOT setting is by Raghuram and colleagues.[8] The investigators reported an IFI rate of 12% despite antifungal prophylaxis and a large percentage of IFIs due to *C parapsilosis*, approximately half of which were fluconazole resistant although typically fluconazole susceptible as a species. These data caution the impact of widespread antifungal prophylaxis on emergence of drug resistance species and also put into question the efficacy of current prophylactic strategies in current era of transplantation.

In addition to the observed change in the spectrum of known candida species, there are reports of global emergence of novel species, such as *C auris*.[34] *C auris* is an emerging pathogen that was first reported from Japan,[35] but since then there have been several reports of health care–associated infections from several countries. The Centers for Disease Control and Infection (CDC) issued an alert regarding the global emergence of this pathogen in 2016, requesting that laboratories and health care facilities report *C auris* infection to the CDC.[36] The significance of this global emerging pathogen is multifold. The first challenge lies in diagnosis of *C auris*, which with commercially available diagnostics is often misidentified as *C haemulonii*. Since this issue was identified, health care practitioners and laboratories have been requested to send isolates that are identified as *C haemulonii* or are unable to be speciated to the CDC for further identification.[35] The second challenge lies in the treatment of *C auris* because in many cases it tends to be multidrug resistant and in some cases, pan-resistance to all available antifungal agents has been seen. In the cases reported in United States, however, most isolates have had lower MIC to echinocandins,[34] making these a potentially effective agent for treatment of these infections. Clinical and Laboratory Standards Institute (CLSI) guidelines, however, for drug susceptibility for this species have not yet been developed. Third, it is clear that *C auris* causes health care–associated outbreaks and there is evidence to suggest that there is nosocomial transmission to patients based on whole-genome sequencing of patient isolates from the same hospital, demonstration of skin and other body site colonization weeks to months after infection, and the presence of *C auris* in environmental samples from the hospital room of a patient with infection.[34] These findings have huge implications on patient care in all settings and, to prevent the emergence of a nosocomial outbreak, health care providers and hospitals must follow recommendations of the CDC on infection prevention and communicate patient history and recommended precautions to other facilities in case of interinstitutional transfer.

C auris infections in the United Sates have been most commonly identified in the blood stream and tend to occur in patients with immunocompromised states. Other sites of infection reported in the United States include urine and ear.[34] The initial report of *C auris* as a novel species came from a patient in Japan with ear infection, hence giving this organism its name.[35] More recently, there was report of donor-derived *C auris* infection in an LTX recipient in Boston, Massachusetts.[37] As anticipated based on recent reports, the identification of the isolate (from recipients bronchoalveolar lavage) proved challenging and it was misidentified as *C haemulonii*. On further testing at the local department of health and at the CDC, the isolate was confirmed *C auris*. Hospital respiratory cultures from the organ donor revealed *C haemulonii* but these were reportedly not tested further for species identification. Whole-genome sequencing of the recipient isolate, however, did show close link to *C auris* isolates from Illinois, which is where the organ donor was from, making donor-derived transmission of infection highly likely. As pointed out in this case report by Azar and colleagues,[37] cases such as this warrant review of current policies and procedures for infection assessment of organ donors. In current practice, isolation of candida in donor specimens other than in the blood are often believed colonizers and are not routinely identified to the species level. This raises the possibility of missed diagnosis and transmission of a potentially drug-resistant pathogen through transplantation. Until better diagnostic methodologies are made available, however, the issue of misidentification of *C auris* remains a real possibility and it is of utmost importance that transplant practitioners remain aware of these issues and seek guidance from transplant infectious diseases experts, local health department, and the CDC in evaluation of isolates that have characteristics suggestive of *C auris*.

Antifungal Prophylaxis in Solid Organ Transplantation

As with risk factors, antifungal prophylaxis for IC in SOT is best described in LT recipients. Several studies have established the role of antifungal prophylaxis for prevention of IFIs after LT.[38–41] As discussed previously, over the past 2 decades there has been an evolution in the traditional risk factors for IC and the spectrum of candida species causing infection. This evolution in fungal species and risk factors plus the implication of universal antifungal prophylaxis in the rise of nonalbicans species led to re-examination of prophylactic strategies. Current American Society of Transplantation (AST) guidelines recommend using a targeted approach with use of antifungal prophy-laxis in high-risk LT, SBT, and PTX, with choice of prophylactic antifungal agent to be targeted to risk factors for IC versus IA, and considering use of a mold-active agent in patients at high risk for IA.[2,42] Withholding antifungal prophylaxis in low-risk LT recip-ients has been studied and shown safe.[43] Despite these data, recent multicenter sur-vey revealed that there remains wide variation in the antifungal prophylactic strategies among institutions, and use of universal prophylaxis remains significant, with flucon-azole remaining the most commonly used prophylactic agent.[44] Studies that have examined echinocandin (anidulafungin and micafungin) versus fluconazole and amphotericin B have not found a statistically significant difference in outcomes.[38,40,41] In addition to systemic antifungals, topical agents are used for prophylaxis after SOT. A randomized controlled study comparing clotrimazole troche with placebo troche in patients with malignancy and KT showed a lower incidence of oral candidiasis in the clotrimazole group.[45] In subsequent years, studies looked at nystatin suspension in comparison with clotrimazole troche in KT[46] and LT patients[47] and found that both were equally effective in preventing oral candidiasis. The use of topical agents for fungal prophylaxis is a common clinical practice after SOT and although data suggest efficacy in prevention of oral mucosal candidiasis, the impact on IC (if any) is unknown and currently there are no international consensus guidelines on the role of these as prophylactic agents.

Use of antifungal prophylaxis after thoracic transplantation is targeted primarily at prevention of IA and has been shown in several studies efficacious in reducing the inci-dence of IFIs.[22,48–50] Because risk factors for IC remain poorly understood in this setting, no standardized guidelines exist and prophylactic regimens remain institu-tion-specific.[48]

It is important to recognize the impact of widespread fluconazole prophylaxis on the observed shift in spectrum of *Candida* species and emergence of antifungal drug resis-tance, which has been highlighted by many experts in the field.[51,52] The use of targeted antifungal prophylaxis and avoidance of universal prophylaxis (as recommended in the current AST guidelines),[2] therefore, is of utmost importance to curtail the risk of further antifungal drug resistance. Furthermore, transplant practitioners must review institu-tional protocols on infection prophylaxis at regular intervals to update their policies in accordance with the latest information on host risk factors and species trends. Individ-ual institutions must take into account local spectrum of fungal species and drug sus-ceptibility profiles and tailor protocol to better target the risk to their patients.[51,52]

INFECTIONS DUE TO *CRYPTOCOCCUS* SPECIES IN SOLID ORGAN TRANSPLANTATION

Cryptococcus is the third most common etiology and accounts for 7% to 8% of IFIs after SOT.[1,53] According to multicenter epidemiologic data (TRANSNET and Prospec-tive Antifungal Therapy Alliance registry), cryptococcal infection is seen most commonly in KT recipients followed by LT and HT.[1,53] It is typically a late-occurring infection (median time to onset: 464–805.5 days; range 4–4826)[1,53,54] that seems to have an earlier onset after LTX, LT, and HT compared with KT.[54,55] Very early-onset cryptococcosis ($\leq$30 days post-transplant) is well documented, with an incidence of 5% to 10% and has been reported most commonly in LT and LTX recipients.[54,56] Risk factors for development of cryptococcosis after SOT are not as well defined as

IC and IA. Cryptococcosis in SOT is primarily considered the result of reactivation of latent or old infection in the setting of iatrogenic immunosuppression. This was shown nicely in a study by Saha and colleagues,[57] where 52% of recipients who developed cryptococcosis post-transplant had serologic evidence of prior infection pretransplant. Furthermore, those who were seropositive developed cryptococcosis earlier post-transplant than those without (5.6 ± 3.4 months vs 40.6 ± 63.8 months, respectively; P = .0011). Cryptococcal serologic testing could prove a useful tool in gauging risk of reactivation cryptococcosis in the post-transplant setting and although available through select commercial laboratories anecdotally does not seem commonly used by most transplant centers. Other mechanisms of pathogenesis include donor-derived infection[56] and primary infection due to environmental exposures, both of which are well documented.[58–60]

Variables Influencing Clinical Manifestations and Mortality—Type of Transplant and Immunosuppression

Cryptococcosis is associated with significant morbidity and mortality in SOT recipients. The reported mortality rate in the literature ranges from 14% in some series to as high as 42%.[55,61] Disseminated cryptococcosis with fungemia and central nervous system (CNS) infection is seen in 55% to 68% of cases[55,61] and is associated with higher risk of mortality compared with localized pulmonary or cutaneous infection. Other than disseminated infection, renal failure in SOT recipients carries an independent significantly higher risk of mortality due to cryptococcosis (OR 16.4; 95% CI, 1.9–143; P = .004)[55] (hazard ratio [HR] 2.99; 95% CI, 1.12–7.98; P = .028).[61]

The clinical manifestations of cryptococcosis in SOT recipients (localized vs disseminated infection) and associated mortality are significantly impacted by the type of immunosuppressive regimen. A study by Husain and colleagues[55] showed that patients receiving tacrolimus-based regimens are at significantly lower risk of CNS infection (78% vs 11%; P = .001) and are more likely to have localized forms of disease (66% vs 21%; P = .006) in comparison with patients receiving non–tacrolimus-based regimens. Singh and colleagues[61] further showed that use of a calcineurin inhibitor (CNI)-based regimen is independently associated with lower mortality (adjusted HR 0.21; P = .008). The protective effect of CNI is attributed to inhibition of binding between cryptococcal protein CB1 and calcineurin.[62] Among CNIs, tacrolimus, which has better penetration of the blood-brain barrier, has been shown associated with lower risk of CNS cryptococcosis in comparison with cyclosporine (11% vs 67%; P = .04).[55] The same study showed the impact of immunosuppressive type on mortality, which was lowest among those who received tacrolimus versus cyclosporine versus azathioprine with mycophenolate mofetil (7.9% vs 20% vs 40%; P = .004).[61] Type of transplant also has an impact on clinical manifestations and mortality in cryptococcosis. It is well established that patients with liver cirrhosis are at higher risk of cryptococcosis.[63–65] The unique risk of cryptococcosis in patients with liver cirrhosis has been attributed to intrinsic immune defects, including impaired chemotaxis and hepatic iron overload.[66,67] After transplantation, the LT recipients remain at significantly higher risk of disseminated cryptococcosis, a risk that is independent of the type of immunosuppression (adjusted HR 6.65; P = .048).[61] LT recipients are also at higher risk of early-onset cryptococcosis (≤12 months of transplant) in comparison with non-LT transplants.[55]

Cryptococcus gattii—An Emerging Pathogen in the United States

Pathogenic cryptococci are divided into 4 capsular serotypes (A, B, C, and D). Cryptococcus gattii comprises serotypes B and C. C gattii has been known as a pathogen in the tropical and subtropical areas of the world for many years but is now also recognized as an emerging pathogen in the Pacific Northwest (PNW) of Canada and the United States.[68,69] Molecular subtyping categorizes *Cryptococcus gattii* into 4 genotypes: VGI to VGIV. Genotype VGII is further subdivided into VGIIa, VGIIb, and VGIIc. *Cryptococcus gattii* VGII has been identified as the most common molecular type in the PNW outbreak.[70] Cases of animal and human infection due to *Cryptococcus gattii* were first recognized in the PNW on Vancouver Island, British Columbia, in 2000. In 2004, the first case of human infection was identified in the United States in Oregon, followed by 13 more cases from 2005 to 2007.[68,69,71] Since 2008, there has been an ongoing joint collaborative effort for active surveillance of *Cryptococcus gattii* infection between British Columbia and the United States, which has contributed significantly to knowledge about this infection.[68,71]

Since recognition of the PNW outbreak, several studies have described clinical manifestations with an attempt to identify key differences between *Cryptococcus gattii* and *Cryptococcus neoformans*.[69,72–75] Key characteristics of *Cryptococcus gattii* infections identified in the PNW outbreak include infection in the immunocompromised host in up to half of the cases (38%–55%),[75,76] tendency to present as a mass lesion (cryptococcoma) more commonly than *Cryptococcus neoformans*,[72,74,75,77] and reduced in vitro susceptibility to antifungal agents.[73,78,79] A comprehensive review of clinical features of all the cases identified in the United States from 2004 to 2011 is provided by Harris and colleagues.[75] Most of these infections (83/96) occurred in persons with a history of travel or residence in the PNW and majority (78/83) were identified as molecular subtype VGII (outbreak strain).[75] Patients with infection not acquired in the PNW were found to have other molecular subtypes (nonoutbreak strain). The study revealed that persons with the infections due to the outbreak strain in comparison with the nonoutbreak stain are more likely to present with respiratory symptoms (38/51 vs 4/11; $P = .03$) and are less likely to present with CNS symptoms (15/41 and 9/10; $P = .008$). The outbreak strain seemed to cause infection more frequently in those with preexisting conditions compared with nonoutbreak strains (47/55 vs 4/13; $P<.0001$); and use of oral steroids in the past year was independently associated with increased risk of mortality (OR 7.1; 95% CI, 1.01–49.3; $P = .048$).[75] Overall, 91% of patients requiring hospitalization and infections were associated with a case fatality ratio of 33%.[75]

Data specific to SOT were published in 2015 by Forrest and colleagues,[73] who reviewed the cases of *Cryptococcus gattii* reported in Oregon with focus on clinical features and outcome in the transplant host. In this series, 11 of 62 patients were SOT recipients. The median post-transplant time to infection was 17.8 months (1 month to 15 years). Six of 11 patients were reported to have disseminated infection, including fungemia and CNS disease.[73] Findings that were seen more commonly among SOT recipients in comparison with non-SOT included radiographic abnormalities on lung imaging (90% vs 5%; $P<.001$) and leptomeningeal enhancement on brain imaging (70% vs 7%; $P = .002$). Cryptococcoma presenting as brain and lung masses were seen more commonly among the non-SOT patients.[73] The median CSF cryptococcal antigen titer was lower among the SOT than the non-SOT cases (1:8 vs 1:1012; $P<.034$), although the difference between serum cryptococcal antigen titer was not statistically different.[73] As reported previously, MIC to fluconazole was elevated for most isolates ranging from 2 μg/mL to 32 μg/mL. Overall, there were 8 deaths in the SOT-group compared with none in the non-SOT group; 90-day mortality among SOT patients was 36%, which as Forrest and colleagues[73] concluded, is significantly higher that the reported mortality for cryptococcosis in SOT (14%).

In a review of current literature on *Cryptococcus gattii*, available data on epidemiology of this outbreak are limited by the fact that most clinical microbiology laboratories do not perform routine subtyping of isolates to species level. Therefore, the reported incidence is likely an underestimation due to misdiagnosis of clinical isolates as *Cryptococcus neoformans*. Also, although there seems reduced susceptibility to antifungal agents on in vitro testing, the clinical significance of this finding is not known because testing methodology is not standardized between laboratories and currently there are no CLSI breakpoints for interpretation.[69,71] Nevertheless, there is a possibility of antifungal resistance especially to fluconazole in the management of *Cryptococcus gattii* cases. Another fact that has come to light through recent studies is that *Cryptococcus gattii*, which was initially believed a pathogen solely of the immunocompetent host, in reality causes disease across a wider spectrum of hosts, including those with HIV and SOT.[73] Although HIV is an uncommon risk factor for *Cryptococcus gattii* (in comparison with *Cryptococcus neoformans*), it is by no means insignificant. As in the review by Harris and colleagues,[75] HIV was present as a risk factor in 5% of the overall cohort with *Cryptococcus gattii* infection and 55% had some form of immunocompromise. Similarly, 38% of the cases in the BC cohort were reported to have some form of immunocompromise.[77]

Cryptococcus-Associated Immune Reconstitution Syndrome

Immune reconstitution syndrome (IRIS) in SOT recipients has been most well described with cryptococcosis. In prospective studies of cryptococcosis in SOT recipients, IRIS was observed in 4.8% to 14% of the patients occurring at a median of 5.5 weeks from time of initiation of antifungal therapy.[80–82] Patients on tacrolimus, mycophenolate mofetil, and prednisone seem at higher risk of IRIS than those who are on other immunosuppressive regimens (4/4 vs 21/83; $P = .007$).[82] Shortly after the initial reports of IRIS in SOT recipients with cryptococcosis, the impact of IRIS on allograft function was realized.[81] In this study of 54 KT recipients with cryptococcosis, a higher incidence of graft loss due to chronic allograft rejection was seen among those with IRIS versus those who did not have IRIS (66% vs 5.9%; $P = .012$,[81] and 15.4% vs 2.6%; $P = .07$).[80]

The critical role of host $CD4^+$ helper T cells (T_H) in the cell-mediated immune response against cryptococcosis is well established.[83] T_H1 response is proinflammatory whereas T_H2 response is characterized as anti-inflammatory. Cryptococcus acts as a mitogen and a potent stimulator of T cells.[84,85] Furthermore, cryptococcus preferentially stimulates T_H2, which suppresses inflammation, weakens host defenses, and aids disease progression.[86–90] Immunosuppressive agents like tacrolimus have the same effect as cryptococcosis with a predominant T_H2 cytokine response.[87,91–93] After initiation of antifungal therapy and withdrawal of immunosuppression, the T_H1-T_H2 ratio is reversed, which leads to a predominant T_H1-based proinflammatory cytokine response. These immunologic changes promote inflammation, which forms the basis of IRIS and allograft loss associated with it.[81,82,87]

IRIS remains a clinical entity because there are no established biomarkers for diagnosis. Heightened awareness among transplant practitioners, therefore, is necessary for timely recognition and management. There are no studies to guide treatment and most of the published data describes clinical experience with management of IRIS in HIV/AIDS patients. Based on existing data and clinical experience, transplant infectious diseases experts have recommended treatment of IRIS with a prolonged steroid taper over 6 weeks to 8 weeks.[94] It is also recommended that in SOT recipients on treatment of cryptococcosis, withdrawal of immunosuppression be gradual and spaced out in relation to time of initiation of antifungal therapy to reduce the risk of IRIS.[94] In regard to this, data on CNIs are noteworthy. Discontinuation of CNI has been identified as an independent risk factor for IRIS in SOT recipients with cryptococcosis with an associated 5-fold increase in the risk of IRIS (adjusted OR 5.11; P = .02).[80] This observation is strengthened by in vitro data on antifungal properties of CNI, including inhibition of binding between cryptococcal protein CB1 and calcineurin,[62] and the presence of synergism with antifungals against cryptococcal isolates.[95] In addition to the impact of CNI discontinuation on IRIS, data have shown that SOT recipients with CNS cryptococcosis carry a higher risk of IRIS.[80] In patients with HIV/AIDS, paucity of inflammation in the CSF at the time of cryptococcal meningitis diagnosis has been associated with higher risk of IRIS but whether this is true for non-HIV patients is not clear.[96] γ-Interferon has been used for treatment of cryptococcal IRIS but data are limited to a few case reports of its use in management in HIV/AIDS, SOT recipients, and patients with other cell-mediated immune deficiencies.[97–99] Until there are more definitive data on this area, the risk of allograft rejection with γ-interferon must be weighed against the benefits of such therapy in each case.

SUMMARY

IC remains the most common IFI in SOT recipients. The risk factors for IC have evolved over the past several years with reduced impact of operative variables; which is in correlation with advancement in transplantation practices. Infection due to candida species is more common in thoracic transplant recipients than commonly perceived, and risk factors for IC in this population remain poorly understood. Impact of widespread universal fluconazole prophylaxis on emergence of resistant species must be better recognized and institutions should use targeted antifungal prophylaxis for high risk patients. Emergence of drug-resistant (potentially pan-resistant) novel species like *C auris* is alarming. Health care practitioners need to be aware of the predilection of *C auris* toward immunosuppressed hosts, such as SOT recipients; tendency to cause infection in the nosocomial setting; and associated diagnostic and therapeutic challenges. Transplant institutions should contact their local health department for help with species confirmation and drug-susceptibility testing in suspected cases. Cryptococcus remains a pathogen associated with significant morbidity and mortality in SOT recipients. Disseminated infection and renal failure are associated with increased mortality whereas CNI-based regimens are associated with localized infection and reduced mortality. *Cryptococcus gattii* is an emerging pathogen in SOT recipients, which should be considered in cases of cryptococcosis with travel to or residence in the PNW of Canada and the United States. Infection due to *Cryptococcus gattii* might be associated with reduced susceptibility to antifungal agents although the true significance of this finding is at this time unclear. Cryptococcosis-associated IRIS remains a clinical entity and heightened awareness is necessary for timely diagnosis and management. Discontinuation of CNI is associated with significant increase in risk of IRIS, and data on optimal treatment are lacking and guidance is based only on expert opinion.

REFERENCES

1. Pappas PG, Alexander BD, Andes DR, et al. Invasive fungal infections among organ transplant recipients: results of the Transplant-Associated Infection Surveillance Network (TRANSNET). Clin Infect Dis 2010;50(8):1101–11.
2. Silveira FP, Kusne S. Candida infections in solid organ transplantation. Am J Transplant 2013;13(Suppl 4):220–7.
3. Andes DR, Safdar N, Baddley JW, et al. The epidemiology and outcomes of invasive Candida infections among organ transplant recipients in the United States:

results of the Transplant-Associated Infection Surveillance Network (TRANSNET). Transpl Infect Dis 2016;18(6):921–31.

4. De Pauw B, Walsh TJ, Donnelly JP, et al. Revised definitions of invasive fungal disease from the European Organization for Research and Treatment of Cancer/Invasive Fungal Infections Cooperative Group and the National Institute of Allergy and Infectious Diseases Mycoses Study Group (EORTC/MSG) Consensus Group. Clin Infect Dis 2008;46(12):1813–21.

5. Collins LA, Samore MH, Roberts MS, et al. Risk factors for invasive fungal infections complicating orthotopic liver transplantation. J Infect Dis 1994;170(3):644–52.

6. Husain S, Tollemar J, Dominguez EA, et al. Changes in the spectrum and risk factors for invasive candidiasis in liver transplant recipients: prospective, multicenter, case-controlled study. Transplantation 2003;75(12):2023–9.

7. Lichtenstern C, Hochreiter M, Zehnter VD, et al. Pretransplant model for end stage liver disease score predicts posttransplant incidence of fungal infections after liver transplantation. Mycoses 2013;56(3):350–7.

8. Raghuram A, Restrepo A, Safadjou S, et al. Invasive fungal infections following liver transplantation: incidence, risk factors, survival, and impact of fluconazole-resistant Candida parapsilosis (2003-2007). Liver Transpl 2012;18(9):1100–9.

9. Saliba F, Delvart V, Ichai P, et al. Fungal infections after liver transplantation: outcomes and risk factors revisited in the MELD era. Clin Transplant 2013;27(4):E454–61.

10. Singh N, Wagener MM, Marino IR, et al. Trends in invasive fungal infections in liver transplant recipients: correlation with evolution in transplantation practices. Transplantation 2002;73(1):63–7.

11. Hadley S, Samore MH, Lewis WD, et al. Major infectious complications after orthotopic liver transplantation and comparison of outcomes in patients receiving cyclosporine or FK506 as primary immunosuppression. Transplantation 1995; 59(6):851–9.

12. Shi SH, Lu AW, Shen Y, et al. Spectrum and risk factors for invasive candidiasis and non-Candida fungal infections after liver transplantation. Chin Med J 2008; 121(7):625–30.

13. Karchmer AW, Samore MH, Hadley S, et al. Fungal infections complicating orthotopic liver transplantation. Trans Am Clin Climatol Assoc 1995;106:38–47 [discussion: 47–8].

14. Florescu DF, Islam KM, Grant W, et al. Incidence and outcome of fungal infections in pediatric small bowel transplant recipients. Transpl Infect Dis 2010;12(6): 497–504.

15. van Hal SJ, Marriott DJ, Chen SC, et al. Candidemia following solid organ transplantation in the era of antifungal prophylaxis: the Australian experience. Transpl Infect Dis 2009;11(2):122–7.

16. Benedetti E, Gruessner AC, Troppmann C, et al. Intra-abdominal fungal infections after pancreatic transplantation: incidence, treatment, and outcome. J Am Coll Surg 1996;183(4):307–16.

17. Fontana I, Bertocchi M, Diviacco P, et al. Infections after simultaneous pancreas and kidney transplantation: a single-center experience. Transplant Proc 2009; 41(4):1333–5.

18. Herrero-Martinez JM, Lumbreras C, Manrique A, et al. Epidemiology, risk factors and impact on long-term pancreatic function of infection following pancreas-kidney transplantation. Clin Microbiol Infect 2013;19(12):1132–9.

19. Rostambeigi N, Kudva YC, John S, et al. Epidemiology of infections requiring hospitalization during long-term follow-up of pancreas transplantation. Transplantation 2010;89(9):1126–33.

20. Rabin AS, Givertz MM, Couper GS, et al. Risk factors for invasive fungal disease in heart transplant recipients. J Heart Lung Transplant 2015;34(2):227–32.

21. Echenique IA, Angarone MP, Gordon RA, et al. Invasive fungal infection after heart transplantation: a 7-year, single-center experience. Transpl Infect Dis 2017;19(1):1–11.

22. Tissot F, Pascual M, Hullin R, et al. Impact of targeted antifungal prophylaxis in heart transplant recipients at high risk for early invasive fungal infection. Transplantation 2014;97(11):1192–7.

23. Berenger BM, Doucette K, Smith SW. Epidemiology and risk factors for nosocomial bloodstream infections in solid organ transplants over a 10-year period. Transpl Infect Dis 2016;18(2):183–90.

24. Horvath J, Dummer S, Loyd J, et al. Infection in the transplanted and native lung after single lung transplantation. Chest 1993;104(3):681–5.

25. Palmer SM, Perfect JR, Howell DN, et al. Candidal anastomotic infection in lung transplant recipients: successful treatment with a combination of systemic and inhaled antifungal agents. J Heart Lung Transplant 1998;17(10):1029–33.

26. Avery RK. Antifungal prophylaxis in lung transplantation. Semin Respir Crit Care Med 2011;32(6):717–26.

27. Dowling RD, Baladi N, Zenati M, et al. Disruption of the aortic anastomosis after heart-lung transplantation. Ann Thorac Surg 1990;49(1):118–22.

28. Mead L, Danziger-Isakov LA, Michaels MG, et al. Antifungal prophylaxis in pediatric lung transplantation: an international multicenter survey. Pediatr Transplant 2014;18(4):393–7.

29. Pilarczyk K, Haake N, Heckmann J, et al. Is universal antifungal prophylaxis mandatory in adults after lung transplantation? A review and meta-analysis of observational studies. Clin Transplant 2016;30(12):1522–31.

30. Pfaller MA, Andes DR, Diekema DJ, et al. Epidemiology and outcomes of invasive candidiasis due to non-albicans species of Candida in 2,496 patients: data from the Prospective Antifungal Therapy (PATH) registry 2004-2008. PLoS One 2014; 9(7):e101510.

31. Trick WE, Fridkin SK, Edwards JR, et al. Secular trend of hospital-acquired candidemia among intensive care unit patients in the United States during 1989-1999. Clin Infect Dis 2002;35(5):627–30.

32. Pfaller MA, Diekema DJ, Gibbs DL, et al. Results from the ARTEMIS DISK Global Antifungal Surveillance Study, 1997 to 2007: a 10.5-year analysis of susceptibilities of Candida Species to fluconazole and voriconazole as determined by CLSI standardized disk diffusion. J Clin Microbiol 2010;48(4):1366–77.

33. Lockhart SR, Wagner D, Iqbal N, et al. Comparison of in vitro susceptibility characteristics of Candida species from cases of invasive candidiasis in solid organ and stem cell transplant recipients: Transplant-Associated Infections Surveillance Network (TRANSNET), 2001 to 2006. J Clin Microbiol 2011;49(7):2404–10.

34. Vallabhaneni S, Kallen A, Tsay S, et al. Investigation of the first seven reported cases of Candida auris, a Globally Emerging Invasive, Multidrug-Resistant Fungus-United States, May 2013-August 2016. Am J Transplant 2017;17(1):296–9.

35. Satoh K, Makimura K, Hasumi Y, et al. Candida auris sp. nov., a novel ascomycetous yeast isolated from the external ear canal of an inpatient in a Japanese hospital. Microbiol Immunol 2009;53(1):41–4.

36. CDC. Clinical Alert to U.S. Healthcare Facilities - June 2016. Global Emergence of Invasive Infections Caused by the Multidrug-Resistant Yeast Candida auris. Available at: https://wwwcdcgov/fungal/diseases/candidiasis/candida-auris-alerthtml. Accessed January 11, 2018.

37. Azar MM, Turbett SE, Fishman JA, et al. Donor-derived transmission of Candida auris during lung transplantation. Clin Infect Dis 2017;65(6):1040–2.

38. Saliba F, Pascher A, Cointault O, et al. Randomized trial of micafungin for the prevention of invasive fungal infection in high-risk liver transplant recipients. Clin Infect Dis 2015;60(7):997–1006.

39. Sun HY, Cacciarelli TV, Singh N. Micafungin versus amphotericin B lipid complex for the prevention of invasive fungal infections in high-risk liver transplant recipients. Transplantation 2013;96(6):573–8.

40. Winston DJ, Limaye AP, Pelletier S, et al. Randomized, double-blind trial of anidulafungin versus fluconazole for prophylaxis of invasive fungal infections in high-risk liver transplant recipients. Am J Transplant 2014;14(12):2758–64.

41. Winston DJ, Pakrasi A, Busuttil RW. Prophylactic fluconazole in liver transplant recipients. A randomized, double-blind, placebo-controlled trial. Ann Intern Med 1999;131(10):729–37.

42. Giannella M, Bartoletti M, Morelli M, et al. Antifungal prophylaxis in liver transplant recipients: one size does not fit all. Transpl Infect Dis 2016;18(4):538–44.

43. Pappas PG, Andes D, Schuster M, et al. Invasive fungal infections in low-risk liver transplant recipients: a multi-center prospective observational study. Am J Transplant 2006;6(2):386–91.

44. Singh N, Wagener MM, Cacciarelli TV, et al. Antifungal management practices in liver transplant recipients. Am J Transplant 2008;8(2):426–31.

45. Owens NJ, Nightingale CH, Schweizer RT, et al. Prophylaxis of oral candidiasis with clotrimazole troches. Arch Intern Med 1984;144(2):290–3.

46. Gombert ME, duBouchet L, Aulicino TM, et al. A comparative trial of clotrimazole troches and oral nystatin suspension in recipients of renal transplants. Use in prophylaxis of oropharyngeal candidiasis. JAMA 1987;258(18):2553–5.

47. Ruskin JD, Wood RP, Bailey MR, et al. Comparative trial of oral clotrimazole and nystatin for oropharyngeal candidiasis prophylaxis in orthotopic liver transplant patients. Oral Surg Oral Med Oral Pathol 1992;74(5):567–71.

48. Dummer JS, Lazariashvilli N, Barnes J, et al. A survey of anti-fungal management in lung transplantation. J Heart Lung Transplant 2004;23(12):1376–81.

49. Munoz P, Valerio M, Palomo J, et al. Targeted antifungal prophylaxis in heart transplant recipients. Transplantation 2013;96(7):664–9.

50. Patel TS, Eschenauer GA, Stuckey LJ, et al. Antifungal prophylaxis in lung transplant recipients. Transplantation 2016;100(9):1815–26.

51. Winston DJ, Busuttil RW, Singh N. Antifungal prophylaxis in liver transplant recipients. Clin Infect Dis 2015;15:1349–50.

52. Huprikar S. Revisiting antifungal prophylaxis in high-risk liver transplant recipients. Am J Transplant 2014;14(12):2683–4.

53. Neofytos D, Fishman JA, Horn D, et al. Epidemiology and outcome of invasive fungal infections in solid organ transplant recipients. Transpl Infect Dis 2010; 12(3):220–9.

54. George IA, Santos CAQ, Olsen MA, et al. Epidemiology of cryptococcosis and cryptococcal meningitis in a large retrospective cohort of patients after solid organ transplantation. Open Forum Infect Dis 2017;4(1):ofx004.

55. Husain S, Wagener MM, Singh N. Cryptococcus neoformans infection in organ transplant recipients: variables influencing clinical characteristics and outcome. Emerg Infect Dis 2001;7(3):375–81.

56. Sun HY, Alexander BD, Lortholary O, et al. Unrecognized pretransplant and donor-derived cryptococcal disease in organ transplant recipients. Clin Infect Dis 2010;51(9):1062–9.

57. Saha DC, Goldman DL, Shao X, et al. Serologic evidence for reactivation of cryptococcosis in solid-organ transplant recipients. Clin Vaccine Immunol 2007; 14(12):1550–4.

58. Kapoor A, Flechner SM, O'Malley K, et al. Cryptococcal meningitis in renal transplant patients associated with environmental exposure. Transpl Infect Dis 1999; 1(3):213–7.

59. Baddley JW, Forrest GN. Cryptococcosis in solid organ transplantation. Am J Transplant 2013;13(Suppl 4):242–9.

60. Nosanchuk JD, Shoham S, Fries BC, et al. Evidence of zoonotic transmission of Cryptococcus neoformans from a pet cockatoo to an immunocompromised patient. Ann Intern Med 2000;132(3):205–8.

61. Singh N, Alexander BD, Lortholary O, et al. Cryptococcus neoformans in organ transplant recipients: impact of calcineurin-inhibitor agents on mortality. J Infect Dis 2007;195(5):756–64.

62. Gorlach J, Fox DS, Cutler NS, et al. Identification and characterization of a highly conserved calcineurin binding protein, CBP1/calcipressin, in Cryptococcus neoformans. EMBO J 2000;19(14):3618–29.

63. Baddley JW, Perfect JR, Oster RA, et al. Pulmonary cryptococcosis in patients without HIV infection: factors associated with disseminated disease. Eur J Clin Microbiol Infect Dis 2008;27(10):937–43.

64. Jean SS, Fang CT, Shau WY, et al. Cryptococcaemia: clinical features and prognostic factors. QJM 2002;95(8):511–8.

65. Lin YY, Shiau S, Fang CT. Risk factors for invasive Cryptococcus neoformans diseases: a case-control study. PLoS One 2015;10(3):e0119090.

66. DeMeo AN, Andersen BR. Defective chemotaxis associated with a serum inhibitor in cirrhotic patients. N Engl J Med 1972;286(14):735–40.

67. Alexander J, Limaye AP, Ko CW, et al. Association of hepatic iron overload with invasive fungal infection in liver transplant recipients. Liver Transplant 2006; 12(12):1799–804.

68. Center of Disease Control and Prevention. Emergence of Cryptococcus gattii– Pacific Northwest, 2004-2010. Am J Transplant 2011;11(9):1989–92.

69. Datta K, Bartlett KH, Baer R, et al. Spread of Cryptococcus gattii into Pacific Northwest region of the United States. Emerg Infect Dis 2009;15(8):1185–91.

70. Byrnes EJ 3rd, Bildfell RJ, Frank SA, et al. Molecular evidence that the range of the Vancouver Island outbreak of Cryptococcus gattii infection has expanded into the Pacific Northwest in the United States. J Infect Dis 2009;199(7):1081–6.

71. Dixit A, Carroll SF, Qureshi ST. Cryptococcus gattii: an emerging cause of fungal disease in North America. Interdiscip Perspect Infect Dis 2009;2009:840452.

72. Chen S, Sorrell T, Nimmo G, et al. Epidemiology and host- and variety-dependent characteristics of infection due to Cryptococcus neoformans in Australia and New Zealand. Australasian Cryptococcal Study Group. Clin Infect Dis 2000; 31(2):499–508.

73. Forrest GN, Bhalla P, DeBess EE, et al. Cryptococcus gattii infection in solid organ transplant recipients: description of Oregon outbreak cases. Transpl Infect Dis 2015;17(3):467–76.

74. Grosse P, Tintelnot K, Sollner O, et al. Encephalomyelitis due to Cryptococcus neoformans var gattii presenting as spinal tumour: case report and review of the literature. J Neurol Neurosurg Psychiatry 2001;70(1):113–6.

75. Harris JR, Lockhart SR, Debess E, et al. Cryptococcus gattii in the United States: clinical aspects of infection with an emerging pathogen. Clin Infect Dis 2011; 53(12):1188–95.

76. MacDougall L, Fyfe M, Romney M, et al. Risk factors for Cryptococcus gattii infection, British Columbia, Canada. Emerg Infect Dis 2011;17(2):193–9.
77. Galanis E, Macdougall L, Kidd S, et al. Epidemiology of Cryptococcus gattii, British Columbia, Canada, 1999-2007. Emerg Infect Dis 2010;16(2):251–7.
78. Chen YC, Chang SC, Shih CC, et al. Clinical features and in vitro susceptibilities of two varieties of Cryptococcus neoformans in Taiwan. Diagn Microbiol Infect Dis 2000;36(3):175–83.
79. Khan ZU, Randhawa HS, Kowshik T, et al. Antifungal susceptibility of Cryptococcus neoformans and Cryptococcus gattii isolates from decayed wood of trunk hollows of Ficus religiosa and Syzygium cumini trees in north-western India. J Antimicrob Chemother 2007;60(2):312–6.
80. Sun HY, Alexander BD, Huprikar S, et al. Predictors of immune reconstitution syndrome in organ transplant recipients with cryptococcosis: implications for the management of immunosuppression. Clin Infect Dis 2015;60(1):36–44.
81. Singh N, Lortholary O, Alexander BD, et al. Allograft loss in renal transplant recipients with cryptococcus neoformans associated immune reconstitution syndrome. Transplantation 2005;80(8):1131–3.
82. Singh N, Lortholary O, Alexander BD, et al. An immune reconstitution syndrome-like illness associated with Cryptococcus neoformans infection in organ transplant recipients. Clin Infect Dis 2005;40(12):1756–61.
83. Kawakami K. Regulation by innate immune T lymphocytes in the host defense against pulmonary infection with Cryptococcus neoformans. Jpn J Infect Dis 2004;57(4):137–45.
84. Mody CH, Wood CJ, Syme RM, et al. The cell wall and membrane of Cryptococcus neoformans possess a mitogen for human T lymphocytes. Infect Immun 1999;67(2):936–41.
85. Mody CH, Sims KL, Wood CJ, et al. Proteins in the cell wall and membrane of Cryptococcus neoformans stimulate lymphocytes from both adults and fetal cord blood to proliferate. Infect Immun 1996;64(11):4811–9.
86. Vecchiarelli A, Retini C, Monari C, et al. Purified capsular polysaccharide of Cryptococcus neoformans induces interleukin-10 secretion by human monocytes. Infect Immun 1996;64(7):2846–9.
87. Sun HY, Singh N. Opportunistic infection-associated immune reconstitution syndrome in transplant recipients. Clin Infect Dis 2011;53(2):168–76.
88. Retini C, Vecchiarelli A, Monari C, et al. Capsular polysaccharide of Cryptococcus neoformans induces proinflammatory cytokine release by human neutrophils. Infect Immun 1996;64(8):2897–903.
89. Lortholary O, Sitbon K, Dromer F. Evidence for human immunodeficiency virus and Cryptococcus neoformans interactions in the pro-inflammatory and anti-inflammatory responses in blood during AIDS-associated cryptococcosis. Clin Microbiol Infect 2005;11(4):296–300.
90. Chaka W, Heyderman R, Gangaidzo I, et al. Cytokine profiles in cerebrospinal fluid of human immunodeficiency virus-infected patients with cryptococcal meningitis: no leukocytosis despite high interleukin-8 levels. University of Zimbabwe Meningitis Group. J Infect Dis 1997;176(6):1633–6.
91. Ferraris JR, Tambutti ML, Cardoni RL, et al. Conversion from cyclosporine A to tacrolimus in pediatric kidney transplant recipients with chronic rejection: changes in the immune responses. Transplantation 2004;77(4):532–7.
92. Spencer CM, Goa KL, Gillis JC. Tacrolimus. An update of its pharmacology and clinical efficacy in the management of organ transplantation. Drugs 1997;54(6):925–75.

93. Thomson AW, Bonham CA, Zeevi A. Mode of action of tacrolimus (FK506): molecular and cellular mechanisms. Ther Drug Monit 1995;17(6):584–91.
94. Singh N, Perfect JR. Immune reconstitution syndrome associated with opportunistic mycoses. Lancet Infect Dis 2007;7(6):395–401.
95. Kontoyiannis DP, Lewis RE, Alexander BD, et al. Calcineurin inhibitor agents interact synergistically with antifungal agents in vitro against Cryptococcus neoformans isolates: correlation with outcome in solid organ transplant recipients with cryptococcosis. Antimicrob Agents Chemother 2008;52(2):735–8.
96. Boulware DR, Bonham SC, Meya DB, et al. Paucity of initial cerebrospinal fluid inflammation in cryptococcal meningitis is associated with subsequent immune reconstitution inflammatory syndrome. J Infect Dis 2010;202(6):962–70.
97. Netea MG, Brouwer AE, Hoogendoorn EH, et al. Two patients with cryptococcal meningitis and idiopathic CD4 lymphopenia: defective cytokine production and reversal by recombinant interferon- gamma therapy. Clin Infect Dis 2004;39(9):e83–7.
98. Pappas PG, Bustamante B, Ticona E, et al. Recombinant interferon- gamma 1b as adjunctive therapy for AIDS-related acute cryptococcal meningitis. J Infect Dis 2004;189(12):2185–91.
99. Summers SA, Dorling A, Boyle JJ, et al. Cure of disseminated cryptococcal infection in a renal allograft recipient after addition of gamma-interferon to anti-fungal therapy. Am J Transplant 2005;5(8):2067–9.

Endemic Mycoses in Solid Organ Transplant Recipients

Jeremy S. Nel, MD, Luther A. Bartelt, MD, David van Duin, MD, PhD,
Anne M. Lachiewicz, MD, MPH*

KEYWORDS

- Solid organ transplant • Endemic mycoses • Histoplasmosis • Blastomycosis
- Coccidioidomycosis

KEY POINTS

- Endemic mycoses are thermally dimorphic fungal pathogens occupying a specific geographic range.
- Histoplasmosis, coccidioidomycosis, and blastomycosis are the chief endemic mycoses in North America.
- Infections with endemic mycoses are uncommon, but can cause serious infection in solid organ transplant recipients.

INTRODUCTION

The endemic mycoses are a group of thermally dimorphic fungal pathogens occupying a specific geographic range. This geographic restriction occurs as a result of the unique environmental requirements that best promote sporulation for each species. In North America, the chief endemic mycoses are histoplasmosis, coccidioidomycosis, and blastomycosis.

GENERAL PRINCIPLES

Although they can cause serious infections, all 3 endemic mycoses are surprisingly rare in solid organ transplant (SOT) recipients (**Table 1**).[1,2] A prospective study

Disclosure Statement: D. van Duin has served as a consultant for Allergan, Achaogen, Shionogi, Tetraphase, Sanofi-Pasteur, Medimmune, and Astellas, and has received research funding from Steris Inc and Scynexis. A.M. Lachiewicz has served as a consultant for Destum Partners and KPB Biosciences, and received research funding from GlaxoSmithKline. J.S. Nel and L.A. Bartelt have no disclosures.
Funding: This work is supported in part by the National Center for Advancing Translational Sciences, National Institutes of Health Grant KL2TR001109 (A.M. Lachiewicz) and National Institutes of Health National Institutes of Health National Institute of Allergy and Infectious Diseases Grant K08-AI108730 (L.A. Bartelt).
Division of Infectious Diseases, University of North Carolina, CB 7030, 130 Mason Farm Road, Chapel Hill, NC 27599, USA
* Corresponding author.
E-mail address: anne_lachiewicz@med.unc.edu

Infect Dis Clin N Am 32 (2018) 667–685
https://doi.org/10.1016/j.idc.2018.04.007
0891-5520/18/© 2018 Elsevier Inc. All rights reserved.

id.theclinics.com

Table 1
Endemic mycoses in SOT recipients

	Histoplasmosis	Blastomycosis	Coccidioidomycosis
Principle North American areas of endemicity	Ohio and Mississippi River Valley areas	Ohio, Mississippi and Tennessee River Valley areas, Great Lakes region	Southwest USA and Northern Mexico
Cases acquired through infected allograft	Yes	No	Yes
Typical clinical presentation	Disseminated disease typically involving lungs, bone marrow, liver and spleen	Severe pulmonary disease ± dissemination often involving skin	Disseminated disease typically involving lungs, skin, bone, joints, meninges
Severity of illness compared to immunocompetent patients	Increased	Increased	Increased
Typical histologic appearance	Small yeast, 2-5 μm in size, with narrow-based budding, often clustered within macrophages	Large yeast, 8–15 μm in size, with broad-based budding and a thick, refractile cell wall	Large (10–100 μm) unique structures called spherules, containing numerous endospores.
Role of antibody detection	Limited role, test insensitive	Insensitive, limited clinical usefulness	Moderately sensitive, but if positive generally indicates current or recent infection. EIA more sensitive but less specific than immunodiffusion tests.
Role of urine antigen detection	Highly sensitive test (≥93%)	Moderately sensitive test (76%–93%)	Relatively insensitive test (≤71%)
Mortality	~10%	~25-38%	~43-62%

Abbreviations: EIA, enzyme-linked immunoassay; SOT, solid organ transplantation.

performed in 15 transplant centers throughout the United States, including in high incidence areas, found only 33 cases of endemic mycoses among 16,806 patients who received a SOT during the 5-year study period; 23 were histoplasmosis, 6 were coccidioidomycosis, and 4 were blastomycosis.[1] By way of contrast, the incidence of invasive candidiasis in SOT recipients is approximately an order of magnitude higher.[3] The incidence of the endemic mycoses is typically greatest in the 12 months after transplant, but the risk period extends for years thereafter.[1,4–7]

Histoplasmosis, coccidioidomycosis, and blastomycosis are all caused by environmental, soil-based fungi that are acquired chiefly, although not exclusively, through inhalation of conidia that have been aerosolized as a result of disturbance of the soil in which they are produced.[8] The causative fungi are all thermally dimorphic, existing initially as a mold in the environment and then once in the body transforming themselves into either yeasts or, in the case of coccidioidomycosis, specialized structures called spherules.[8,9] The fungi typically establish themselves initially in the lung, although whether this is clinically apparent or not depends on a balance between the burden of disease and the state of the host immune system. Clinical disease can also occur when immunosuppression causes a loss of containment of a previously controlled infection, such as occurs from antirejection medication.[10,11] Dissemination of the fungus can occur throughout the body if the immune system is unable to control the infection within the lungs. In the case of histoplasmosis and coccidioidomycosis, rare cases of disease acquired by an infected allograft have also been described; there are no reports of this with blastomycosis to date.[1,12–15] There is typically a median of 2 weeks from symptoms onset until the diagnosis is ultimately made.[5,7] In general, SOT recipients have been found to have more severe disease and a higher disease-related mortality from the endemic mycoses than immunocompetent patients.[2–6]

Currently, no single diagnostic test has optimal sensitivity and specificity to reliably diagnose any of the endemic mycoses. Thus, in situations where histoplasmosis, blastomycosis, or coccidioidomycosis are considered, multiple different tests should be used. In general, microscopy, culture, antigen detection, and antibody assays are well-established for all the endemic mycoses, although with important differences in their limitations that vary by species. Polymerase chain reaction testing is less well-established and often not commercially available, but offers the potential to complement the existing diagnostic armamentarium.

The agents used for treatment of the endemic mycoses are the polyenes (with liposomal amphotericin B now preferred) and the azoles (chiefly itraconazole or fluconazole). In general, mild infections can be treated with an azole alone, but more severe and/or disseminated disease (as occurs frequently in SOT recipients) requires initial therapy with amphotericin B and transition to an azole once clinical improvement occurs.[16–18] Most SOT recipients with histoplasmosis, blastomycosis, and coccidioidomycosis generally require at least 12 months of treatment along with a temporary decrease in immunosuppression regimens if possible. A risk of recrudescence or relapse exists for all of the endemic mycoses. However, the role and benefit of secondary prophylaxis is unclear and much debated.

HISTOPLASMOSIS
Epidemiology

Mycelial growth in histoplasmosis is favored in soil in climates with moderate temperatures (between 15°C and 40°C), high relative humidity and a soil pH of greater than 5.5, although spores can survive for many years in less favorable environmental conditions.[19] Bird and bat guano provides a high nitrogen, phosphorus, and organic matter content that is especially advantageous for histoplasmosis' sporulation, allowing for mycelial growth even in the absence of soil.[20] Typical risk factors for histoplasmosis acquisition in endemic areas include spelunking, farming, cleaning up bird droppings, refurbishing buildings that have been inhabited by birds or bats, such as barns, or other activities that disturb the soil.[19,21]

In the United States, studies from the 1950s to the 1970s identified areas of endemicity on the basis of positive histoplasmin skin test reactivity. Within North America, these areas are centered around the Mississippi and Ohio River valleys (**Fig. 1**). Outside the United States, areas in Central and South America, and large parts of Africa and Australasia, are also considered endemic.[21,22] However, it is likely that histoplasmosis can at least occasionally be acquired from a much wider range of environments than previously thought, especially in immunocompromised hosts.[23,24]

Pathogenesis

Infection with *Histoplasma capsulatum* is typically acquired when aerosolized microconidia are inhaled, because these infectious particles are small enough to reach the alveoli.[10,21] Once in the lung, the microcondia transform into yeasts and are phagocytosed by macrophages, within which they initially proliferate and may be transported throughout the reticuloendothelial system. Approximately 1 to 2 weeks are required before sufficient Th1 cell-mediated immune response is generated to either kill or control the fungi in a quiescent state, driven by cytokines including interleukin-12, tumor necrosis factor-α, and interferon-γ.[25] This process may be impaired in SOT recipients. In addition, previous immunologic control of the fungus can be lost in patients who later receive immunosuppressant medication.[10]

Histoplasmosis in SOT recipients can thus be acquired in 1 of 2 main ways: as a new (primary) infection or via reactivation of a previously controlled infection. A surprisingly low baseline incidence in endemic areas (usually <0.5%) combined with dramatic

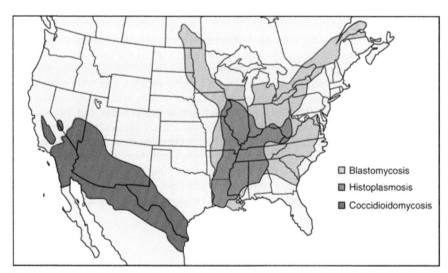

Fig. 1. Geographic distribution of endemic fungal infections in the North America. (*From* Ryan KJ. The systemic fungal pathogens: cryptococcus, histoplasma, blastomyces, coccidioides, paracoccidioides. In: Ryan KJ, editor. Sherris medical microbiology. 7th edition. New York: McGraw-Hill; 2018. p. 750; with permission.)

increases seen during community outbreaks argue that primary infection may be the dominant mode of acquisition.[5,26–28] Rarely, histoplasmosis can also rarely be transmitted via an infected allograft, although only a handful of confirmed cases of this have been published to date.[12,13]

Clinical Presentation

In hosts with intact immunity, histoplasmosis is usually confined to the lungs, with a diverse array of presentations, including acute and chronic pneumonias, isolated pulmonary nodules, fibrosing mediastinitis, and broncholithiasis. In SOT recipients, however, presentation is mostly that of progressive disseminated disease.[5,6,28] As may be expected from the pathogenesis of histoplasmosis, pulmonary involvement is extremely common (>80%, although this may be subclinical and detectable only on chest computed tomography scans), and thereafter the sites most likely to be involved are lymphoid-rich tissues: bone marrow, liver, spleen, and gastrointestinal tract.[5,28] Typical symptoms include fever, fatigue, nonproductive cough, and diarrhea, and typical signs include hepatomegaly, splenomegaly, lymphadenopathy, and sometimes oral ulcers. Central nervous system (CNS) disease (<10%) and skin (<5%) involvement seem to be relatively uncommon. Almost any site can ultimately be involved however; rare cases of histoplasmosis in SOT recipients are reported involving the adipose tissue and tonsils.[5,29] Patients can also present with an undifferentiated sepsis picture.

Diagnosis

No single test is sufficiently sensitive to reliably diagnose histoplasmosis in SOT recipients, so a strategy using multiple diagnostic modalities simultaneously is recommended (**Table 2**). The single most sensitive test is a urine *Histoplasma* antigen test, which is positive in approximately 93% of cases when the newer generation assays are used. The test's sensitivity correlates positively with disease severity.[6,30] However, the assay's specificity is limited by cross-reactions to antigens from *Blastomyces*, *Paracoccidioides*, and *Penicillium* species.[30–32] Blood, bone marrow, and bronchoalveolar lavage cultures are all moderately sensitive in disseminated disease, but typically take several weeks to become positive.[33] A bronchoscopic lung biopsy or cytology is positive in approximately three-quarters of cases.[6] *Histoplasma capsulatum's* distinctive histologic appearance is that of a yeast, 2 to 5 μm in size, with narrow-based budding, often clustered within macrophages.[34] The least sensitive test seems to be serum antibodies, with an overall sensitivity in SOT recipients of just 36% in 1 large series.[6] Of note, false-positive *Aspergillus galactomannan* results have been

Table 2
Approximate sensitivities of histoplasmosis diagnostic tests in solid-organ transplant recipients

Test	Approximate Sensitivity (%)
Urine antigen	≥93
Serum antigen	80
Antibody	35
Blood culture	50–70
Bronchoalveolar lavage culture	60–72
Lung biopsy or cytology	77

Data from Refs.[2,5,6,28,86]

reported in SOT recipients who had histoplasmosis.[35] This finding should be borne in mind in SOT patients from histoplasmosis-endemic areas.

Treatment

Even without clear evidence of dissemination, SOT recipients with histoplasmosis should generally be treated as if they have disseminated disease.[21] Liposomal amphotericin B is preferred over both itraconazole and amphotericin B deoxycholate for initial treatment in moderate and severe cases of disseminated disease.[16,36,37] Liposomal amphotericin B has a lower rate of associated toxicities than the deoxycholate form, and is also possibly more potent in disseminated histoplasmosis.[36] Liposomal amphotericin B should even be considered in cases complicated by renal disease despite the potential for additional nephrotoxicity; in many cases, as the disease comes under control, renal function improves rather than worsens.[21] Liposomal amphotericin B is generally given for 1 to 2 weeks, followed by oral itraconazole for at least a year (**Table 3**). All azoles have some activity in histoplasmosis, although posaconazole is possibly the best alternative to itraconazole in cases of drug intolerance or clinical failure.[21] Rising minimum inhibitory concentrations to both fluconazole and voriconazole have been observed while on therapy (whereas this has not been demonstrated with posaconazole), and there is limited clinical experience with isavuconazole.[38] There is no role for echinocandin therapy in histoplasmosis.[31]

Once the diagnosis of histoplasmosis is made, immunosuppressive medication should be reduced, although the optimal timing and strategy in this regard is unknown. Azole treatment can probably be stopped after 12 months if there is no evidence of active infection. Ideally, the urine and blood antigen tests should be negative by that point, although they may remain positive at a low level for years after clinical

Table 3
Typical therapeutic regimens for endemic fungi in SOT recipients

	Mild Disease	Severe Disease	CNS Disease
Histoplasmosis	Itraconazole 200 mg every 8 hours for 3 d and then twice daily for 12 mo	Liposomal amphotericin B (3 mg/kg) for 1–2 wk then itraconazole 200 mg twice daily for 12 mo	Liposomal amphotericin B (5 mg/kg) for 4–6 wk then itraconazole 200 mg twice daily for 12 mo
Blastomycosis	Itraconazole 200 mg every 8 hours for 3 d and then twice daily for 12 mo (but consider treating as for severe disease in all immunosuppressed patients)	Liposomal amphotericin B (3 mg/kg) for 1–2 wk then itraconazole 200 mg twice daily for 12 mo	Liposomal amphotericin B (5 mg/kg) for 4–6 wk then a triazole for 12 mo (optimal triazole unclear)
Coccidioidomycosis	Fluconazole 400 mg/d for at least 12 mo	Liposomal amphotericin B (5 mg/kg) for 1–2 wk then fluconazole 400 mg/d for at least 12 mo	Fluconazole 400–1200 mg/d, continued indefinitely

Abbreviations: CNS, central nervous system; SOT, solid organ transplantation.

resolution of disease. Therapy should not be prolonged merely because of this low-level antigenemia. After completion of treatment, long-term suppressive azole therapy in SOT recipients may be considered, but there is little evidence to endorse this practice, and the risk of disease relapse after completion of therapy is less than 5% when adequate initial therapy is given.[6] In addition, in high-risk patients (eg, patients in whom no significant reduction of immunosuppression was possible), relapses can be screened for by serial urine antigen testing.[16] Thus, chronic suppressive therapy may be unnecessary for the majority of SOT recipients.

Prognosis

The mortality from histoplasmosis acquired after SOT is approximately 10%.[1,6,28] In the largest study, 72% of the deaths occurred within 1 month after diagnosis, and on multivariate analysis those who died from histoplasmosis were statistically more likely to be older and to have had severe disease, as might be expected.[6]

BLASTOMYCOSIS

Epidemiology

A recent phylogenetic analysis has revealed that *Blastomyces dermatitidis,* the sole cause of blastomycosis, is in fact 2 distinct species, *B dermatitidis* and *Blastomyces gilchristii*.[39] The natural habitat of *Blastomyces* is largely unknown, partly because, unlike other dimorphic fungi, it is extremely difficult to culture the organism from soil samples. Interesting new phylogeographic work has found a strong association of blastomycosis with freshwater basins, which complements earlier findings that suggested that *Blastomyces* conidiophores required exposure to water before their conidia could be dispersed by air currents.[40,41] In North America, endemic regions seem to be the US and Canadian areas bordering the Mississippi, Ohio, Tennessee, and Nelson River drainage basins, and a small area in the northeast surrounding the St Lawrence River (see **Fig. 1**). A detailed history usually reveals occupational or recreational activities that have disrupted the soil in these regions, such as construction, boating, fishing, cutting trees, or clearing brush. As with all endemic mycoses, however, cases can occasionally be seen outside these endemic regions (see **Table 1**).[42]

Pathogenesis

In a similar manner to other endemic fungi, *Blastomyces* conidia must generally be inhaled to acquire the infection. Once inside the lung, the conidia transform into the yeast phase, and can survive within macrophages. Both innate and cell-mediated immunity play vital roles in controlling blastomycosis, whereas the humoral immune system plays no clear role.[43] Unlike histoplasmosis and coccidiomycosis, no cases of blastomycosis acquired via infected allograft have been reported.[1]

Clinical Presentation

In immunocompetent individuals, approximately one-half of blastomycosis infections are asymptomatic and, of the symptomatic cases, pulmonary infection occurs in approximately 80% and disseminated disease occurs in 25% to 40%—a far higher rate than seen with other endemic mycoses.[17,44] Interestingly, from the limited number of cases published to date, the chief difference in presentation among SOT recipients is not necessarily a greater propensity for disseminated disease, but rather more severe pulmonary disease, with a higher consequent mortality.[2,3,7] Lung involvement in SOT recipients more frequently progresses to acute respiratory distress syndrome and respiratory failure. In disseminated cases, the same typical sites are involved as with immunocompetent individuals. The skin is the most frequently involved extrapulmonary site, although multiple pustules or ulcers are more common than the classic verrucous lesions seen in immunocompetent patients.[45,46] Bone (lytic lesions), genitourinary (prostatitis or epididymitis), and CNS (meningitis or abscess) involvement are the next most common manifestations.

Diagnosis

Blastomycosis has a distinctive appearance on histologic specimens, namely that of a large yeast, 8 to 15 μm in size, with broad-based budding and a thick refractile cell wall.[34] This characteristic appearance permits a rapid diagnosis to be provisionally made directly from sputum, bronchoalveolar lavage specimens, and tissue biopsies. This property is especially useful considering the frequent involvement of the skin, which provides an easily accessible biopsy site. A definitive diagnosis requires culturing the organism, but like the other endemic fungi this usually takes 1 to 4 weeks. Blastomycosis antigen enzyme-linked immunoassay tests can be performed on urine, blood, and cerebrospinal fluid samples, with urine having the greatest sensitivity (76%–93%).[47,48] Like the urine histoplasmosis antigen test, this also suffers from a lack of specificity, principally owing to cross-reaction with other endemic fungi.[43,47] Unlike histoplasmosis and coccidiomycosis, commercially available serologic testing in blastomycosis has poor sensitivity and therefore little clinical usefulness.[49]

Treatment

In immunocompetent patients, milder non-CNS forms of blastomycosis may be treated entirely with an azole, typically itraconazole. However, because of the greater propensity for severe disease, it is recommended that blastomycosis cases in SOT recipients generally be treated with amphotericin B for 1 to 2 weeks initially, or until improvement is noted.[17,43] Thereafter, as with histoplasmosis, approximately 12 months of oral itraconazole should be given. Itraconazole is probably more efficacious than fluconazole, and considerably more clinical experience exists with itraconazole than with any other of the azoles in the treatment of blastomycosis (see **Table 3**).[50]

Prognosis

The limited numbers of cases of blastomycosis in SOT recipients reported in the literature makes assessing outcomes with any precision difficult, but mortality in SOT recipients with blastomycosis seems to be in the 35% to 38% range (although the rate directly attributable to blastomycosis itself is likely closer to 25%).[2,7] This mortality rate is higher than that seen in immunocompetent patients, though lower than seen in patients with malignancies or AIDS.[7]

COCCIDIODOMYCOSIS
Epidemiology

Coccidiodomycosis is caused by 1 of 2 species: *Coccidioides immitis* or *Coccidioides posadasii*.[51] Unlike *Histoplasma* and *Blastomyces*, *Coccidioides* is found exclusively within in hot, dry climates, in arid and semiarid soil.[52] Specifically, *Coccidioides* is found in the southwestern United States, in the San Joaquin Valley, southern California, Texas, Arizona, and New Mexico, together with northern Mexico and noncontiguous areas in South America (see **Fig. 1**).[53,54] *C immitis* is found predominantly within California and *C posadasii* is found in the remainder of the endemic areas in the Western hemisphere. Drought conditions are associated with a higher incidence of reported coccidioidomycosis the following year, possibly because *Coccidioides* is relatively more tolerant of such conditions than competing organisms, and because dry conditions favor spore distribution.[54] In endemic areas, sandstorms, military exercises, and outdoor construction work are recognized risk factors for disease acquisition.[55]

Pathogenesis

Maturing mycelial cells develop within the soil into arthroconidia, which are prone to be aerosolized by air currents or other disruptions of the soil. When inhaled, the arthroconidia form unique structures called spherules. Each of these develops to contain viable spores that can form further spherules when the original spherule ruptures, thereby quickly generating an exponential increase in fungal burden if unchecked. T-cell immunity is the principal form of control required for coccidioidomycosis, which may otherwise spread to extrapulmonary locations. Disseminated coccidioidomycosis is associated with a failure to generate an interferon-γ–led delayed-type hypersensitivity response to coccidioidal antigens.[56] In a similar manner to histoplasmosis and blastomycosis, coccidioidomycosis can either be acquired de novo or be reactivate from a dormant state if the patient loses prior immunologic control of the organism owing to immunosuppression.[11] Rarely, coccidioidomycosis can be transmitted via infected allograft.[14,15]

Clinical Manifestations

In immunocompetent hosts, approximately 60% of disease is asymptomatic and the vast majority of the remainder manifests as isolated pulmonary disease, with only less than 0.5% of patients having disseminated infection.[55] In immunocompromised hosts, such as SOT recipients, the rates of disease dissemination increase markedly, causing an increase in mortality and morbidity. Pulmonary disease mimics community-acquired pneumonia and can range from minimally symptomatic to fulminant disease. Apart from the lung, common sites for dissemination are the CNS, liver, spleen, kidney, skin, and joints.[4,57]

Diagnosis

The spherule is pathognomonic for coccidioidomycosis, and thus identification of it from any sample establishes the diagnosis. *Coccidioides* cultures readily on most media in approximately 1 week.[4] Laboratory personnel should be warned that coccidioidomycosis is suspected, because biocontainment procedures are required for safety when working with cultures. In tissue samples, spherules may be surrounded by either a granulomatous or a suppurative inflammatory response.[4] The sensitivity of serologic tests is lessened in SOT recipients, who may not mount as robust an antibody response.[4,58] Furthermore, a detectable serologic response may take 3 or more weeks to develop, causing false-negative results in early infection. However, because antibody levels generally decrease to undetectable levels with successful clearance of infection, a positive result typically represents either recent or active infection.[59] Overall, enzyme-linked immunoassays are more sensitive but less specific than immunodiffusion tests; thus, the immunodiffusion tests are often used as confirmation tests for positive enzyme-linked immunoassay results. Urine or serum antigen testing is insensitive but most likely to be positive in disseminated disease. Cross-reaction with *Histoplasma* antigen test occurs.[60,61]

Treatment

As with the treatment of other endemic fungi in SOT recipients, mild pulmonary forms of the disease can be treated with azoles alone, but severe or disseminated cases generally require intravenous amphotericin B therapy initially, followed by azole therapy for approximately 12 months (see **Table 3**). Fluconazole and itraconazole are the most commonly used azoles, with fluconazole generally being preferred on the basis of more reliable absorption and less severe drug–drug interactions. A randomized, controlled trial comparing the 2 azoles failed to find a statistically significant difference in clinical response or relapse rate between them, although there was a trend toward itraconazole superiority.[62]

Fluconazole is the recommended first-line treatment for CNS infections, in contrast with histoplasmosis and blastomycosis, where the initial treatment for infections involving the CNS should be with amphotericin B. Immunosuppression should be lessened when possible, at least until the infection has begun to improve.[59] The risk of recrudescent infection in SOT recipients with evidence of prior coccidioidomycosis may be substantial, and is far higher than seen with the other endemic mycoses.[4,57,59] Thus, patients with a history of coccidioidomycosis should receive preemptive therapy after transplantation. Many experts also tend to preemptively treat all SOT recipients in endemic areas, regardless of the evidence for prior coccidioidomycosis.[59] In either case, the usual duration of therapy is 6 to 12 months. Furthermore, after successful treatment of SOT recipients, indefinite secondary prophylaxis with fluconazole is often necessary for as long as the patient takes immunosuppressive medications, because the rate of relapse is otherwise unacceptably high.

Prognosis

Although heterogeneous, the mortality rate in SOT recipients who develop coccidioidomycosis is substantial, and higher than seen with the other endemic mycosis. Early reports from the 1980s showed mortality rates of up to 62%, and a large-scale study 2 decades later highlighted a 43% mortality attributable to coccidioidomycosis.[1,4] Mortality rates are higher with disseminated disease than localized pulmonary disease.

TREATMENT ISSUES IN SOLID ORGAN TRANSPLANT RECIPIENTS

The primary agents available to treat the endemic mycoses are amphotericin B and the triazole antifungals. The echinocandins have poor in vitro activity against the dimorphic fungi and should not be considered as treatment options for them.[16,17,59,63] Amphotericin B is only available intravenously, in either a deoxycholate or a liposomal form. When the drug is required, the liposomal formulation is preferred owing to its lower toxicity, particularly nephrotoxicity. In a randomized controlled trial of disseminated histoplasmosis in patients with AIDS, there was also a trend toward a higher clinical success rate and a lower mortality rate with the liposomal amphotericin B.[36] Common side effects include nephrotoxicity, hypokalemia, and hypomagnesemia, as well as infusion-related chills. Severe disease from the endemic mycoses is often accompanied by a degree of renal impairment, but renal dysfunction should not necessarily dissuade clinicians from using amphotericin B, because it is preferred over the azoles in most cases of severe disease.[16–18,21] Although the CNS penetration of amphotericin B is poor (<3%), amphotericin B has demonstrable efficacy and is recommended first-line therapy for meningitis in both histoplasmosis and blastomycosis, although not coccidioidomycosis.[16–18]

Of the triazoles, the bulk of clinical experience lies with the first-generation agents, itraconazole and fluconazole. Voriconazole, posaconazole, and isavuconazole are less well-studied despite their demonstrable in vitro activity, and their clinical evidence base primarily consists of small case series, often as salvage therapy, and with varying degrees of success.[28,64–67] Fluconazole has oral bioavailability of more than 90%, and absorption is not significantly affected by food or gastric acidity.[68] The reliability of its absorption precludes the need to check plasma levels routinely. Fluconazole has the best CNS penetration of any of the available antifungal drugs (approximately 75%) and is used as an agent of first choice for coccidioidomycosis meningitis.[18,69]

Itraconazole is available both as a capsule or a solution. The solution formulation is preferred because of greater bioavailability, although gastrointestinal tolerability can be more problematic. Importantly, instructions to maximize bioavailability are opposite depending on the formulation. Food and an acidic gastric pH improve absorption of the capsule form of the drug (and so proton pump inhibitors, H_2-antagonists, and antacids are contraindicated, whereas acidic cola beverages can improve absorption).[70,71] By contrast, the oral solution is best absorbed on an empty stomach, and gastric pH has no effect.[72] The erratic absorption of either form of the drug makes checking blood levels mandatory.[73] A further important limitation of itraconazole is its poor CNS penetration, although successful treatment of meningitis is nonetheless achievable.[69] Despite these disadvantages, itraconazole seems to be more efficacious than fluconazole in histoplasmosis and possibly in blastomycosis as well, accounting for its preference as the azole of choice for these conditions.[50,74]

Drug–drug interactions between commonly used immunosuppressive medications in SOT recipients and the antifungal medications discussed are essentially limited to the triazole class. These agents all target the fungal cytochrome P450-dependent enzyme lanosterol 14-α-demethylase, thereby inhibiting fungal ergosterol production.[75] However, all the azoles have varying degrees of affinity for various human cytochrome P450 enzyme system isoforms as well, and this property accounts for the bulk of the drug–drug interactions witnessed.[76] In general, fluconazole has the least potent inhibition of cytochrome P450, and thus the fewest drug–drug interactions. The other mechanism of drug–drug interactions is via P-glycoprotein, an efflux pump for xenobiotics, which the triazoles similarly can inhibit and/or be a substrate of.[76,77]

It takes approximately 1 week after starting a triazole antifungal for the full effect of the enzyme inhibition to be felt. Conversely, when the triazole therapy is discontinued, the enzyme inhibition can last for up to a month thereafter.[76] Close attention to azoles and immunosuppressive drug levels and dosage adjustments should be taken, particularly around these times. The effects of the antifungal drugs on commonly used immunosuppressive medications are summarized in **Table 4**. In general, drug levels of the calcineurin inhibitors (eg, tacrolimus) and mammalian target of rapamycin inhibitors (eg, sirolimus) almost always require dose reduction when triazoles are used. Of the listed antifungals, only isavuconazole has been documented to alter mycophenolate levels. The data for increased prednisone exposure with azoles that are strong CYP3A4 inhibitors (itraconazole, voriconazole, posaconazole, and ketoconazole) are contradictory, and so monitoring for steroid side effects is recommended.[78–81] There is no evidence of significant drug–drug interactions with prednisone and any of the other antifungals.

Reductions in immunosuppressive drug exposure can cause an immune reconstitution syndrome (IRS) with any of the endemic fungi. This syndrome is manifest by an immunologically mediated worsening of the symptoms and signs of the infection, and may be hard to distinguish from treatment failure.[82] Clues to IRS include clinical deterioration despite adequate antifungal therapy, a failure to culture viable organisms from involved body sites, and stable or decreasing antigen levels for the endemic mycoses despite the clinical worsening.[83] Management is on a case-by-case basis, and depends on delicately navigating the trade-off between the need to control the infection and to maintain an adequate level of immunosuppression to prevent organ rejection. Mild cases of IRS usually settle without intensifying immunosuppression, but IRS

Table 4
Therapeutic agents for the treatment of endemic mycoses

Drug	Common Side Effects	CSF Penetration	Tacrolimus Dose Requirement	Cyclosporine Dose Requirement	Mycophenolate Dose Requirement	Sirolimus Dose Requirement	Prednisone Dose Requirement
Liposomal amphotericin B	Nephrotoxicity, hypokalemia, hypomagnesemia, infusion-related chills.	Poor (<3%) but often clinically effective nonetheless[69]	No significant change	No significant change	No significant change	No significant change	No significant change
Fluconazole	Generally well-tolerated. Can cause transaminitis occasionally.	Good (50%–94%)[69]	Decreased by 40%–60%[87,88]	Decreased by 21%–50%[76,89]	No significant change	No significant change	No significant change
Itraconazole	Nausea, vomiting. Can cause transaminitis occasionally.	Poor (<10%), but clinical efficacy may be achieved nonetheless[69]	Decreased by 40%–60% in general, but highly variable[76,90]	Decreased by 50%–66%[76,91]	No significant change	Decreased by 50%–90%[92,93]	Unclear; monitor for side effects
Voriconazole	Visual disturbances, occasional transaminitis	Moderate (38%–68%)[69]	Decreased by 66%[94,95]	Decreased by 50%[96]	No significant change	Decreased by 66%–90%[93]	Unclear; monitor for side effects
Posaconazole	Generally well-tolerated. Can cause transaminitis occasionally.	Poor, but clinical efficacy may be achieved nonetheless[97]	Decreased by 66%[98,99]	Decreased by 25%–29%[98]	No significant change	Decreased by 90%[100]	Unclear; monitor for side effects
Isavuconazole	Headache, nausea, vomiting, shortened QTc, transaminitis	Unclear	Decreased by 23%[101]	Decreased, mildly[102]	Decreased, moderately[102]	Decreased, moderately[102]	No significant change

Abbreviation: CSF, cerebrospinal fluid.

reactions can be life threatening, especially if they occur in sites such as the CNS, and these more severe instances usually mandate temporarily increasing the level of immunosuppression again.

PROPHYLAXIS REGIMENS IN SOLID ORGAN TRANSPLANT RECIPIENTS: AN UNRESOLVED ISSUE

A donor known with active disease with any of the endemic fungi is not considered a suitable candidate until (in the case of living donors) several months of therapy have controlled the infection.[84] Nonetheless, active donor infection is sometimes only discovered after transplantation has occurred, in which case primary prophylaxis of the recipient is indicated (**Table 5**). The other definite indication for peritransplant prophylaxis is in SOT recipients with evidence of prior coccidioidomycosis. This evidence may include positive serologic tests or thin-walled cavities seen on chest radiographs or computed tomography scans. Equivocal cases required specialist assessment, although many experts give prophylaxis to all SOT recipients if they reside in a coccidioidomycosis-endemic area, regardless of prior coccidioidomycosis or not.[59] There is only limited evidence for this practice, however. Primary prophylaxis in patients living in areas endemic for histoplasmosis or blastomycosis, and secondary

Table 5
Suggested prophylactic regimens for endemic fungi in SOT recipients

	Recipient Peritransplant Prophylaxis	Secondary Prophylaxis for Recipients After Completion of Treatment Course
Histoplasmosis	Donor with localized pulmonary disease: itraconazole 200 mg once or twice daily for 3–6 mo Donor with disseminated disease: itraconazole 200 mg once or twice daily for 12 mo[84]	Not routinely indicated. Can monitor urine antigen level every 3 mo to determine need. If required, consider itraconazole 200 mg/d.[16,84]
Blastomycosis	Donor with localized pulmonary disease: itraconazole 200 mg once or twice daily for 3–6 mo Donor with disseminated disease: itraconazole 200 mg once or twice daily for 12 mo	Not routinely indicated. If required, consider itraconazole 200 mg/d.[17]
Coccidioidomycosis	Donor with isolated pulmonary disease: fluconazole 400 mg/d for 3–12 mo (non-lung recipients) or lifelong (lung recipients). Donor with positive serology or extrapulmonary disease: fluconazole 400 mg/d lifelong.[84] Recipient with positive serology or history of coccidioidomycosis: fluconazole 200 mg/d for 6–12 mo. Recipient living in a Coccidioides-endemic area: fluconazole 200 mg/d for 6–12 mo.[59]	Fluconazole 400 mg/d indefinitely.[59]

Abbreviation: SOT, solid organ transplantation.

prophylaxis in patients with a history of prior histoplasmosis or blastomycosis is probably unnecessary. This probably includes patients living in endemic areas who have computed tomography evidence of calcified granulomas in lungs, liver, spleen, lymph nodes, or other organs, because the risk of reinfection in this case seems low to nonexistent.[16,26,85]

There is a similar lack of definitive evidence to guide secondary prophylaxis in SOT recipients after completion of a treatment course. The relapse rate after treatment completion in coccidioidomycosis is particularly high in SOT recipients, and so consensus opinion is that all such patients should receive life-long secondary prophylaxis.[59] The role of secondary prophylaxis for histoplasmosis and blastomycosis is less clear, and should probably be limited to cases at high risk of relapse only (see **Table 5**).[16,84] These high-risk scenarios would include patients in whom immunosuppression was not able to be lessened.

SUMMARY

Histoplasmosis, blastomycosis, and coccidioidomycosis are all relatively rare in SOT recipients, even those from endemic areas. However, they are more difficult to diagnose than many other infections that plague this population and can cause significant morbidity and mortality if they are not identified early. Therapy for the endemic mycoses is typically given for at least a year and is frequently complicated by drug–drug interactions between the triazoles and antirejection medications that requires close monitoring of immunosuppressive drug levels both when the triazoles are started and when they are stopped again after treatment completion.

REFERENCES

1. Kauffman CA, Freifeld AG, Andes DR, et al. Endemic fungal infections in solid organ and hematopoietic cell transplant recipients enrolled in the Transplant-Associated Infection Surveillance Network (TRANSNET). Transpl Infect Dis 2014;16(2):213–24.
2. Grim SA, Proia L, Miller R, et al. A multicenter study of histoplasmosis and blastomycosis after solid organ transplantation. Transpl Infect Dis 2012;14(1):17–23.
3. Pappas PG, Alexander BD, Andes DR, et al. Invasive fungal infections among organ transplant recipients: results of the Transplant-Associated Infection Surveillance Network (TRANSNET). Clin Infect Dis 2010;50(8):1101–11.
4. Blair JE, Logan JL. Coccidioidomycosis in solid organ transplantation. Clin Infect Dis 2001;33(9):1536–44.
5. Cuellar-Rodriguez J, Avery RK, Lard M, et al. Histoplasmosis in solid organ transplant recipients: 10 years of experience at a large transplant center in an endemic area. Clin Infect Dis 2009;49(5):710–6.
6. Assi M, Martin S, Wheat LJ, et al. Histoplasmosis after solid organ transplant. Clin Infect Dis 2013;57(11):1542–9.
7. Gauthier GM, Safdar N, Klein BS, et al. Blastomycosis in solid organ transplant recipients. Transpl Infect Dis 2007;9(4):310–7.
8. Kauffman CA. Endemic mycoses: blastomycosis, histoplasmosis, and sporotrichosis. Infect Dis Clin North Am 2006;20(3):645–62, vii.
9. Malcolm TR, Chin-Hong PV. Endemic mycoses in immunocompromised hosts. Curr Infect Dis Rep 2013;15(6):536–43.
10. Woods JP. Revisiting old friends: developments in understanding Histoplasma capsulatum pathogenesis. J Microbiol 2016;54(3):265–76.

11. Benedict K, Thompson GR 3rd, Deresinski S, et al. Mycotic infections acquired outside areas of known endemicity, United States. Emerg Infect Dis 2015; 21(11):1935–41.
12. Limaye AP, Connolly PA, Sagar M, et al. Transmission of Histoplasma capsulatum by organ transplantation. N Engl J Med 2000;343(16):1163–6.
13. Schwenk HT, Vo P, Moffitt K, et al. Allograft-transmitted Histoplasma capsulatum infection in a solid organ transplant recipient. J Pediatric Infect Dis Soc 2013; 2(3):270–3.
14. Dierberg KL, Marr KA, Subramanian A, et al. Donor-derived organ transplant transmission of coccidioidomycosis. Transpl Infect Dis 2012;14(3):300–4.
15. Nelson JK, Giraldeau G, Montoya JG, et al. Donor-derived Coccidioides immitis endocarditis and disseminated infection in the setting of solid organ transplantation. Open Forum Infect Dis 2016;3(3):ofw086.
16. Wheat LJ, Freifeld AG, Kleiman MB, et al. Clinical practice guidelines for the management of patients with histoplasmosis: 2007 update by the Infectious Diseases Society of America. Clin Infect Dis 2007;45(7):807–25.
17. Chapman SW, Dismukes WE, Proia LA, et al. Clinical practice guidelines for the management of blastomycosis: 2008 update by the Infectious Diseases Society of America. Clin Infect Dis 2008;46(12):1801–12.
18. Galgiani JN, Ampel NM, Blair JE, et al. Executive summary: 2016 Infectious Diseases Society of America (IDSA) clinical practice guideline for the treatment of coccidioidomycosis. Clin Infect Dis 2016;63(6):717–22.
19. Mott DF. The opposite end of the spectrum–managing nongame species that are prospering. In: Proceedings of the Workshop on Management of Nongame Species and Ecological Communities. Kensington (KY), June 11–12, 1985. p. 151–8.
20. Krzysik AJ. Birds in human modified environments and bird damage control: social, economic, and health implications. Washington, DC: US Construction Engineering Research Laboratory; 1989.
21. Wheat LJ, Azar MM, Bahr NC, et al. Histoplasmosis. Infect Dis Clin North Am 2016;30(1):207–27.
22. Kauffman CA. Histoplasmosis. Clin Chest Med 2009;30(2):217–25, v.
23. Bahr NC, Antinori S, Wheat LJ, et al. Histoplasmosis infections worldwide: thinking outside of the Ohio River valley. Curr Trop Med Rep 2015;2(2):70–80.
24. Centers for Disease Control and Prevention. Histoplasmosis in a state where it is not known to be endemic–Montana, 2012-2013. MMWR Morb Mortal Wkly Rep 2013;62(42):834–7.
25. Horwath MC, Fecher RA, Deepe GS Jr. Histoplasma capsulatum, lung infection and immunity. Future Microbiol 2015;10(6):967–75.
26. Vail GM, Young RS, Wheat LJ, et al. Incidence of histoplasmosis following allogeneic bone marrow transplant or solid organ transplant in a hyperendemic area. Transpl Infect Dis 2002;4(3):148–51.
27. Wheat LJ, Smith EJ, Sathapatayavongs B, et al. Histoplasmosis in renal allograft recipients. Two large urban outbreaks. Arch Intern Med 1983;143(4):703–7.
28. Freifeld AG, Iwen PC, Lesiak BL, et al. Histoplasmosis in solid organ transplant recipients at a large Midwestern university transplant center. Transpl Infect Dis 2005;7(3–4):109–15.
29. Dufresne SF, LeBlanc RE, Zhang SX, et al. Histoplasmosis and subcutaneous nodules in a kidney transplant recipient: erythema nodosum versus fungal panniculitis. Transpl Infect Dis 2013;15(2):E58–63.

30. Hage CA, Ribes JA, Wengenack NL, et al. A multicenter evaluation of tests for diagnosis of histoplasmosis. Clin Infect Dis 2011;53(5):448–54.
31. Kauffman CA. Histoplasmosis: a clinical and laboratory update. Clin Microbiol Rev 2007;20(1):115–32.
32. Wheat J, Wheat H, Connolly P, et al. Cross-reactivity in Histoplasma capsulatum variety capsulatum antigen assays of urine samples from patients with endemic mycoses. Clin Infect Dis 1997;24(6):1169–71.
33. Assi MA, Sandid MS, Baddour LM, et al. Systemic histoplasmosis: a 15-year retrospective institutional review of 111 patients. Medicine (Baltimore) 2007; 86(3):162–9.
34. Guarner J, Brandt ME. Histopathologic diagnosis of fungal infections in the 21st century. Clin Microbiol Rev 2011;24(2):247–80.
35. Vergidis P, Walker RC, Kaul DR, et al. False-positive Aspergillus galactomannan assay in solid organ transplant recipients with histoplasmosis. Transpl Infect Dis 2012;14(2):213–7.
36. Johnson PC, Wheat LJ, Cloud GA, et al. Safety and efficacy of liposomal amphotericin B compared with conventional amphotericin B for induction therapy of histoplasmosis in patients with AIDS. Ann Intern Med 2002;137(2):105–9.
37. Wheat LJ, Cloud G, Johnson PC, et al. Clearance of fungal burden during treatment of disseminated histoplasmosis with liposomal amphotericin B versus itraconazole. Antimicrob Agents Chemother 2001;45(8):2354–7.
38. Wheat LJ, Connolly P, Smedema M, et al. Activity of newer triazoles against Histoplasma capsulatum from patients with AIDS who failed fluconazole. J Antimicrob Chemother 2006;57(6):1235–9.
39. Brown EM, McTaggart LR, Zhang SX, et al. Phylogenetic analysis reveals a cryptic species Blastomyces gilchristii, sp. nov. within the human pathogenic fungus Blastomyces dermatitidis. PLoS One 2013;8(3):e59237.
40. McDonough ES, Wisniewski TR, Penn LA, et al. Preliminary studies on conidial liberation of Blastomyces dermatitidis and Histoplasma capsulatum. Sabouraudia 1976;14(2):199–204.
41. McTaggart LR, Brown EM, Richardson SE. Phylogeographic analysis of Blastomyces dermatitidis and Blastomyces gilchristii reveals an association with North American Freshwater Drainage Basins. PLoS One 2016;11(7):e0159396.
42. Baddley JW, Winthrop KL, Patkar NM, et al. Geographic distribution of endemic fungal infections among older persons, United States. Emerg Infect Dis 2011; 17(9):1664–9.
43. McBride JA, Gauthier GM, Klein BS. Clinical manifestations and treatment of blastomycosis. Clin Chest Med 2017;38(3):435–49.
44. Klein BS, Vergeront JM, Weeks RJ, et al. Isolation of Blastomyces dermatitidis in soil associated with a large outbreak of blastomycosis in Wisconsin. N Engl J Med 1986;314(9):529–34.
45. Kauffman CA, Miceli MH. Histoplasmosis and blastomycosis in solid organ transplant recipients. J Fungi 2015;1(2):94–106.
46. Levy AL, Wilkin N, Poh-Fitzpatrick MB, et al. Verrucous nodules on the toes of a renal transplant recipient. Cutaneous blastomycosis. Arch Dermatol 2007; 143(5):653–8.
47. Durkin M, Witt J, Lemonte A, et al. Antigen assay with the potential to aid in diagnosis of blastomycosis. J Clin Microbiol 2004;42(10):4873–5.
48. Frost HM, Novicki TJ. Blastomyces antigen detection for diagnosis and management of blastomycosis. J Clin Microbiol 2015;53(11):3660–2.

49. Wheat LJ. Antigen detection, serology, and molecular diagnosis of invasive mycoses in the immunocompromised host. Transpl Infect Dis 2006;8(3):128–39.

50. Pappas PG, Bradsher RW, Kauffman CA, et al. Treatment of blastomycosis with higher doses of fluconazole. The National Institute of Allergy and Infectious Diseases Mycoses Study Group. Clin Infect Dis 1997;25(2):200–5.

51. Hector RF, Laniado-Laborin R. Coccidioidomycosis–a fungal disease of the Americas. PLoS Med 2005;2(1):e2.

52. Fisher FS, Bultman MW, Johnson SM, et al. Coccidioides niches and habitat parameters in the southwestern United States: a matter of scale. Ann N Y Acad Sci 2007;1111:47–72.

53. Lauer A, Talamantes J, Castanon Olivares LR, et al. Combining forces–the use of Landsat TM satellite imagery, soil parameter information, and multiplex PCR to detect Coccidioides immitis growth sites in Kern County, California. PLoS One 2014;9(11):e111921.

54. Coopersmith EJ, Bell JE, Benedict K, et al. Relating coccidioidomycosis (valley fever) incidence to soil moisture conditions. Geohealth 2017;1:51–63.

55. Hage CA, Knox KS, Wheat LJ. Endemic mycoses: overlooked causes of community acquired pneumonia. Respir Med 2012;106(6):769–76.

56. Ampel NM, Christian L. In vitro modulation of proliferation and cytokine production by human peripheral blood mononuclear cells from subjects with various forms of coccidioidomycosis. Infect Immun 1997;65(11):4483–7.

57. Blair JE. Coccidioidomycosis in liver transplantation. Liver Transpl 2006;12(1):31–9.

58. Blair JE, Coakley B, Santelli AC, et al. Serologic testing for symptomatic coccidioidomycosis in immunocompetent and immunosuppressed hosts. Mycopathologia 2006;162(5):317–24.

59. Galgiani JN, Ampel NM, Blair JE, et al. 2016 Infectious Diseases Society of America (IDSA) clinical practice guideline for the treatment of coccidioidomycosis. Clin Infect Dis 2016;63(6):e112–46.

60. Kuberski T, Myers R, Wheat LJ, et al. Diagnosis of coccidioidomycosis by antigen detection using cross-reaction with a Histoplasma antigen. Clin Infect Dis 2007;44(5):e50–4.

61. Durkin M, Connolly P, Kuberski T, et al. Diagnosis of coccidioidomycosis with use of the Coccidioides antigen enzyme immunoassay. Clin Infect Dis 2008; 47(8):e69–73.

62. Galgiani JN, Catanzaro A, Cloud GA, et al. Comparison of oral fluconazole and itraconazole for progressive, nonmeningeal coccidioidomycosis. A randomized, double-blind trial. Mycoses Study Group. Ann Intern Med 2000;133(9):676–86.

63. Espinel-Ingroff A. Comparison of In vitro activities of the new triazole SCH56592 and the echinocandins MK-0991 (L-743,872) and LY303366 against opportunistic filamentous and dimorphic fungi and yeasts. J Clin Microbiol 1998; 36(10):2950–6.

64. Thompson GR 3rd, Rendon A, Ribeiro Dos Santos R, et al. isavuconazole treatment of cryptococcosis and dimorphic mycoses. Clin Infect Dis 2016;63(3): 356–62.

65. Catanzaro A, Cloud GA, Stevens DA, et al. Safety, tolerance, and efficacy of posaconazole therapy in patients with nonmeningeal disseminated or chronic pulmonary coccidioidomycosis. Clin Infect Dis 2007;45(5):562–8.

66. Stevens DA, Rendon A, Gaona-Flores V, et al. Posaconazole therapy for chronic refractory coccidioidomycosis. Chest 2007;132(3):952–8.

67. Restrepo A, Tobon A, Clark B, et al. Salvage treatment of histoplasmosis with posaconazole. J Infect 2007;54(4):319–27.

68. Brammer KW, Farrow PR, Faulkner JK. Pharmacokinetics and tissue penetration of fluconazole in humans. Rev Infect Dis 1990;12(Suppl 3):S318–26.
69. Kethireddy S, Andes D. CNS pharmacokinetics of antifungal agents. Expert Opin Drug Metab Toxicol 2007;3(4):573–81.
70. Jaruratanasirikul S, Kleepkaew A. Influence of an acidic beverage (Coca-Cola) on the absorption of itraconazole. Eur J Clin Pharmacol 1997;52(3):235–7.
71. Jaruratanasirikul S, Sriwiriyajan S. Effect of omeprazole on the pharmacokinetics of itraconazole. Eur J Clin Pharmacol 1998;54(2):159–61.
72. Vyas KS, Bariola JR, Bradsher RW Jr. Treatment of endemic mycoses. Expert Rev Respir Med 2010;4(1):85–95.
73. Prentice AG, Glasmacher A. Making sense of itraconazole pharmacokinetics. J Antimicrob Chemother 2005;56(Suppl 1):i17–22.
74. McKinsey DS, Kauffman CA, Pappas PG, et al. Fluconazole therapy for histoplasmosis. The National Institute of Allergy and Infectious Diseases Mycoses Study Group. Clin Infect Dis 1996;23(5):996–1001.
75. Ghannoum MA, Rice LB. Antifungal agents: mode of action, mechanisms of resistance, and correlation of these mechanisms with bacterial resistance. Clin Microbiol Rev 1999;12(4):501–17.
76. Dodds-Ashley E. Management of drug and food interactions with azole antifungal agents in transplant recipients. Pharmacotherapy 2010;30(8):842–54.
77. Lin JH, Yamazaki M. Role of P-glycoprotein in pharmacokinetics: clinical implications. Clin Pharmacokinet 2003;42(1):59–98.
78. Lebrun-Vignes B, Archer VC, Diquet B, et al. Effect of itraconazole on the pharmacokinetics of prednisolone and methylprednisolone and cortisol secretion in healthy subjects. Br J Clin Pharmacol 2001;51(5):443–50.
79. Yamashita SK, Ludwig EA, Middleton E Jr, et al. Lack of pharmacokinetic and pharmacodynamic interactions between ketoconazole and prednisolone. Clin Pharmacol Ther 1991;49(5):558–70.
80. Varis T, Kivisto KT, Neuvonen PJ. The effect of itraconazole on the pharmacokinetics and pharmacodynamics of oral prednisolone. Eur J Clin Pharmacol 2000;56(1):57–60.
81. Zurcher RM, Frey BM, Frey FJ. Impact of ketoconazole on the metabolism of prednisolone. Clin Pharmacol Ther 1989;45(4):366–72.
82. Gupta AO, Singh N. Immune reconstitution syndrome and fungal infections. Curr Opin Infect Dis 2011;24(6):527–33.
83. Jazwinski A, Naggie S, Perfect J. Immune reconstitution syndrome in a patient with disseminated histoplasmosis and steroid taper: maintaining the perfect balance. Mycoses 2011;54(3):270–2.
84. Singh N, Huprikar S, Burdette SD, et al. Donor-derived fungal infections in organ transplant recipients: guidelines of the American Society of Transplantation, infectious diseases community of practice. Am J Transplant 2012;12(9):2414–28.
85. Straub M, Schwarz J. The healed primary complex in histoplasmosis. Am J Clin Pathol 1955;25(7):727–41.
86. Hage C, Kleiman MB, Wheat LJ. Histoplasmosis in solid organ transplant recipients. Clin Infect Dis 2010;50(1):122–3 [author reply: 123–4].
87. Manez R, Martin M, Raman D, et al. Fluconazole therapy in transplant recipients receiving FK506. Transplantation 1994;57(10):1521–3.
88. Lumlertgul D, Noppakun K, Rojanasthien N, et al. Pharmacokinetic study of the combination of tacrolimus and fluconazole in renal transplant patients. J Med Assoc Thai 2006;89(Suppl 2):S73–8.

89. Canafax DM, Graves NM, Hilligoss DM, et al. Interaction between cyclosporine and fluconazole in renal allograft recipients. Transplantation 1991;51(5):1014–8.
90. Mori T, Aisa Y, Kato J, et al. Drug interaction between oral solution itraconazole and calcineurin inhibitors in allogeneic hematopoietic stem cell transplantation recipients: an association with bioavailability of oral solution itraconazole. Int J Hematol 2009;90(1):103–7.
91. Kramer MR, Marshall SE, Denning DW, et al. Cyclosporine and itraconazole interaction in heart and lung transplant recipients. Ann Intern Med 1990; 113(4):327–9.
92. Kuypers DR, Claes K, Evenepoel P, et al. Drug interaction between itraconazole and sirolimus in a primary renal allograft recipient. Transplantation 2005;79(6):737.
93. Sadaba B, Campanero MA, Quetglas EG, et al. Clinical relevance of sirolimus drug interactions in transplant patients. Transplant Proc 2004;36(10):3226–8.
94. Mori T, Aisa Y, Kato J, et al. Drug interaction between voriconazole and calcineurin inhibitors in allogeneic hematopoietic stem cell transplant recipients. Bone Marrow Transplant 2009;44(6):371–4.
95. Venkataramanan R, Zang S, Gayowski T, et al. Voriconazole inhibition of the metabolism of tacrolimus in a liver transplant recipient and in human liver microsomes. Antimicrob Agents Chemother 2002;46(9):3091–3.
96. Romero AJ, Le Pogamp P, Nilsson LG, et al. Effect of voriconazole on the pharmacokinetics of cyclosporine in renal transplant patients. Clin Pharmacol Ther 2002;71(4):226–34.
97. Lazowski J, Radzikowska B, Zadrozynska E. Determination of blood level of diphenylhydantoin in the treatment of epilepsy. The need for monitoring. Wiad Lek 1977;30(20):1613–6 [in Polish].
98. Sansone-Parsons A, Krishna G, Martinho M, et al. Effect of oral posaconazole on the pharmacokinetics of cyclosporine and tacrolimus. Pharmacotherapy 2007; 27(6):825–34.
99. Berge M, Chevalier P, Benammar M, et al. Safe management of tacrolimus together with posaconazole in lung transplant patients with cystic fibrosis. Ther Drug Monit 2009;31(3):396–9.
100. Merck & Co. Inc. Noxafil® (posaconazole) injection 18 mg/mL Noxafil® (posaconazole) delayed-release tablets 100 mg Noxafil® (posaconazole) oral suspension 40 mg/mL. 2015.
101. Rivosecchi RM, Clancy CJ, Shields RK, et al. Effects of isavuconazole on the plasma concentrations of tacrolimus among solid-organ transplant patients. Antimicrob Agents Chemother 2017;61(9) [pii:e00970-17].
102. Groll AH, Desai A, Han D, et al. Pharmacokinetic assessment of drug-drug interactions of isavuconazole with the immunosuppressants cyclosporine, mycophenolic acid, prednisolone, sirolimus, and tacrolimus in healthy adults. Clin Pharmacol Drug Dev 2017;6(1):76–85.

Mold Infections in Solid Organ Transplant Recipients

Tracy L. Lemonovich, MD

KEYWORDS

- Antifungal • Aspergillosis • Invasive fungal infections • Fusariosis • Mucormycosis
- Transplant

KEY POINTS

- Mold infections in solid organ transplant (SOT) recipients are a significant cause of morbidity with a high 12-week mortality of 29%.
- The most common and serious mold infections in SOT recipients include invasive aspergillosis, mucormycosis, fusariosis, scedosporiosis, and phaeohyphomycosis.
- Diagnosis of mold infections can be challenging and usually requires histopathologic and/or microbiologic criteria, often obtained by biopsy and culture of affected tissues. Blood cultures are positive in about half of the patients with disseminated *Fusarium* species or *Lomentospora prolificans* infections.
- Treatment of mold infections often necessitates combined antifungal therapy and surgical excision or debridement for localized disease.

INTRODUCTION

Mold infections are an important cause of morbidity and mortality in the solid organ transplant (SOT) population. These infections carry a significant clinical and economic burden.[1–3] Mold infections include invasive aspergillosis (IA) and other emerging fungal pathogens, such as mucormycosis (zygomycosis), *Fusarium*, *Scedosporium*, and the dematiaceous fungi (dark molds), among others. Diagnosis and management of these patients are challenging, often requiring invasive diagnostic methodologies and a multidisciplinary approach to treatment. IA is the most common mold infection and second most common invasive fungal infection (IFI) (after *Candida*) in SOT recipients, accounting for 19% to 25% of all IFIs, with non-Aspergillus molds making up 7% to 10%.[4–7] Risk factors for infection include immunosuppressive therapy, loss of skin or mucosal integrity, and risks specific to organ transplant type, such as chronic lung disease or anatomic disruptions.[6,8] The 12-week overall mortality of mold infections in SOT recipients is overall high at 29% but varies by organ transplant type, with the

Disclosure Statement: The author has served on a medical affairs advisory board for Allergan.
Department of Medicine, Division of Infectious Diseases and HIV Medicine, UH Cleveland Medical Center, Case Western Reserve University School of Medicine, 11100 Euclid Avenue, Cleveland, OH 44106, USA
E-mail address: tracy.lemonovich@UHhospitals.org

Infect Dis Clin N Am 32 (2018) 687–701
https://doi.org/10.1016/j.idc.2018.04.006
0891-5520/18/© 2018 Elsevier Inc. All rights reserved.

highest mortality in liver transplant recipients.[5,9] This article reviews the epidemiology, risk factors, microbiology, diagnostic, and treatment approach to mold infections in SOT recipients.

ASPERGILLOSIS

IA is generally acquired via inhalation of conidia, making pulmonary infection the most common site of infection. Infections may be localized (pulmonary or extrapulmonary including surgical wound infections) or disseminated. Lung transplant recipients can be at risk for tracheobronchitis or infection of the bronchial anastomosis. IA occurs in 1% to 15% of SOT recipients.[10] Mortality in a recent series of SOT recipients was reported at 22%, which appears improved from historical cohorts, wherein mortality has been as high as 92% in some SOT populations.[11–13] The most common species causing human disease is *Aspergillus fumigatus*; *Aspergillus flavus*, *Aspergillus niger*, and *Aspergillus terreus* are also frequently encountered.

Diagnosis of IA, like other IFI, requires microbiologic and/or histopathologic criteria to define proven infection by European Organization for Research and Treatment of Cancer/Mycoses Study Group revised definitions.[14] Acquisition of adequate specimens is crucial for early diagnosis; bronchoscopy with bronchoalveolar lavage (BAL) is recommended for patients with suspected invasive pulmonary aspergillosis (IPA) with consideration of transbronchial biopsy or percutaneous needle biopsy depending on radiographic site of lesion.[15] Staining shows narrow septate hyphae with acute angle branching (**Fig. 1**). Recommended radiographic imaging should include chest computerized tomography (CT) scan for suspected IPA. Typical CT findings include nodules, consolidative lesions, or wedge-shaped infarcts. The classic halo sign, a nodule surrounded by a perimeter of ground glass opacity reflecting hemorrhage, may be seen particularly in neutropenic patients. An air crescent, or cavity in a mass or nodule, is usually a late CT finding.[15] Biomarkers such galactomannan (GM) and (1-3)-β-D-glucan from the serum may be considered but have low sensitivity in SOT recipients. Serum GM sensitivity has been reported to be only 20% to 30% in SOT populations.[16,17] However, testing of BAL for GM may improve sensitivity to 67% to 100% in SOT recipients.[10] Molecular testing with Aspergillus polymerase chain reaction (PCR) shows promise with high sensitivity for diagnosis of IA in some studies,

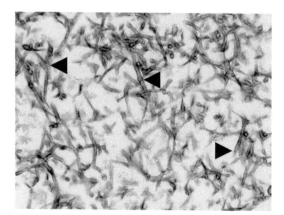

Fig. 1. *Aspergillus* narrow septate hyphae (*arrowheads*) (GMS stain, oil magnification ×1000). (*Courtesy of* Dr Daniel Rhoads and Dr Wissam Dahoud, UH Cleveland Medical Center, Cleveland, OH; with permission.)

out its exact role in diagnosis and management of SOT recipients (and other patient populations) is still not established.[15,18] Blood cultures with *Aspergillus* species usually are consistent with contamination and are rarely associated with IA even in high-risk patients.[19]

Early initiation of antifungal treatment of strongly suspected IA is recommended while conducting diagnostic testing to limit progression of disease.[15] Voriconazole, a triazole, is considered the drug of choice for primary therapy in all patient populations, including SOT recipients. This recommendation is based on a randomized trial of voriconazole compared with amphotericin B deoxycholate for treatment of IA in mostly hematopoietic stem cell transplant recipients and patients with hematologic malignancies showing improved survival with voriconazole[20] and has been supported by additional studies of voriconazole treatment, including those in SOT recipients.[10] Alternative antifungal therapies include liposomal or other lipid formulations of amphotericin and isavuconazole. A randomized trial showed noninferiority of isavuconazole compared with voriconazole in the treatment of IPA.[21] In general, *Aspergillus* azole resistance in the United States is low (<3%), and routine antifungal susceptibility testing (AFST) for initial infection is not recommended except in the patient in whom azole resistance is suspected or who is unresponsive to antifungal therapy.[15] Resistance to the echinocandins is also uncommon, as is amphotericin resistance with the exception of particular species such as *A terreus*.[15] Combination therapy (usually voriconazole plus an echinocandin) appears promising particularly for use in severe disease and has shown reduced mortality in some SOT recipients.[22] Tracheobronchial aspergillosis (TBA) occurs primarily in lung transplant recipients, affecting 4% to 6% of this patient population usually within 3 to 6 months posttransplant.[15,23] Risk factors for TBA include exposure of the lung allograft to the environment, *Aspergillus* colonization pretransplant and posttransplant, high degree of immune suppression, impaired mucociliary clearance, and pulmonary denervation.[24] Recommended treatment of TBA includes a mold-active triazole and adjunctive inhaled amphotericin, given associated anastomotic endobronchial ischemia or ischemic reperfusion injury due to airway ischemia.[15] Duration of therapy is usually 6 to 12 weeks for IPA depending on disease response to treatment and degree of immune suppression, at least 3 months for TBA or until resolution of infection.[10,15] Adjunctive therapies for IA include reduction in immune suppression, surgery for localized disease, and colony-stimulating factors or granulocyte infusions for neutropenic patients.[15] Although an optimal prophylaxis strategy has not been defined for SOT recipients, prophylaxis for IA is indicated for certain high-risk SOT populations. **Table 1** summarizes a prophylaxis strategy for high-risk SOT recipients.

MUCORMYCOSIS

Invasive mucormycosis (IM) is caused by Zygomycetes (order Mucorales) and is rare, making up only 2% of fungal infections in SOT recipients with overall incidence of 0.07% at 1 year posttransplant.[25] However, this infection has a high fatality rate with 90-day survival of only 50% to 60%.[26] Traditional risk factors for IM include uncontrolled diabetes mellitus, corticosteroids, and neutropenia as well as renal failure, reactivation of immunomodulating herpesviruses, malnutrition, and prior voriconazole and/or caspofungin use in SOT recipients.[27,28] Clinically important species of Zygomycetes include *Rhizopus, Mucor, Rhizomucor, Cunninghamella, Absidia, Apophysomyces*, and *Myocladus*.[7] Clinical disease spectrum includes pulmonary disease as the most common, but can also include rhino-sino-orbital (including extension to the brain), disseminated, gastrointestinal, and primary cutaneous

Table 1
Prophylaxis recommendations for invasive aspergillosis in solid organ transplant recipients

Organ Type	Risk Factors	Antifungal Prophylaxis	Duration
Lung	• Colonization with Aspergillus pretransplant or posttransplant • Mold infection in explanted lungs • Fungal infections in the sinuses • Single lung recipients	• Systemic triazole (voriconazole or itraconazole) OR inhaled amphotericin B product • For patients with listed risk factors, systemic voriconazole or itraconazole is preferred	• 3–4 mo posttransplant • Reinitiation of antifungal prophylaxis should occur if receiving thymoglobulin, aletuzumab, or high-dose corticosteroids
Liver	• Retransplantation • Renal failure, particularly requiring dialysis • Transplantation for fulminant hepatic failure • Reoperation	• Lipid formulation of amphotericin B OR an echinocandin	• Initial hospital stay or 4 wk posttransplant
Heart	• Pretransplant Aspergillus colonization • Reoperation • Cytomegalovirus disease • Posttransplant renal failure requiring hemodialysis • Presence of IA in the transplant program within 2 mo or transplant	• Itraconazole OR voriconazole	• 50–150 d

Adapted from Singh N, Husain S. AST infectious diseases community of practice. Aspergillosis in solid organ transplantation. Am J Transplant 2013;13(suppl 4):230; with permission.

disease.[6,29,30] Lung infection may present with consolidation/mass lesions, nodules, or cavities.[29] Disseminated infection can involve essentially any organ, including the lungs, heart, brain, liver, esophagus, stomach, small and large bowel, kidney, retroperitoneum, thyroid, and skin.[7] Primary cutaneous infection can occur at sites of surgical incisions or drains, intravenous catheter sites, and after skin trauma. Lesions may present with black necrosis with surrounding cellulitis, thrombophlebitis, or extension to deeper structures.[28] Lung and liver transplant recipients appear to be at highest risk for IM with infections occurring at a median of 6 months after transplant, but may occur as early as the first month post-ransplant in liver transplant recipients.[29]

Diagnosis typically requires an invasive procedure such as biopsy, fine-needle aspiration, bronchoscopy, endoscopy, or surgical exploration.[28] CT chest imaging may show a reverse halo sign, an area of ground glass opacity with a ring of consolidation. Staining shows broad, ribbonlike, nonseptate hyphae with irregular walls and 90° angle branching (**Figs. 2** and **3**). Diagnosis may be made by histology, culture, or both.[28,31] PCR testing is being increasingly used for diagnosis of mucormycosis and appears to be highly sensitive.[32] PCR testing of circulating DNA in serum may be a useful tool for both early detection and treatment monitoring.[33,34] Treatment of

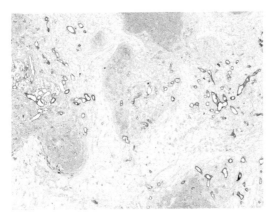

Fig. 2. Zygomycete in sinus vessel (GMS stain, magnification ×200). (*Courtesy of* Dr Daniel Rhoads and Dr Wissam Dahoud, UH Cleveland Medical Center, Cleveland, OH; with permission.)

mucormycosis often requires surgical treatment with excision or debridement of necrotic tissues combined with antifungal therapy. Recommended induction therapy is with lipid formulation amphotericin B.[35] Isavuconazole is also now a first-line treatment option based on a recent single-arm open-label trial with case-control analysis showing efficacy similar to amphotericin B.[36] Use of combination therapy with an echinocandin and lipid amphotericin B has been described in animal models and retrospective reports.[37–39] The combination of isavuconazole with micafungin has also been recently studied in murine models and in vitro studies showing synergy.[40,41] Posaconazole can be used for salvage therapy in patients intolerant to or failing amphotericin B or as maintenance antifungal therapy.[42–44] Isavuconazole can also be considered for maintenance and salvage therapy and has been reported to be successfully used for salvage in SOT patients.[45–47]

Fusarium

Fusariosis accounts for less than 1% of IFIs in SOT recipients and may occur late in the posttransplant period with a median time to infection of 365 days.[7,8] *Fusarium solani* is the most common species causing infection; other common species include *Fusarium oxysporum* and *Fusarium verticillioides*.[48] Exposure to fungi occurs by inhalation of airborne conidia or direct contact with contaminated material, such as soil, plants, or other organic matter.[7] The clinical spectrum of fusariosis includes superficial cutaneous infection, localized infections especially of the respiratory tract and sinuses, and disseminated infection.[49,50] Risk of infection can vary by transplant type, but lung transplant recipients appear particularly vulnerable to pulmonary fusariosis.[51] Primary skin infection due to direct inoculation may present with skin nodules, ulcers, cellulitis, or subcutaneous abscesses that can resemble ecthyma gangrenosum.[49] Localized infections are most common in the respiratory tract and sinuses, but can also include septic arthritis, endophthalmitis, osteomyelitis, cystitis, and brain abscess.[52] Disseminated infection occurs when 2 or more noncontiguous sites/organs are affected and may involve the gastrointestinal tract, liver, heart valves, kidneys, lungs, central nervous system (CNS), and skin.[7] Disseminated infection often is associated with characteristic skin lesions that may appear as targetoid red or violaceous painful nodules, which often ulcerate with an eschar.[52,53]

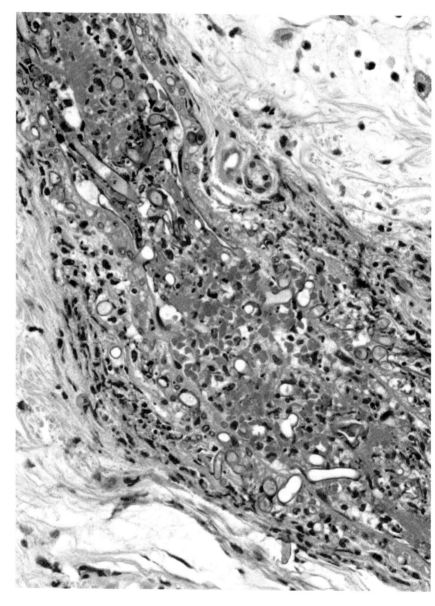

Fig. 3. Zygomycete in sinus vessel (hematoxylin and eosin stain, magnification ×400). (*Courtesy of* Dr Daniel Rhoads and Dr Wissam Dahoud, UH Cleveland Medical Center, Cleveland, OH; with permission.)

Diagnoses of fusariosis can be made by skin biopsy in cases of cutaneous involvement. Unlike many other mold infections, *Fusarium* frequently grows from blood cultures in disseminated infections and has been reported to be positive in 40% of cases.[54] Histopathologic appearance is similar to *Aspergillus* with acute branching septate hyphae. Culture testing should involve identification to the species level and AFST whenever possible to help guide therapy.[55,56] Nonculture biomarkers, such as GM and (1-3)-β-D-glucan, may be helpful adjuncts to diagnosis, but their exact role has not been defined.[7,57] Molecular PCR testing appears promising but has not been standardized for diagnosis.[55] Treatment of fusariosis depends on the site and extent of infection, the specific *Fusarium* species and its antifungal susceptibilities, as well as underlying host factors.[51] Surgical excision or debridement should be considered when feasible particularly for primary cutaneous and localized infections. Antifungal therapy is often guided based on species and antifungal susceptibilities. Amphotericin B, including lipid formulations and voriconazole, is first-line therapy for fusariosis; *F solani* appears to be more susceptible to amphotericin than the triazoles.[51] Posaconazole also has been used for primary and salvage therapy.[58,59] Combination therapy with amphotericin B and voriconazole or another triazole should be considered while awaiting identification and susceptibility data and/or in severe infection.[6,60] Overall mortality of fusariosis remains high with estimates ranging from 44% to 67% in various series, but lung transplant recipients appear to have a higher mortality at 67%.[48,51,61] SOT recipients with localized infection tend to have a better outcome than patients with hematological malignancies or bone marrow transplant.[50]

Scedosporium/Pseudallescheria

Scedosporium and *Pseudallescheria* species are found in soil and water, with infections usually occurring by inhalation of spores or by direct contact. Predominant species causing infection include *Scedosporium apiospermum*, *Pseudalleschia boydii*, and *L prolificans*. *S apiospermum* had previously been considered the asexual state of *P boydii* but is now considered a distinct species.[62] Lung transplant recipients are at risk for infection, particularly in cystic fibrosis (CF) patients, who are often colonized before transplant.[63,64] Other SOT recipients can also be affected, with clinical spectrum including localized infections of respiratory tract, sinuses, surgical site, and skin as well as disseminated infections involving the brain/CNS, eye, blood vessels, heart, bone, and joints.[65–67] Median time to infection after transplant is reported to be 4 months.[67] Diagnosis is by biopsy of affected tissues with culture and pathology, and histopathologic appearance is similar to *Aspergillus*.[6] Blood cultures may be positive in greater than 50% of *L prolificans* disseminated infections due to hematogenous spread.[55] Antifungal treatment of scedosporiosis should be directed by species identification and AFST of clinical isolates due to variable susceptibility to antifungal agents, with many species resistant to amphotericin B.[55,68] Voriconazole is usually considered first-line therapy and appears to be associated with better survival in transplant recipients than other therapies.[55,69,70] Surgical debridement should be considered whenever feasible and may be the primary therapy in *L prolificans* infections in which the organism may be resistant to all antifungals.[71] Combination therapy of voriconazole plus an echinocandin or terbinafine should be considered in severe or resistant infections.[55,72] CF patients known to be colonized with *Scedosporium* pre–lung transplant should be given antifungal prophylaxis, usually with a triazole.[64] Mortality from scedosporiosis is high, ranging from 58% to 72% in transplant recipients.[67,69]

Table 2
Summary of important fungal pathogens in solid organ transplant recipients

Fungal Pathogen	Important Species	Risk Factors/Transplant Type	Clinical Manifestations	Diagnosis	Treatment
Aspergillus	*A fumigatus, A flavus, A niger, A terreus*	Neutropenia Lung, liver, heart	IPA (most common) TBA (lung transplant) Disseminated	Narrow, septate hyphae with acute angle branching	Voriconazole
Zygomycetes	Rhizopus, Mucor, Rhizomucor, Absidia, Cunninghamella, Apophysomyces, Myocladus	Uncontrolled DM Corticosteroids Neutropenia Renal failure Immunomodulating viruses Malnutrition Prior voriconazole/caspofungin use Liver, lung, kidney	Pulmonary (most common) Rhino-sino-orbital Disseminated Primary cutaneous Gastrointestinal Bronchial anastomosis (lung transplant)	Broad, ribbonlike, nonseptate hyphae Molecular testing	Lipid formulation amphotericin Surgical debridement when feasible
Fusarium	*F solani, F oxysporum, F verticillioides*	Lung, liver	Pulmonary Primary cutaneous Disseminated (often involving skin) Sinusitis Osteomyelitis/septic arthritis Endophthalmitis Brain abscess	Histopathology similar to Aspergillus Blood cultures may be positive	Amphotericin B or voriconazole Surgical debridement when feasible

Scedosporium/ pseudallescheria	S apiospermum, P boydii, Lomentospora prolificans	Lung	Pulmonary Sinusitis Surgical site Skin Disseminated	Histopathology similar to Aspergillus Blood cultures may be positive with L prolificans	Voriconazole Combination therapy Surgical debridement when feasible
Dematiaceous fungi (dark molds)	Alternaria, Exophiala, Curvularia, Cladosporium, Ochroconis, Bipolaris	All SOT types	Skin (nodules, abscesses, ulcers) Pulmonary Disseminated	Septate hyphae with GMS silver stain Fontana-Masson staining with melanin	Surgical excision of cutaneous lesions Triazoles
Paecilomyces		Heart, lung	Skin and soft tissue Peritonitis Sternal wound infection	Irregular septate hyphae	Voriconazole or posaconazole Surgical debridement when feasible

Abbreviation: DM, diabetes mellitus.
Adapted from Refs.[6,7,10]

Dematiaceous Fungi (Dark Molds)

The dematiaceous, or dark-pigmented, molds can cause the invasive infections phaeohyphomycosis, chromoblastomycosis, or mycetoma.[73] Primary cutaneous infections are the most common clinical presentation in SOT recipients and can cause subcutaneous nodules, abscesses, pustules, or purulent ulcerations.[6,74] Other sites of infection include the lungs and disseminated infection with CNS involvement. The most important pathogens causing infection in this group include *Alternaria, Exophiala, Curvularia, Cladosporium, Ochroconis,* and *Bipolaris.*[7,73] Time to infection posttransplant can be long, ranging from 2 months to 11 years with a median of 685 days.[73,74] Diagnosis is usually by biopsy with histopathology and culture; septate hyphae are present with silver stain, and Fontana-Masson staining can demonstrate the presence of melanin.[6] Surgical excision is the mainstay of treatment of primary cutaneous lesions and may not require antifungal therapy.[75] AFST should be used to guide therapy. First-line antifungal treatment includes voriconazole, posaconazole, and itraconazole; echinocandins and amphotericin B may also be useful.[7,76] Combination antifungal therapy may be considered for CNS or disseminated infections.[76]

PAECILOMYCES

Paecilomyces is a rare pathogen in SOT recipients and tends to cause localized skin and soft tissue infections, sometimes associated with other fungi or mycobacteria.[77–79] Case reports have also described peritonitis in a liver transplant recipient and sternal wound infection in a lung transplant recipient.[80,81] Histopathology of tissues may show irregular septate hyphae with Periodic acid-Schiff or Grocott's methenamine silver (GMS) stains but may appear similar to other molds.[6] Surgical excision and debridement are recommended and may be sufficient for cutaneous infection; voriconazole or posaconazole can be used for more extensive disease, but antifungal susceptibilities may help guide therapy.[6,7]

OTHER FUNGI

Numerous other fungi are rare but potentially emerging causes of mold infection in SOT recipients. These fungi include *Scopulariopsis, Trichoderma,* and *Acremonium* species in which various localized and disseminated infections have been described.[82–84] Treatment generally involves surgical excision when possible and antifungal therapy based on susceptibility testing.[6,7]

   Table 2 summarizes the clinical manifestations, diagnosis, and treatment of important mold infections in SOT recipients.

SUMMARY

Mold infections remain an important cause of infection in SOT recipients, and a high level of clinical suspicion and vigilance are required for diagnosis and management. Advancements in diagnostics, such as molecular testing, may improve diagnosis in the future. The role of routine AFST for mold infections and the microbiologic definitions of antifungal resistance are still being determined. More data are needed regarding a correlation between antifungal susceptibilities and clinical outcomes.[85] The role of newer antifungal therapies, such as isavuconazole, in primary and salvage treatment is still evolving. Further research into the epidemiology, clinical manifestations, diagnosis, approach to prophylaxis, treatment, and outcomes of these infections is needed.

REFERENCES

1. Kontoyiannis DP, Yang H, Song J, et al. Prevalence, clinical and economic burden of mucormycosis-related hospitalizations in the United States: a retrospective study. BMC Infect Dis 2016;16(1):730–5.
2. Menzin J, Meyers JL, Friedman M, et al. The economic costs to United States hospitals of invasive fungal infections in transplant patients. Am J Infect Control 2011;39(4):e15–20.
3. Menzin J, Meyers JL, Friedman M, et al. Mortality, length of hospitalization, and costs associated with invasive fungal infections in high-risk patients. Am J Health Syst Pharm 2009;66(19):1711–7.
4. Pappas PG, Alexander BD, Andes DR, et al. Invasive fungal infections among organ transplant recipients: results of the Transplant-Associated Infection Surveillance Network (TRANSNET). Clin Infect Dis 2010;50(8):1101–11.
5. Neofytos D, Fishman JA, Horn D, et al. Epidemiology and outcome of invasive fungal infections in solid organ transplant recipients. Transpl Infect Dis 2010; 12(3):220–9.
6. Huprikar S, Shoham S, AST Infectious Diseases Community of Practice. Emerging fungal infections in solid organ transplantation. Am J Transplant 2013;13(Suppl 4):262–71.
7. Shoham S. Emerging fungal infections in solid organ transplant recipients. Infect Dis Clin North Am 2013;27(2):305–16.
8. Crabol Y, Lortholary O. Invasive mold infections in solid organ transplant recipients. Scientifica (Cairo) 2014;2014:821969.
9. Neofytos D, Treadway S, Ostrander D, et al. Epidemiology, outcomes, and mortality predictors of invasive mold infections among transplant recipients: a 10-year, single-center experience. Transpl Infect Dis 2013;15(3):233–42.
10. Singh N, Husain S, AST Infectious Diseases Community of Practice. Aspergillosis in solid organ transplantation. Am J Transpl 2013;13(Suppl 4):228–41.
11. Steinbach WJ, Marr KA, Anaissie EJ, et al. Clinical epidemiology of 960 patients with invasive aspergillosis from the PATH Alliance registry. J Infect 2012;65(5): 453–64.
12. Morgan J, Wannemuehler KA, Marr KA, et al. Incidence of invasive aspergillosis following hematopoietic stem cell and solid organ transplantation: interim results of a prospective multicenter surveillance program. Med Mycol 2005;43(Suppl 1): S49–58.
13. Singh N, Arnow PM, Bonham A, et al. Invasive aspergillosis in liver transplant recipients in the 1990s. Transplantation 1997;64(5):716–20.
14. De Pauw B, Walsh TJ, Donnelly JP, et al. Revised definitions of invasive fungal disease from the European Organization for Research and Treatment of Cancer/Invasive Fungal Infections Cooperative Group and the National Institute of Allergy and Infectious Diseases Mycoses Study Group (EORTC/MSG) Consensus Group. Clin Infect Dis 2008;46:1813–21.
15. Patterson TF, Thompson GR 3rd, Denning DW, et al. Practice guidelines for the diagnosis and management of aspergillosis: 2016 update by the Infectious Diseases Society of America. Clin Infect Dis 2016;63(4):e1–60.
16. Husain S, Kwak EJ, Obman A, et al. Prospective assessment of Platelia Aspergillus galactomannan antigen for the diagnosis of invasive aspergillosis in lung transplant recipients. Am J Transpl 2004;4:796–802.
17. Pfeiffer CD, Fine JP, Safdar N. Diagnosis of invasive aspergillosis using a galactomannan assay: a meta-analysis. Clin Infect Dis 2006;42:1417–27.

18. Imbert S, Gauthier L, Joly I, et al. Aspergillus PCR in serum for the diagnosis, follow-up and prognosis of invasive aspergillosis in neutropenic and nonneutropenic patients. Clin Microbiol Infect 2016;22(6):562.e1-8.

19. Simoneau E, Kelly M, Labbe AC, et al. What is the clinical significance of positive blood cultures with Aspergillus sp in hematopoietic stem cell transplant recipients? A 23 year experience. Bone Marrow Transpl 2005;35(3):303–6.

20. Herbrecht R, Denning DW, Patterson TF, et al. Voriconazole versus amphotericin B for primary therapy of invasive aspergillosis. N Engl J Med 2002;347:408–15.

21. Maertens JA, Raad II, Marr KA, et al. Isavuconazole versus voriconazole for primary treatment of invasive mould disease caused by Aspergillus and other filamentous fungi (SECURE): a phase 3, randomised-controlled, non-inferiority trial. Lancet 2016;387:760–9.

22. Singh N, Limaye AP, Forrest G, et al. Combination of voriconazole and caspofungin as primary therapy for invasive aspergillosis in solid organ transplant recipients: a prospective, multicenter, observational study. Transplantation 2006;81: 320–6.

23. Husain S, Paterson DL, Studer S, et al. Voriconazole prophylaxis in lung transplant recipients. Am J Transpl 2006;6:3008–16.

24. Horvath J, Dummer S, Loyd J, et al. Infection in the transplanted and native lung after single lung transplantation. Chest 1993;104:681–5.

25. Park BJ, Pappas PG, Wannemuehler KA, et al. Invasive non-Aspergillus mold infections in transplant recipients, United States, 2001–2006. Emerg Infect Dis 2011;17(10):1855–64.

26. Abidi MZ, Sohail MR, Cummins N, et al. Stability in the cumulative incidence, severity and mortality of 101 cases of invasive mucormycosis in high-risk patients from 1995 to 2011: a comparison of eras immediately before and after the availability of voriconazole and echinocandin-amphotericin combination therapies. Mycoses 2014;57(11):687–98.

27. Singh N, Aguado JM, Bonatti H, et al. Zygomycosis in solid organ transplant recipients: a prospective, matched case-control study to assess risks for disease and outcome. J Infect Dis 2009;200(6):1002–11.

28. Almyroudis NG, Sutton DA, Linden P, et al. Zygomycosis in solid organ transplant recipients in a tertiary transplant center and review of the literature. Am J Transpl 2006;6(10):2365–74.

29. Sun HY, Aguado JM, Bonatti H, et al, Zygomycosis Transplant Study Group. Pulmonary zygomycosis in solid organ transplant recipients in the current era. Am J Transpl 2009;9(9):2166–71.

30. Sun HY, Forrest G, Gupta KL, et al. Rhino-orbital-cerebral zygomycosis in solid organ transplant recipients. Transplantation 2010;90(1):85–92.

31. Song Y, Qiao J, Giovanni G, et al. Mucormycosis in renal transplant recipients: review of 174 reported cases. BMC Infect Dis 2017;17(1):283–8.

32. Salehi E, Hedayati MT, Zoll J, et al. Discrimination of aspergillosis, mucormycosis, fusariosis, and scedosporiosis in formalin-fixed paraffin-embedded tissue specimens by use of multiple real-time quantitative PCR assays. J Clin Microbiol 2016; 54(11):2798–803.

33. Millon L, Larosa F, Lepiller Q, et al. Quantitative polymerase chain reaction detection of circulating DNA in serum for early diagnosis of mucormycosis in immunocompromised patients. Clin Infect Dis 2013;56(10):e95–101.

34. Millon L, Herbrecht R, Grenouillet F, et al, French Mycosis Study Group. Early diagnosis and monitoring of mucormycosis by detection of circulating DNA in serum: retrospective analysis of 44 cases collected through the French

Surveillance Network of Invasive Fungal Infections (RESSIF). Clin Microbiol Infect 2016;22(9):810.e1-e8.

35. Cornely OA, Arikan-Akdagli S, Dannaoui E, et al, European Society of Clinical Microbiology and Infectious Diseases Fungal Infection Study Group, European Confederation of Medical Mycology. ESCMID and ECMM joint clinical guidelines for the diagnosis and management of mucormycosis 2013. Clin Microbiol Infect 2014;20(Suppl 3):5–26.

36. Marty FM, Ostrosky-Zeichner L, Cornely OA, et al, VITAL and FungiScope Mucormycosis Investigators. Isavuconazole treatment for mucormycosis: a single-arm open-label trial and case-control analysis. Lancet Infect Dis 2016;16(7):828–37.

37. Reed C, Bryant R, Ibrahim AS. Combination polyene-caspofungin treatment of rhino-orbital-cerebral mucormycosis. Clin Infect Dis 2008;47(3):364–71.

38. Ibrahim AS, Gebremariam T, Fu Y, et al. Combination echinocandin-polyene treatment of murine mucormycosis. Antimicrob Agents Chemother 2008;52(4):1556–8.

39. Spellberg B, Fu Y, Edwards JE Jr, et al. Combination therapy with amphotericin B lipid complex and caspofungin acetate of disseminated zygomycosis in diabetic ketoacidotic mice. Antimicrob Agents Chemother 2005;49(2):830–2.

40. Gebremariam T, Wiederhold NP, Alqarihi A, et al. Monotherapy or combination therapy of isavuconazole and micafungin for treating murine mucormycosis. J Antimicrob Chemother 2017;72(2):462–6.

41. Katragkou A, McCarthy M, Meletiadis J, et al. In vitro combination of isavuconazole with micafungin or amphotericin B deoxycholate against medically important molds. Antimicrob Agents Chemother 2014;58(11):6934–7.

42. Kim JH, Benefield RJ, Ditolla K. Utilization of posaconazole oral suspension or delayed-released tablet salvage treatment for invasive fungal infection. Mycoses 2016;59(11):726–33.

43. Vehreschild JJ, Birtel A, Vehreschild MJ, et al. Mucormycosis treated with posaconazole: review of 96 case reports. Crit Rev Microbiol 2013;39(3):310–24.

44. Alexander BD, Perfect JR, Daly JS, et al. Posaconazole as salvage therapy in patients with invasive fungal infections after solid organ transplant. Transplantation 2008;86(6):791–6.

45. Miceli MH, Kauffman CA. Isavuconazole: a new broad-spectrum triazole antifungal agent. Clin Infect Dis 2015;61(10):1558–65.

46. Natesan SK, Chandrasekar PH. Isavuconazole for the treatment of invasive aspergillosis and mucormycosis: current evidence, safety, efficacy, and clinical recommendations. Infect Drug Resist 2016;9:291–300.

47. Martin MS, Smith AA, Lobo M, et al. Successful treatment of recurrent pulmonary mucormycosis in a renal transplant patient: a case report and literature review. Case Rep Transplant 2017;2017:1925070.

48. Muhammed M, Anagnostou T, Desalermos A, et al. Fusarium infection: report of 26 cases and review of 97 cases from the literature. Medicine (Baltimore) 2013;92(6):305–16.

49. Halpern M, Balbi E, Carius L, et al. Cellulitis and nodular skin lesions due to Fusarium spp in liver transplant: case report. Transplant Proc 2010;42(2):599–600.

50. Sampathkumar P, Paya CV. Fusarium infection after solid-organ transplantation. Clin Infect Dis 2001;32(8):1237–40.

51. Carneiro HA, Coleman JJ, Restrepo A, et al. Fusarium infection in lung transplant patients: report of 6 cases and review of the literature. Medicine (Baltimore) 2011;90(1):69–80.

52. Gupta AK, Baran R, Summerbell RC. Fusarium infections of the skin. Curr Opin Infect Dis 2000;13(2):121–8.
53. Nucci M, Anaissie E. Fusarium infections in immunocompromised patients. Clin Microbiol Rev 2007;20(4):695–704.
54. Dignani MC, Anaissie E. Human fusariosis. Clin Microbiol Infect 2004;10(Suppl 1):67–75.
55. Tortorano AM, Richardson M, Roilides E, et al, European Society of Clinical Microbiology and Infectious Diseases Fungal Infection Study Group, European Confederation of Medical Mycology. ESCMID and ECMM joint guidelines on diagnosis and management of hyalohyphomycosis: Fusarium spp., Scedosporium spp. and others. Clin Microbiol Infect 2014;20(Suppl 3):27–46.
56. Espinel-Ingroff A, Colombo AL, Cordoba S, et al. International evaluation of MIC distributions and epidemiological cutoff value (ECV) definitions for fusarium species identified by molecular methods for the CLSI broth microdilution method. Antimicrob Agents Chemother 2015;60(2):1079–84.
57. Tortorano AM, Esposto MC, Prigitano A, et al. Cross-reactivity of Fusarium spp. in the Aspergillus galactomannan enzyme-linked immunosorbent assay. J Clin Microbiol 2011;50:1051–3.
58. Horn DL, Freifeld AG, Schuster MG, et al. Treatment and outcomes of invasive fusariosis: review of 65 cases from the PATH Alliance(®) registry. Mycoses 2014;57(11):652–8.
59. Raad II, Hachem RY, Herbrecht R, et al. Posaconazole as salvage treatment for invasive fusariosis in patients with underlying hematologic malignancy and other conditions. Clin Infect Dis 2006;42(10):1398–403.
60. Liu JY, Chen WT, Ko BS, et al. Combination antifungal therapy for disseminated fusariosis in immunocompromised patients: a case report and literature review. Med Mycol 2011;49(8):872–8.
61. Stempel JM, Hammond SP, Sutton DA, et al. Invasive fusariosis in the voriconazole era: single-center 13-year experience. Open Forum Infect Dis 2015;2(3):ofv099.
62. Lackner M, de Hoog GS, Yang L, et al. Proposed nomenclature for Pseudallescheria, Scedosporium and related genera. Fungal Divers 2014;1:1–10.
63. Abela IA, Murer C, Schuurmans MM, et al. A cluster of scedosporiosis in lung transplant candidates and recipients: the Zurich experience and review of the literature. Transpl Infect Dis 2018;20(1):12792–810.
64. Parize P, Boussaud V, Poinsignon V, et al. Clinical outcome of cystic fibrosis patients colonized by Scedosporium species following lung transplantation: a single-center 15-year experience. Transpl Infect Dis 2017;19(5):12738–44.
65. Johnson LS, Shields RK, Clancy CJ. Epidemiology, clinical manifestations, and outcomes of Scedosporium infections among solid organ transplant recipients. Transpl Infect Dis 2014;16(4):578–87.
66. Troke P, Aguirrebengoa K, Arteaga C, et al, Global Scedosporium Study Group. Treatment of scedosporiosis with voriconazole: clinical experience with 107 patients. Antimicrob Agents Chemother 2008;52(5):1743–50.
67. Castiglioni B, Sutton DA, Rinaldi MG, et al. Pseudallescheria boydii (Anamorph Scedosporium apiospermum). Infection in solid organ transplant recipients in a tertiary medical center and review of the literature. Medicine (Baltimore) 2002;81(5):333–48.
68. Lackner M, de Hoog GS, Verweij PE, et al. Species-specific antifungal susceptibility patterns of Scedosporium and Pseudallescheria species. Antimicrob Agents Chemother 2012;56(5):2635–42.

69. Husain S, Muñoz P, Forrest G, et al. Infections due to Scedosporium apiospermum and Scedosporium prolificans in transplant recipients: clinical characteristics and impact of antifungal agent therapy on outcome. Clin Infect Dis 2005; 40(1):89–99.

70. Schwartz S, Reisman A, Troke PF. The efficacy of voriconazole in the treatment of 192 fungal central nervous system infections: a retrospective analysis. Infection 2011;39(3):201–10.

71. Cortez KJ, Roilides E, Quiroz-Telles F, et al. Infections caused by Scedosporium spp. Clin Microbiol Rev 2008;21(1):157–97.

72. Rodríguez MM, Calvo E, Serena C, et al. Effects of double and triple combinations of antifungal drugs in a murine model of disseminated infection by Scedosporium prolificans. Antimicrob Agents Chemother 2009;53(5):2153–5.

73. Schieffelin JS, Garcia-Diaz JB, Loss GE Jr, et al. Phaeohyphomycosis fungal infections in solid organ transplant recipients: clinical presentation, pathology, and treatment. Transpl Infect Dis 2014;16(2):270–8.

74. McCarty TP, Baddley JW, Walsh TJ, et al. Phaeohyphomycosis in transplant recipients: results from the Transplant Associated Infection Surveillance Network (TRANSNET). Med Mycol 2015;53(5):440–6.

75. Santos DW, Camargo LF, Gonçalves SS, et al. Melanized fungal infections in kidney transplant recipients: contributions to optimize clinical management. Clin Microbiol Infect 2017;23(5):333.e9-e14.

76. Chowdhary A, Meis JF, Guarro J, et al, European Society of Clinical Microbiology and Infectious Diseases Fungal Infection Study Group, European Confederation of Medical Mycology. ESCMID and ECMM joint clinical guidelines for the diagnosis and management of systemic phaeohyphomycosis: diseases caused by black fungi. Clin Microbiol Infect 2014;20(Suppl 3):47–75.

77. Muñoz P, Maddalena G, Vena A, et al. Mold infections in solid organ transplant recipients. In: Ljungman P, Snydman D, Boeckh M, editors. Transplant infections. 4th edition. Switzerland: Springer International Publishing; 2016. p. 719–56.

78. Lavergne RA, Cassaing S, Nocera T, et al. Simultaneous cutaneous infection due to Paecilomyces lilacinus and Alternaria in a heart transplant patient. Transpl Infect Dis 2012;14(6):E156–60.

79. Kim JE, Sung H, Kim MN, et al. Synchronous infection with Mycobacterium chelonae and Paecilomyces in a heart transplant patient. Transpl Infect Dis 2011; 13(1):80–3.

80. Polat M, Kara SS, Tapısız A, et al. Successful treatment of Paecilomyces variotii peritonitis in a liver transplant patient. Mycopathologia 2015;179(3–4):317–20.

81. Lee J, Yew WW, Chiu CS, et al. Delayed sternotomy wound infection due to Paecilomyces variotii in a lung transplant recipient. J Heart Lung Transplant 2002; 21(10):1131–4.

82. Pate MJ, Hemmige V, Woc-Colburn L, et al. Successful eradication of invasive Scopulariopsis brumptii in a liver transplant recipient. Transpl Infect Dis 2016; 18(2):275–9.

83. Chouaki T, Lavarde V, Lachaud L, et al. Invasive infections due to Trichoderma species: report of 2 cases, findings of in vitro susceptibility testing, and review of the literature. Clin Infect Dis 2002;35(11):1360–7.

84. Geyer AS, Fox LP, Husain S, et al. Acremonium mycetoma in a heart transplant recipient. J Am Acad Dermatol 2006;55(6):1095–100.

85. Eschenauer GA, Carver PL. The evolving role of antifungal susceptibility testing. Pharmacotherapy 2013;33(5):465–75.

Prevention and Management of Tuberculosis in Solid Organ Transplant Recipients

David J. Epstein, MD, Aruna K. Subramanian, MD*

KEYWORDS

- Solid organ transplantation • Tuberculosis • Latent tuberculosis infection
- Opportunistic infections • Donor derived infections

KEY POINTS

- Solid organ transplant recipients are at increased risk for tuberculosis reactivation owing to immunosuppression. Some candidates have risk factors for tuberculosis reactivation even pretransplantation.
- Screening for latent tuberculosis infection involves a detailed history, a tuberculin skin test or tuberculosis interferon-gamma release assay, and a chest radiograph.
- Isoniazid for 9 months is the preferred therapy for patients with rifamycin drug interactions. Rifamycins may be preferred for patients at risk of hepatotoxicity from isoniazid.
- Tuberculosis occurs months or years after transplantation. Patients can present with typical features of tuberculosis or with unusual or nonspecific manifestations.
- Tuberculosis treatment in solid organ transplant recipients may be complicated by drug interactions and adverse drug reactions and requires close monitoring.

INTRODUCTION
History and Importance

Because immune suppression to prevent allograft rejection is a cornerstone of solid organ transplantation (SOT), infections occur with relative frequency and often with increased severity. Given the ubiquity of tuberculosis (TB), it is not surprising that this infection has been reported in patients undergoing SOT since the 1960s and 1970s.[1,2]

SOT candidates and recipients contend with unique challenges in TB diagnosis and treatment. They are at high risk for TB reactivation after transplantation, and many enter transplantation with conditions such as end-stage renal disease, diabetes mellitus, or iatrogenic immunosuppression predisposing them to TB reactivation. The

Disclosure Statement: None.
Division of Infectious Diseases and Geographic Medicine, Department of Medicine, Stanford University, 300 Pasteur Drive, Lane Building, Mail Code 5107, Stanford, CA 94305, USA
* Corresponding author.
E-mail address: asubram2@stanford.edu

Infect Dis Clin N Am 32 (2018) 703–718
https://doi.org/10.1016/j.idc.2018.05.002
0891-5520/18/© 2018 Elsevier Inc. All rights reserved.

id.theclinics.com

signs or symptoms of their underlying end-stage organ failure may overlap with the protean manifestations of TB, including weight loss, cough, and malaise. Given their comorbid conditions and medications, they may be at increased risk of adverse drug reactions (ADRs) from antituberculous therapy (ATT), including neuropathy, hepatotoxicity, and gout, and may contend with multiple drug interactions. Finally, posttransplant TB has been associated with allograft loss and increased mortality.[3,4]

Pathogenesis

The pathways through which SOT recipients may develop active TB are several, and can differ from those relevant to non-SOT recipients. SOT candidates may present with latent TB infection (LTBI; **Fig. 1**A) or active TB (**Fig. 1**D). After SOT, those with LTBI may or may not reactivate; those with active TB would be expected to have disease progression. Although difficult to prove, most SOT recipients who develop active TB presumably do so as a reactivation in the context of prior LTBI, especially in countries with low rates of TB endemicity where there is less likelihood of exposure after SOT. Previously uninfected SOT recipients may develop de novo infection through exposure to someone with infectious (typically pulmonary or laryngeal) TB (**Fig. 1**C), but, uniquely, may also contract TB as a donor-derived infection (**Fig. 1**B). TB bacilli may exist in transplanted organs in a spectrum of metabolic activity from quiescent infection in an otherwise healthy donor to florid infection that may have gone unrecognized.[5] Some of these donor-derived infections may be controlled by the recipient's immune system, but many of these recipients will likely develop clinically apparent TB disease.

The most obvious mechanism by which SOT recipients are at increased risk for TB reactivation involves intensive iatrogenic suppression of the immune system. In nearly all cases, SOT recipients are treated with combinations of corticosteroids, antimetabolites, calcineurin inhibitors (CNIs), and mammalian target of rapamycin inhibitors. Initial induction immunosuppression and treatment for rejection often involve administration of antibodies resulting in T-lymphocyte depletion or signaling impairment, including alemtuzumab, antithymocyte globulin, and basiliximab. Additionally, corticosteroids, CNIs, and mechanistic target of rapamycin inhibitors predispose to posttransplant diabetes mellitus, a known risk factor for TB reactivation. Patients can also develop other risk factors for TB reactivation posttransplant, such as end-stage renal disease owing to CNIs or significant weight loss.

Epidemiology

SOT has long been recognized as a strong risk factor for TB reactivation and testing and treating for LTBI has been recommended in these patients in guidelines dating back several decades.[6,7] Several recent studies have established that SOT recipients have a substantially increased risk of TB, with an incidence of at least 4 times that of the general population, and in some studies nearly 30 times that of the general population.[8–11] TB incidence is increased at least 2-fold, even when SOT recipients are matched closely with patients with end-organ disease who did do not ultimately undergo transplantation.[12] Some of these studies included patients who were screened and treated for LTBI, suggesting the incidence comparisons discussed may underestimate the natural history of the disease. Although high-quality data on the incidence of TB among SOT recipients in the United States are not available, the TB incidence among diverse SOT recipients in Spain, a country with a similar although slightly higher TB incidence, was found to be markedly elevated at more than 400 cases per 100,000 person-years.[8,13] Data are insufficient to address whether recipients of some organs are at greater risk than others, with the exception of lung transplantation, which confers a particularly high risk of TB.[8]

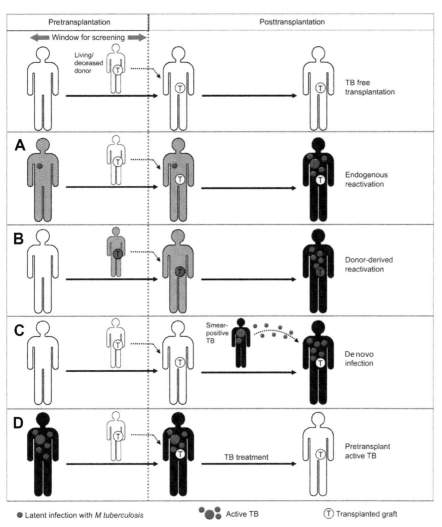

Fig. 1. The 4 different scenarios for infection with *Mycobacterium tuberculosis* in the transplant setting. (*A*) Endogenous reactivation owing to latent infection with *M tuberculosis* (LTBI) in the candidate recipient. (*B*) Donor-derived reactivation owing to LTBI in a living or deceased donor. (*C*) De novo exposure and infection posttransplantation. (*D*) When a patient with active TB urgently requires a transplant (ie, urgent liver transplantation). White, gray, and black figures represent uninfected individuals, individuals with LTBI, and individuals with active TB, respectively. (*Reproduced from* Bumbacea D, Arend SM, Eyuboglu F, et al. The risk of tuberculosis in transplant candidates and recipients: a TBNET consensus statement. Eur Respir J 2012;40(4):992; with permission from the ©ERS 2018.)

PREVENTION OF TUBERCULOSIS

Pretransplant Evaluation for Latent Tuberculosis Infection and Chemoprophylaxis to Prevent Reactivation of Latent Tuberculosis in the Recipient or from the Donor

LTBI has been defined as evidence of immunologic sensitization to TB based on a test for LTBI in those without active disease. Immunologic assays have traditionally involved tuberculin skin tests (TSTs), most commonly using purified protein derivative. More recently,

Mycobacterium tuberculosis (MTB) interferon-gamma release assays (IGRAs) have been used, based on either enzyme-linked immunosorbent assay or enzyme-linked immunospot techniques. This definition of LTBI is problematic because an acquired immune response to TB may result in a positive test for LTBI even though TB bacilli have been eliminated; alternatively, viable TB bacilli may be present despite a false-negative test.[5] Furthermore, the distinction between latent and active infection is somewhat arbitrary, and depends in part on how aggressively evidence is sought for replicating bacilli.[5] Tests for LTBI have been approved for clinical use based on their ability to predict active disease and their correlation with epidemiologic risk factors for TB infection.

These immunologic tests for LTBI—namely, TST, enzyme-linked immunosorbent assay, and enzyme-linked immunospot—correlate only fairly to moderately with each other, highlighting flaws in their validity.[14–21] MTB IGRAs occasionally yield indeterminate results, most commonly in patients with impaired cellular immunity whose lymphocytes fail to sufficiently respond to the mitogen in the positive control tube.[14–21] Although indeterminate test results of IGRAS confound their interpretation, the lack of positive controls in TSTs as typically performed could theoretically provide false reassurance that LTBI is not present in those with immunologic impairment. When comparing the results of a test for LTBI with clinical, epidemiologic, and radiographic evidence of TB exposure, IGRAs may be more sensitive than TSTs with at least similar specificity, and likely greater specificity among those who were vaccinated with the Bacillus Calmette-Guérin vaccine.[22,23] Both the TST and MTB IGRA have been demonstrated to predict the risk of TB after transplantation.[9,24] Therefore, although the MTB IGRA is likely the preferred initial test, those who test negative but have an increased likelihood of having LTBI based on epidemiologic, clinical, or radiographic features should potentially be tested with a TST as well.[23] Those with known LTBI from a previous testing do not need to undergo repeat testing, but should be evaluated to determine whether they have received adequate therapy and whether they may have been reinfected since treatment (**Fig. 2** illustrates these authors' approach to LTBI evaluation in SOT candidates).

In fact, rather than relying solely on TSTs or IGRAs, the most accurate approach to diagnosing LTBI likely involves evaluating a patient's prior TB contact and chest imaging features suggestive of prior TB infection, in addition to querying immunologic evidence of prior TB infection. For example, a study of liver and kidney transplant recipients in China demonstrated that SOT recipients with any of multiple risk factors—positive TST or IGRA, chest radiographs suggestive of prior TB, or recent TB contact—were at increased risk for development of posttransplant TB.[25] Another study of South Korean liver transplant recipients found that those with linear scars or calcified nodules on pretransplant chest radiographs, which likely represent prior TB infection in this epidemiologic setting, were more likely to develop posttransplant TB.[26] In this same study, pretransplant computed tomography (CT) scans of the chest were able to identify evidence of healed or prior TB—such as irregular lines, calcified and noncalcified nodules, and fibrosis—that predicted development of posttransplant TB even in those with normal chest radiographs.[26] Another study confirmed the predictive value of chest CT scans in patients before undergoing lung transplantation to identify those with LTBI at risk for reactivation.[13] Therefore, SOT candidates without recent chest radiographs in the prior 3 to 6 months should generally have them performed, even if they have negative test for LTBI.[25,26] Similarly, a CT scan should be considered among those patients with negative test for LTBI but with high-risk clinical or epidemiologic features for LTBI.[13,25,26]

As is the case for all patients, all those with a positive test for LTBI should undergo a chest radiograph and a careful history and examination to rule out active TB before considering treatment for LTBI (and before pursing transplantation and attendant

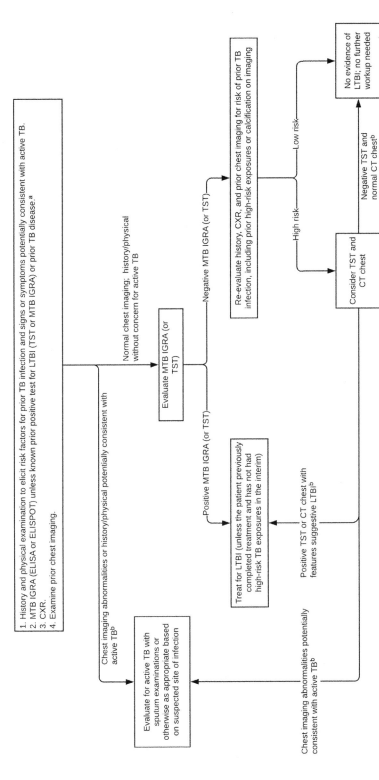

Fig. 2. Algorithm for evaluation of tuberculosis (TB) and latent TB infection (LTBI) among solid organ transplant candidates. CT, computed tomography; CXR, chest radiograph; ELISA, enzyme-linked immunosorbent assay; ELISPOT, enzyme-linked immunospot; IGRA, interferon-gamma release assay; MTB, *Mycobacterium tuberculosis*; TST, tuberculin skin test. [a] Those with prior TB who successfully completed treatment should generally not undergo further testing or treatment for LTBI, except in cases of known high-risk exposures occurring after TB treatment completed. [b] Chest radiographs, CT scans, and other studies showing only fully calcified pulmonary nodules, calcified hilar lymph nodes, or apical pleural scarring do not suggest active disease and these patients generally do not need to be evaluated for active TB based on these features alone.

immunosuppression). Diligence in ruling out active TB is key both to avoid promoting drug-resistant TB by treating active disease with monotherapy, and to defer intensive immunosuppression in the face of an active and uncontrolled pulmonary infection, apart from public health concerns. In those with a chest radiograph showing features potentially consistent with pulmonary after primary or reactivation TB—especially upper lobe infiltrates or cavities—at least 3 induced or expectorated sputum samples, collected 8 hours apart with 1 collected in the early morning should be obtained for MTB polymerase chain reaction testing, acid-fast bacilli smear, and acid-fast bacilli culture. In these cases, a CT scan of the chest can reveal the pattern and extent of disease for diagnostic and prognostic purposes, although it should be noted that pulmonary (and thoracic extrapulmonary) TB can have protean radiographic manifestations, including lobar consolidations, pleural effusions, lymphadenopathy, and osseous involvement. Because chest radiographs can occasionally be normal in those with active pulmonary TB, particularly in patients with immune impairment before transplantation, those with signs or symptoms suggestive of pulmonary TB, such as fever, cough, dyspnea, or chest pain, should undergo further evaluation with serial sputum examinations as detailed and a CT scan.[27] Perhaps with the exception of solitary micronodules stable over several months or features (such as fully calcified nodules or lymph nodes or apical pleural scarring), incidentally discovered pulmonary parenchymal abnormalities on prior scans should similarly prompt collection of sputum to rule out active disease and other workup as appropriate. Finally, those with positive test for LTBI and signs or symptoms that could be consistent with extrapulmonary TB should undergo appropriate workup based on the nature of these localizing features.

The treatment of LTBI, once active disease is ruled out, typically consists of several months of treatment with 1 or more drugs active against MTB. LTBI treatment is intended to decrease the risk of development of active TB by sterilizing bacilli before they become metabolically active and cause clinically apparent disease. Ideal regimens for LTBI treatment, apart from clinical efficacy, would be safe, well-tolerated, of short duration, and without significant drug interactions. In the uncommon situation that the SOT candidate is a known contact of someone with a drug-resistant isolate of TB, antimicrobial susceptibility testing results of the contact will determine in part the best LTBI treatment regimen.[7]

These authors' approach to LTBI treatment is largely similar to patients who are not SOT candidates. **Table 1** provides treatment options for LTBI.[28–34] Nine months of isoniazid (INH [9H]) has been traditionally the treatment of choice for LTBI, and its use in SOT candidates and recipients is supported by more clinical experience and

Table 1
Regimens used for treatment of LTBI

First-line regimens:	Alternative regimens with disadvantages relative to first-line regimens:	Regimens not typically recommended owing to concerns about safety or efficacy and/or limited data:
• 9H (INH ×9 months)[28] • 4R (RIF ×4 months)[28] • 3HP (weekly INH/RPT ×12 doses via DOT)[28]	• 6H (INH ×6 months)[28] • RFB ×4 mo[28] • 3HR (INH/RIF ×3 months)[29,30] • 4HR (INH/RIF ×4 months)[30]	• 2RZ (RIF/PZA ×2 months)[28] • FQ ± EMB, ETO, or PZA ×6-12 mo[31–33] • PZA ± EMB or ETO ×12 mo[33,34] • ETO/CS ×12 mo[34]

Abbreviations: CS, cycloserine; DOT, directly observed therapy; EMB, ethambutol; ETO, ethionamide; FQ, fluoroquinolone; INH, isoniazid; LTBI, latent tuberculosis infection; PZA, pyrazinamide; RFB, rifabutin; RIF, rifampin; RPT, rifapentine.

evidence than other regimens.[35] A particular advantage of this regimen is that it can be started pretransplant and usually continued after transplantation, owing to the lack of significant drug interactions. If transplantation is needed urgently, this regimen is particularly attractive. Still, in the wider population of LTBI patients, clinicians and public health programs are increasingly choosing 4 months of rifampin (RIF [4R]) as a preferred regimen given emerging evidence of better adherence, increased tolerability, and fewer ADRs, particularly hepatotoxicity, compared with 9H.[36–39] Three months of weekly INH and rifapentine (3HP) is an alternative regimen with a shorter duration, potentially allowing completion of LTBI therapy before transplantation, although it is disadvantaged by relatively high rates of ADRs.[40] Another disadvantage of the 3HP regimen is the typical requirement that it be administered via directly observed therapy, although newer data support self-administration.[41] The decision of which of these 3 regimens to use should be based on drug interactions, risk of ADRs, and patient and provider preference. In general, rifamycins should be avoided for LTBI treatment after transplantation given the significant drug interactions with CNIs such as tacrolimus and cyclosporine used for immunosuppression. RIF and rifapentine are potent inducers of cytochrome P450 enzymes,[42] and because the pharmacokinetic effects of chronically administered rifamycins can persist for weeks or longer after the drug is discontinued, 4R should generally not be started unless SOT will be unlikely to occur in the next 6 months.

Liver transplant candidates with LTBI constitute a unique group whom clinicians have sometimes avoided treating given concern for drug-induced liver injury. Fig. 3 provides these authors' approach to LTBI treatment in liver transplant candidates or others with liver disease or who are at increased risk of hepatotoxicity. Treatment for LTBI should be deferred for those with decompensated cirrhosis or acute hepatitis. The risks and benefits of treatment should be considered carefully for other patients with significant liver disease, including those with a baseline alanine transaminase value of more than 3 times the upper limit of normal or bilirubin greater than 2 mg/dL.[43] Sometimes, liver disease stabilizes sufficiently before transplantation to allow LTBI treatment. Often, however, treatment can be deferred until after liver transplantation occurs, when liver function stabilizes. Patients without such severe hepatic dysfunction that treatment is entirely precluded could likely receive 4R. A randomized clinical trial comparing 9H and 4R in a population with high rates of viral hepatitis and baseline transaminase abnormalities showed that none of the RIF-treated patients developed biochemical hepatitis requiring treatment

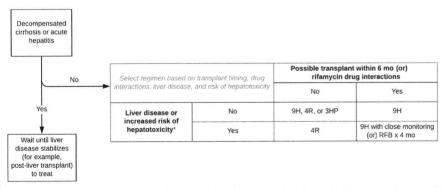

Fig. 3. Algorithm for treatment of latent tuberculosis infection (LTBI) in liver transplant candidates and other organ transplant candidates with liver disease or at increased risk of hepatotoxicity. 3HP, 3 months of weekly isoniazid and rifapentine via directly-observed therapy; 4R, rifampin ×4 months; 9H, isoniazid ×9 months; RFB, rifabutin. [a] See text for risk stratification.

discontinuation, compared with more than 5% of the INH-treated patients.[37] However, patients with compensated cirrhosis who are not eligible for 4R or 3HP can still often tolerate treatment with 9H with close monitoring. Several case series report the successful treatment with 9H of patients with cirrhosis before undergoing liver transplantation without significant ADRs but with the occasional need to interrupt therapy owing to transaminase elevations.[44–46] Another option for patients who are unable to take RIF owing to drug interactions or potential SOT transplantation in the near future is rifabutin.[7,47] Rifabutin is highly active against MTB and similarly less hepatotoxic than INH, but with significantly less (although still significant) cytochrome P450 induction.[47] Its use as a substitute for RIF as treatment for TB and LTBI has been established over many years among patients with human immunodeficiency virus infection taking protease inhibitors.[7]

Issues related to patient monitoring and treatment interruption are generally handled similarly to other patients with LTBI. Patients should be seen by the treating health care provider monthly to assess for signs or symptoms of hepatitis or other ADRs, medication adherence, and in rare cases evidence of development of active TB.[7] Patients should be instructed to immediately stop medications and contact the provider should they develop signs or symptoms potentially concerning for hepatitis or other significant ADRs.[7] Laboratory testing should at a minimum include liver tests (including transaminases and bilirubin) at baseline before treatment, and every 2 to 4 weeks thereafter.[43] Those with significant liver disease should likely have baseline and periodic monitoring of prothrombin time and International Normalized Ratio as well.[43] Those being treated with rifamycin-containing regimens should likely be monitored with a complete blood count with a white blood cell differential given that cytopenias are occasionally reported with long-term rifamycin use.[7] Patients who undergo SOT midtreatment should generally have medications withheld in the immediate peritransplant period until they are tolerating oral medications and clinically stable. Liver transplant recipients should generally wait a few weeks after SOT until liver function stabilizes. Fortunately, interruptions are permitted without requiring therapy to be started anew. For example, patients treated on 9H must complete 9 months of INH (or 270 doses) within 12 months, 120 doses of RIF in 4R treatment must be completed within 6 months, and 11 or 12 doses of 3HP must be completed within 16 weeks.[7,48]

Fluoroquinolones have been appealing candidates for LTBI treatment regimens owing to their in vitro activity against MTB, efficacy as a part of multidrug therapy for active TB, and perceived tolerability and favorable ADR profile. Levofloxacin, particularly, has been suggested as a possible treatment option for LTBI in those with cirrhosis, given the relatively low rates of hepatotoxicity and potentially greater efficacy and safety relative to other minimally hepatotoxic ATT drugs (such as ethambutol [EMB], cycloserine, and aminoglycosides). Unfortunately, an open-label randomized clinical trial comparing levofloxacin with INH for treatment of LTBI among liver transplant candidates was stopped early when nearly 20% of patients in the levofloxacin arm developed tenosynovitis.[31] This experience has been countered by others who report good tolerability of fluoroquinolones for LTBI treatment in this population.[49] Perhaps most important, fluoroquinolones, particularly as monotherapy, have never been demonstrated by reasonable quality evidence to be effective in reducing rates of TB reactivation. Fluoroquinolone-based regimens have been used for LTBI treatment among those exposed to patients with INH-resistant or RIF-resistant TB strains, and a metaanalysis estimated this approach has an efficacy of slightly more than 60%.[33] Although this approach may be reasonable in patients with no other choice, it should not be used for SOT recipients who have treatment alternatives.

Prevention of Donor-Derived Infections

Donor-derived TB has been infrequently described; however, it may have devastating consequences for recipients of multiple organs from the same donor.[50–55] Moreover, such cases may erode confidence in the safety of SOT with programmatic and public health consequences. In other cases, donor-derived TB infection may be mistakenly diagnosed as reactivation TB. Compared with data addressing diagnosis and treatment of LTBI among SOT candidates, interventions to prevent donor-derived infections have sparse data to guide recommendations. Our recommendations herein conform with those proffered by a consensus conference report.[56] Two obvious challenges exist in this arena. First, TST or MTB IGRAs are in vivo and ex vivo tests, respectively, and there are theoretic concerns about their performance in deceased (including brain dead) donors; these assays have not been meaningfully tested on deceased donors. Second, although heart and particularly lung transplants are likely associated with a greater risk of donor-derived TB infection, the risk of abdominal organs less well-known, although documented instances of donor-derived infection through both thoracic and abdominal SOT are well-described.[50–55] Countries of intermediate TB endemicity often do not treat for LTBI when donors are latently infected and this approach does not seem to be associated with high rates of donor-derived TB.[57,58] Still, given the pathophysiology of TB involving early hematogenous and lymphatic spread, we favor treating the recipient for known LTBI, regardless of the organ involved.

Prevention of deceased donor-derived infections involves questioning family members of the potential donor for a known history of LTBI, TB exposure, or risks associated with TB exposure. Rarely, a deceased donor may have a known diagnosis of LTBI, which should not preclude donation unless this individual was a known recent contact of someone with multidrug-resistant TB. Rather, in these cases the recipient should be treated for LTBI after transplantation in case metabolically inactive bacilli present are present in the donated organ or accompanying lymphoid tissue. In other cases, deceased donor LTBI may be suspected based on a history of known exposure or high-risk interactions, potentially accompanied by otherwise unexplained calcified granulomas visualized on imaging, in which case treatment of the recipient for LTBI could be considered on a case-by-case basis. Although donors with known active TB are excluded, lungs of a donor with undiagnosed active pulmonary TB may occasionally be transplanted when routine acid-fast bacilli cultures grow TB weeks later, in which case the recipient should be treated for active disease as described elsewhere in this article.

We favor testing living donors for LTBI according to an algorithm similar to that applied to SOT recipients and treating either the donor or recipient. This approach is particularly important for heart and even more so lung transplants, although we endorse its use for abdominal organ transplants as discussed. Presumably, treating the donor before SOT or the recipient after SOT would be similarly effective; however, because the donor may benefit from treatment and because the recipient may be more at risk from ADRs associated with LTBI therapy, treating the donor rather than recipient may be optimal.

DIAGNOSIS AND TREATMENT OF ACTIVE TUBERCULOSIS
Tuberculosis Diagnosis in Solid Organ Transplant Candidates and Recipients

As in other patients with active TB, SOT recipients with TB disease frequently present with cough, fever, and other constitutional signs and symptoms.[10,59–64] Still, these typical manifestations of TB are not universal, and recipients may have blunted inflammatory responses owing to immunosuppression. Additionally, when SOT recipients present with cough, parenchymal consolidations, or other clinical findings, the differential diagnosis may be more expansive than in other patients, complicating the diagnosis.

Notably, SOT patients commonly present with disseminated and extrapulmonary disease, perhaps at rates higher than in the general population.[3,4,8,10,11,25,59–61,63–69] Radiographic presentations of pulmonary TB are highly varied in SOT patients. Patients may present with normal chest radiographs, or with interstitial opacities or lobar consolidations; cavitary disease is less common, although as in immunocompetent patients with pulmonary TB, lesions commonly affect the upper lobes.[59,64]

TB after SOT is generally a late phenomenon, with large studies reporting median times to TB diagnosis of 5 to 26 months after transplantation (and most studies reporting medians of 8–14 months).[3,10,11,25,60,61,63–67,69,70] Cases of TB diagnosed within 1 month of SOT have been described, but diagnosis this early raises the possibility that at least some of these patients may have had TB that was already active but undiagnosed before transplantation. Notably, the late onset of TB in SOT recipients contrasts sharply with the generally rapid tempo of TB reactivation in the context of tumor necrosis factor-alpha inhibitor use, with a median time to TB reactivation of 12 weeks reported with use of infliximab.[71]

Uniquely, SOT recipients who develop donor-derived TB often present with disease manifestations particular to the type of allograft received. Recipients of infected kidneys, for example, may develop increased creatinine; SOT recipients may also develop wound dehiscence, abscesses, or other surgical site infections owing to TB.[51,54,72] Disseminated infection may be more likely in the case of donor-derived infections as well.[51,54,72]

Tuberculosis Treatment in Solid Organ Transplant Candidates and Recipients

With some exceptions and caveats related to unique circumstances of SOT candidates and recipients, treatment of drug-susceptible TB should generally adhere to recently published guidelines for the general population.[73] Particular features of SOT recipients include immunosuppression with a relatively high risk for progressive or disseminated disease, suggesting early empiric treatment for TB when this diagnosis is seriously considered pending confirmation with microbiologic or other testing.[73] Daily rather than intermittent dosing of ATT and use of directly observed therapy are preferred given their established benefits and to minimize irregular drug interactions with immunosuppressive medications.[73] Additionally, pyridoxine should be universally administered to SOT candidates and recipients, given the multiple comorbidities intrinsic to this population that may increase risk of INH-associated neuropathy.[73] Those being treated for active TB should be evaluated at least monthly in person by the treating provider; more frequent follow-up may be needed.[73] These patients should be monitored at least monthly with complete blood counts, liver tests (including bilirubin and transaminases), and potentially creatinine.[73]

Drug interactions pose a significant challenge to ATT in SOT recipients and candidates. Similar to LTBI, as discussed, rifabutin can be used in place of RIF given less potent induction of hepatic enzymes with less disruption of CNI dosing.[73,74] Even with use of rifabutin, therapeutic levels of CNIs can sometimes be difficult to achieve.[47] All rifamycins also significantly reduce serum levels of mold-active azoles, which undergo significant hepatic metabolism.[42] When concomitant mold-active antifungal therapy is required, isavuconazole may be a more difficult choice given lack of widely available therapeutic drug monitoring (TDM); itraconazole and posaconazole suspension should likely be avoided given the difficulties achieving therapeutic levels. Posaconazole delayed release tablets and voriconazole could be considered when needed with appropriate TDM, although both agents substantially increase rifabutin levels; these bidirectional interactions are particularly challenging.[42] Still, because rifamycins are the most active drugs against TB and form the backbone of ATT, rifamycin-sparing regimens should be used only in the rarest of circumstances because they may be less effective and require a minimum of 12 months of therapy (or 18 months if no injectable agent is used in the first 2 months).[34,75]

Furthermore, renal insufficiency is relatively common among SOT recipients. Among first-line drugs, EMB and pyrazinamide (in addition to rifabutin) undergo varying degrees of renal clearance.[73] TDM of these drugs should be considered for patients with renal insufficiency.[73] Some experts avoid EMB altogether in those with profound renal insufficiency, including those on renal replacement therapy, given unpredictable pharmacokinetics, replacing it with levofloxacin or moxifloxacin. TDM of ATT medications should also be considered in patients who have impaired absorption owing to gastroparesis, malabsorption, or diarrhea.[73]

Patients on ATT with significant liver disease on multiple potentially hepatotoxic agents, including INH and pyrazinamide, should undergo close monitoring, with blood tests every 1 to 4 weeks.[73] For patients with decompensated cirrhosis or acute hepatitis, options for ATT include starting a standard TB regimen with close monitoring, eliminating pyrazinamide (and potentially replacing it with levofloxacin before antimicrobial susceptibility testing results have returned) and extending therapy for pulmonary disease from 6 to 9 months, or treating the patient with exclusively nonhepatotoxic drugs (typically a combination of an aminoglycoside or capreomycin, EMB, cycloserine, and levofloxacin), at least until the patient's liver disease stabilizes.[34,73]

Uncontrolled infection is typically considered a contraindication to SOT.[76] Sparse data exist to support decision making regarding timing of SOT in organ transplant candidates with active TB. Those with kidney failure evaluated for renal transplantation and those with non–life-threatening liver disease should likely defer SOT until they complete TB treatment. Case series have demonstrated the feasibility of liver transplantation in patients with active TB and acute liver failure owing to drug-induced liver injury from ATT.[77] For these and other patients, including those with life-threatening heart or lung failure, decisions about timing should be individualized.

SUMMARY

TB and LTBI are relatively common conditions with frequent diagnostic and management challenges. The unique circumstances of SOT candidates and recipients complicate evaluation and treatment of these diseases further. Particular challenges surround diagnosis and management of LTBI, diagnostic delays and confusion in patients with end organ disease, and avoidance and management of ADRs and drug interactions.

CONTROVERSIES AND AREAS FOR FUTURE STUDY

Despite innumerable publications on issues related to TB and LTBI in SOT candidates and recipients, very few high-quality interventional studies have been performed to answer outstanding questions. High priority should be given to randomized clinical trials evaluating the optimal approach to TB and LTBI diagnosis and treatment, specifically optimal testing algorithms for LTBI and the safety and efficacy of fluoroquinolone-containing regimens and newer ATT medications still in development.

REFERENCES

1. Hill RB Jr, Dahrling BE 2nd, Starzl TE, et al. Death after transplantation; an analysis of sixty cases. Am J Med 1967;42(3):327–34.
2. Neff TA, Hudgel DW. Miliary tuberculosis in a renal transplant recipient. Am Rev Respir Dis 1973;108(3):677–8.

3. Ou SM, Liu CJ, Teng CJ, et al. Impact of pulmonary and extrapulmonary tuberculosis infection in kidney transplantation: a nationwide population-based study in Taiwan. Transpl Infect Dis 2012;14(5):502–9.

4. Joo DJ, Kim BS, Kim SJ, et al. Risk factors and characteristics of post-transplant tuberculosis in an endemic area. Ann Transplant 2013;18:163–73.

5. Barry CE 3rd, Boshoff HI, Dartois V, et al. The spectrum of latent tuberculosis: rethinking the biology and intervention strategies. Nat Rev Microbiol 2009; 7(12):845–55.

6. Screening for tuberculosis and tuberculosis infection in high-risk populations. Recommendations of the advisory council for the elimination of tuberculosis. MMWR Recomm Rep 1995;44(RR-11):19–34.

7. Targeted tuberculin testing and treatment of latent tuberculosis infection. American Thoracic Society. MMWR Recomm Rep 2000;49(RR-6):1–51.

8. Torre-Cisneros J, Doblas A, Aguado JM, et al. Tuberculosis after solid-organ transplant: incidence, risk factors, and clinical characteristics in the RESITRA (Spanish Network of Infection in Transplantation) cohort. Clin Infect Dis 2009; 48(12):1657–65.

9. Jung JY, Joo DJ, Lee CH, et al. Pre-transplant risk factors for tuberculosis after kidney transplant in an intermediate burden area. Int J Tuberc Lung Dis 2012; 16(2):248–54.

10. Marques ID, Azevedo LS, Pierrotti LC, et al. Clinical features and outcomes of tuberculosis in kidney transplant recipients in Brazil: a report of the last decade. Clin Transplant 2013;27(2):E169–76.

11. Jeong JC, Koo TY, Jeon HJ, et al. Utility of QuantiFERON-TB assay for prediction of tuberculosis development in kidney transplant patients in an intermediate-tuberculosis-burden country: lack of evidence for enhanced prediction for short-term tuberculosis development. Transplant Proc 2014;46(2):583–7.

12. Chen CY, Liu CJ, Feng JY, et al. Incidence and risk factors for tuberculosis after liver transplantation in an endemic area: a nationwide population-based matched cohort study. Am J Transplant 2015;15(8):2180–7.

13. Guirao-Arrabal E, Santos F, Redel-Montero J, et al. Risk of tuberculosis after lung transplantation: the value of pretransplant chest computed tomography and the impact of mTOR inhibitors and azathioprine use. Transpl Infect Dis 2016;18(4):512–9.

14. Manuel O, Humar A, Preiksaitis J, et al. Comparison of quantiferon-TB gold with tuberculin skin test for detecting latent tuberculosis infection prior to liver transplantation. Am J Transplant 2007;7(12):2797–801.

15. Richeldi L, Losi M, D'Amico R, et al. Performance of tests for latent tuberculosis in different groups of immunocompromised patients. Chest 2009;136(1):198–204.

16. Kim SH, Lee SO, Park IA, et al. Diagnostic usefulness of a T cell-based assay for latent tuberculosis infection in kidney transplant candidates before transplantation. Transpl Infect Dis 2010;12(2):113–9.

17. Soysal A, Toprak D, Koc M, et al. Diagnosing latent tuberculosis infection in haemodialysis patients: T-cell based assay (T-SPOT.TB) or tuberculin skin test? Nephrol Dial Transplant 2012;27(4):1645–50.

18. Ahmadinejad Z, Azmoudeh Ardalan F, Razzaqi M, et al. QuantiFERON-TB Gold In-Tube test for diagnosis of latent tuberculosis (TB) infection in solid organ transplant candidates: a single-center study in an area endemic for TB. Transpl Infect Dis 2013;15(1):90–5.

19. Kim SY, Jung GS, Kim SK, et al. Comparison of the tuberculin skin test and interferon-gamma release assay for the diagnosis of latent tuberculosis infection before kidney transplantation. Infection 2013;41(1):103–10.

20. Sester M, van Leth F, Bruchfeld J, et al. Risk assessment of tuberculosis in immunocompromised patients. A TBNET study. Am J Respir Crit Care Med 2014; 190(10):1168–76.
21. Edathodu J, Varghese B, Alrajhi AA, et al. Diagnostic potential of interferon-gamma release assay to detect latent tuberculosis infection in kidney transplant recipients. Transpl Infect Dis 2017;19(2):1–5.
22. Ferguson TW, Tangri N, Macdonald K, et al. The diagnostic accuracy of tests for latent tuberculosis infection in hemodialysis patients: a systematic review and meta-analysis. Transplantation 2015;99(5):1084–91.
23. Mazurek GH, Jereb J, Vernon A, et al. Updated guidelines for using interferon gamma release assays to detect mycobacterium tuberculosis infection - United States, 2010. MMWR Recomm Rep 2010;59(RR-5):1–25.
24. Kim SH, Lee SO, Park JB, et al. A prospective longitudinal study evaluating the usefulness of a T-cell-based assay for latent tuberculosis infection in kidney transplant recipients. Am J Transplant 2011;11(9):1927–35.
25. Liu J, Yan J, Wan Q, et al. The risk factors for tuberculosis in liver or kidney transplant recipients. BMC Infect Dis 2014;14:387.
26. Lyu J, Lee SG, Hwang S, et al. Chest computed tomography is more likely to show latent tuberculosis foci than simple chest radiography in liver transplant candidates. Liver Transpl 2011;17(8):963–8.
27. Lee SW, Jang YS, Park CM, et al. The role of chest CT scanning in TB outbreak investigation. Chest 2010;137(5):1057–64.
28. Centers for Disease Control and Prevention: Division of tuberculosis elimination. Latent tuberculosis infection: a guide for primary health care providers, treatment of latent TB infection. 2016. Available at: http://www.cdc.gov/tb/publications/ltbi/treatment.htm Accessed February 12, 2017.
29. Guirao-Arrabal E, Santos F, Redel J, et al. Efficacy and safety of short-term treatment with isoniazid and rifampicin for latent tuberculosis infection in lung transplant candidates. Clin Transplant 2017;31(3):1–3.
30. Spyridis NP, Spyridis PG, Gelesme A, et al. The effectiveness of a 9-month regimen of isoniazid alone versus 3- and 4-month regimens of isoniazid plus rifampin for treatment of latent tuberculosis infection in children: results of an 11-year randomized study. Clin Infect Dis 2007;45(6):715–22.
31. Torre-Cisneros J, San-Juan R, Rosso-Fernandez CM, et al. Tuberculosis prophylaxis with levofloxacin in liver transplant patients is associated with a high incidence of tenosynovitis: safety analysis of a multicenter randomized trial. Clin Infect Dis 2015;60(11):1642–9.
32. Bamrah S, Brostrom R, Dorina F, et al. Treatment for LTBI in contacts of MDR-TB patients, Federated States of Micronesia, 2009-2012. Int J Tuberc Lung Dis 2014; 18(8):912–8.
33. Marks SM, Mase SR, Morris SB. Systematic review, meta-analysis, and cost-effectiveness of treatment of latent tuberculosis to reduce progression to multidrug-resistant tuberculosis. Clin Infect Dis 2017;64(12):1670–7.
34. New York City Department of Health and Mental Hygiene: Bureau of Tuberculosis Control. Clinical Policies and Protocols. 2008. Available at: http://www1.nyc.gov/assets/doh/downloads/pdf/tb/tb-protocol.pdf. Accessed March 12, 2017.
35. Adamu B, Abdu A, Abba AA, et al. Antibiotic prophylaxis for preventing post solid organ transplant tuberculosis. Cochrane Database Syst Rev 2014;(3):CD008597.
36. Menzies D, Long R, Trajman A, et al. Adverse events with 4 months of rifampin therapy or 9 months of isoniazid therapy for latent tuberculosis infection: a randomized trial. Ann Intern Med 2008;149(10):689–97.

37. Chan PC, Yang CH, Chang LY, et al. Latent tuberculosis infection treatment for prison inmates: a randomised controlled trial. Int J Tuberc Lung Dis 2012;16(5): 633–8.
38. Sharma SK, Sharma A, Kadhiravan T, et al. Rifamycins (rifampicin, rifabutin and rifapentine) compared to isoniazid for preventing tuberculosis in HIV-negative people at risk of active TB. Cochrane Database Syst Rev 2013;(7):CD007545.
39. Stagg HR, Zenner D, Harris RJ, et al. Treatment of latent tuberculosis infection: a network meta-analysis. Ann Intern Med 2014;161(6):419–28.
40. Sterling TR, Moro RN, Borisov AS, et al. Flu-like and other systemic drug reactions among persons receiving weekly rifapentine plus isoniazid or daily isoniazid for treatment of latent tuberculosis infection in the PREVENT tuberculosis study. Clin Infect Dis 2015;61(4):527–35.
41. Belknap R, Holland D, Feng PJ, et al. Self-administered versus directly observed once-weekly isoniazid and rifapentine treatment of latent tuberculosis infection: a randomized trial. Ann Intern Med 2017;167(10):689–97.
42. Finch CK, Chrisman CR, Baciewicz AM, et al. Rifampin and rifabutin drug interactions: an update. Arch Intern Med 2002;162(9):985–92.
43. Saukkonen JJ, Cohn DL, Jasmer RM, et al. An official ATS statement: hepatotoxicity of antituberculosis therapy. Am J Respir Crit Care Med 2006;174(8):935–52.
44. Jahng AW, Tran T, Bui L, et al. Safety of treatment of latent tuberculosis infection in compensated cirrhotic patients during transplant candidacy period. Transplantation 2007;83(12):1557–62.
45. Singh N, Wagener MM, Gayowski T. Safety and efficacy of isoniazid chemoprophylaxis administered during liver transplant candidacy for the prevention of posttransplant tuberculosis. Transplantation 2002;74(6):892–5.
46. Moon HH, Park SY, Kim JM, et al. Isoniazid prophylaxis for latent tuberculosis infections in liver transplant recipients in a tuberculosis-endemic area. Ann Transplant 2017;22:338–45.
47. Hickey MD, Quan DJ, Chin-Hong PV, et al. Use of rifabutin for the treatment of a latent tuberculosis infection in a patient after solid organ transplantation. Liver Transpl 2013;19(4):457–61.
48. Centers for Disease Control and Prevention. Recommendations for use of an isoniazid-rifapentine regimen with direct observation to treat latent Mycobacterium tuberculosis infection. MMWR Morb Mortal Wkly Rep 2011;60(48):1650–3.
49. Tien V, Robilotti E, Callister D, et al. Tolerability of fluoroquinolones in management of latent tuberculosis in liver transplant candidates. Clin Infect Dis 2015; 61(10):1631–2.
50. Graham JC, Kearns AM, Magee JG, et al. Tuberculosis transmitted through transplantation. J Infect 2001;43(4):251–4.
51. Edathodu J, Alrajhi A, Halim M, et al. Multi-recipient donor-transmitted tuberculosis. Int J Tuberc Lung Dis 2010;14(11):1493–5.
52. Weile J, Eickmeyer H, Dreier J, et al. First case of Mycobacterium tuberculosis transmission by heart transplantation from donor to recipient. Int J Med Microbiol 2013;303(8):449–51.
53. Jensen TO, Darley DR, Goeman EE, et al. Donor-derived tuberculosis (TB): isoniazid-resistant TB transmitted from a lung transplant donor with inadequately treated latent infection. Transpl Infect Dis 2016;18(5):782–4.
54. Bucher JN, Schoenberg MB, Freytag I, et al. Donor-derived tuberculosis after solid organ transplantation in two patients and a staff member. Infection 2016; 44(3):365–70.

55. Mortensen E, Hellinger W, Keller C, et al. Three cases of donor-derived pulmonary tuberculosis in lung transplant recipients and review of 12 previously reported cases: opportunities for early diagnosis and prevention. Transpl Infect Dis 2014;16(1):67–75.

56. Morris MI, Daly JS, Blumberg E, et al. Diagnosis and management of tuberculosis in transplant donors: a donor-derived infections consensus conference report. Am J Transplant 2012;12(9):2288–300.

57. Hernandez-Hernandez E, Alberu J, Gonzalez-Michaca L, et al. Screening for tuberculosis in the study of the living renal donor in a developing country. Transplantation 2006;81(2):290–2.

58. Jambaldorj E, Han M, Jeong JC, et al. Poor predictability of QuantiFERON-TB assay in recipients and donors for tuberculosis development after kidney transplantation in an intermediate-TB-burden country. BMC Nephrol 2017;18(1):88.

59. Bodro M, Sabe N, Santin M, et al. Clinical features and outcomes of tuberculosis in solid organ transplant recipients. Transplant Proc 2012;44(9):2686–9.

60. Imai S, Ito Y, Hirai T, et al. Clinical features and risk factors of tuberculosis in living-donor liver transplant recipients. Transpl Infect Dis 2012;14(1):9–16.

61. Yoo JW, Jo KW, Kim SH, et al. Incidence, characteristics, and treatment outcomes of mycobacterial diseases in transplant recipients. Transpl Int 2016;29(5):549–58.

62. Queipo JA, Broseta E, Santos M, et al. Mycobacterial infection in a series of 1261 renal transplant recipients. Clin Microbiol Infect 2003;9(6):518–25.

63. Costa SD, de Sandes-Freitas TV, Jacinto CN, et al. Tuberculosis after kidney transplantation is associated with significantly impaired allograft function. Transpl Infect Dis 2017;19(5):1–7.

64. Chen SY, Wang CX, Chen LZ, et al. Tuberculosis in southern Chinese renal-transplant recipients. Clin Transplant 2008;22(6):780–4.

65. Meinerz G, da Silva CK, Goldani JC, et al. Epidemiology of tuberculosis after kidney transplantation in a developing country. Transpl Infect Dis 2016;18(2):176–82.

66. Canet E, Dantal J, Blancho G, et al. Tuberculosis following kidney transplantation: clinical features and outcome. A French multicentre experience in the last 20 years. Nephrol Dial Transplant 2011;26(11):3773–8.

67. Lopez de Castilla D, Schluger NW. Tuberculosis following solid organ transplantation. Transpl Infect Dis 2010;12(2):106–12.

68. Atasever A, Bacakoglu F, Toz H, et al. Tuberculosis in renal transplant recipients on various immunosuppressive regimens. Nephrol Dial Transplant 2005;20(4):797–802.

69. Guida JP, Bignotto Rosane D, Urbini-Santos C, et al. Tuberculosis in renal transplant recipients: a Brazilian center registry. Transplant Proc 2009;41(3):883–4.

70. Ha YE, Joo EJ, Park SY, et al. Tacrolimus as a risk factor for tuberculosis and outcome of treatment with rifampicin in solid organ transplant recipients. Transpl Infect Dis 2012;14(6):626–34.

71. Keane J, Gershon S, Wise RP, et al. Tuberculosis associated with infliximab, a tumor necrosis factor alpha-neutralizing agent. N Engl J Med 2001;345(15):1098–104.

72. Kay A, Barry PM, Annambhotla P, et al. Solid organ transplant-transmitted tuberculosis linked to a community outbreak - California, 2015. MMWR Morb Mortal Wkly Rep 2017;66(30):801–5.

73. Nahid P, Dorman SE, Alipanah N, et al. Official American Thoracic Society/Centers for Disease Control and Prevention/Infectious Diseases Society of America

Clinical Practice Guidelines: treatment of drug-susceptible tuberculosis. Clin Infect Dis 2016;63(7):e147–95.

74. Hebert MF, Fisher RM, Marsh CL, et al. Effects of rifampin on tacrolimus pharmacokinetics in healthy volunteers. J Clin Pharmacol 1999;39(1):91–6.

75. Drug-resistant tuberculosis: a survival guide for clinicians. 3rd edition. 2016. Available at: http://www.currytbcenter.ucsf.edu/products/drug-resistant-tuberculosis-survivalguide-clinicians-3rd-edition. Accessed March 12, 2017.

76. Steinman TI, Becker BN, Frost AE, et al. Guidelines for the referral and management of patients eligible for solid organ transplantation. Transplantation 2001; 71(9):1189–204.

77. Lee YT, Hwang S, Lee SG, et al. Living-donor liver transplantation in patients with concurrent active tuberculosis at transplantation. Int J Tuberc Lung Dis 2010; 14(8):1039–44.

Management of Mycobacterium Other than Tuberculosis in Solid Organ Transplantation

Maricar F. Malinis, MD

KEYWORDS

- Mycobacterium other than tuberculosis • Solid organ transplantation • Treatment

KEY POINTS

- Owing to immunosuppressive agents, impairment of host defenses in solid organ transplant recipients increases the risk of infections owing to mycobacteria other than tuberculosis.
- Mycobacteria other than tuberculosis is uncommon, but carries significant morbidity and mortality in the solid organ transplant population.
- Lung transplant recipients are at higher risk compared with other solid organ transplant recipients.
- Treatment of mycobacteria other than tuberculosis requires appropriate selection of antimicrobial agents, management of side effects, and consideration of drug–drug interactions.

INTRODUCTION

Mycobacteria other than tuberculosis (MOTT) are ubiquitous in the environment. To date, there are more than 150 different species of MOTT that have been described as a result of improved culturing and sequencing techniques and differentiation of species.[1] Owing to impaired T-cell–mediated immunity, solid organ transplant (SOT) recipients are at an increased risk for MOTT. The incidence of MOTT in SOT is low; however, it is essential to recognize the complexity of diagnosis and treatment of MOTT in this population. The latter involves awareness of drug combinations specific for MOTT species and drug–drug interactions between antimycobacterial drugs and immunosuppressive medications. This review focuses on relevant MOTT infections in SOT recipients and its management.

Disclosure Statement: No Disclosures.
Section of Infectious Diseases, Yale School of Medicine, PO Box 208022, New Haven, CT 06520-8022, USA
E-mail address: maricar.malinis@yale.edu

Infect Dis Clin N Am 32 (2018) 719–732
https://doi.org/10.1016/j.idc.2018.04.011
0891-5520/18/© 2018 Elsevier Inc. All rights reserved.
id.theclinics.com

OVERVIEW OF MYCOBACTERIUM OTHER THAN TUBERCULOSIS

Only about one-half of the MOTT infections can potentially cause disease in humans and animals. MOTT are classified by growth rate and colony pigmentation in culture media. MOTT are found in the soil, water, plant material, animals, and birds.[2] Only a few species that are known to cause disease have been recovered from the environment.[3,4] Tap water is considered a common reservoir for common human MOTT pathogens. Biofilm in pipes allows growth of MOTT and may render them less susceptible to disinfectants and antibacterial therapy.[5,6] MOTT have been implicated in healthcare-acquired outbreaks. A recent outbreak of *Mycobacterium abscessus* has shown that more than one-half of the patients who developed an infection or colonization were SOT recipients, with the majority being lung transplant recipients.[7] Person-to-person[8] and donor-derived transmission of MOTT are rare.[9,10]

SOT recipients with prior colonization or environmental exposure are at increased risk for clinical disease progression owing to T-cell–mediated immunity impairment and an overall net state of immunosuppression. **Table 1** summarizes the MOTT reported in SOT recipients. There are limited data on the incidence of infections owing to MOTT in SOT. The incidence is higher compared with the general population. He incidence of MOTT varies depending on type of organ transplanted, which are as follows: 0.1% in liver transplantation,[11] 0.16% to 0.55% in kidney transplantation,[12–20] 0.24% to 2.80% in heart transplant,[21,22] and 0.46% to 4.40% in lung transplantation.[23–26] To date, the incidence in the pancreas and small bowel transplant recipients is unknown. Lung transplant recipients, as expected, have a higher overall risk estimated at 1.1 per 100 person-years in contrast with non–lung transplant recipients at 0.02 per 100 person-years.[27] Factors that may predispose lung transplant recipients

Table 1
Mycobacterium species other than tuberculosis that cause infection in solid organ transplant recipients

Slow-Growing Mycobacteria (Growth >7 d)	Rapid-Growing Mycobacteria (Growth <7 d)
M asiaticum	M abscessus[a]
M avium complex (includes avium and intracellulare)[a]	M boletti
	M fortuitum[a]
M celatum	M chelonae[a]
M gastri	M mageritense
M genavense	M massiliense
M gordonae (commonly a contaminant)	M mucogenicum
M haemophilum	M neoaurum
M kansasii[a]	
M malmoense	
M marinum[a]	
M scrofulaceium	
M simiae	
M szulgai	
M terrae	
M triplex	
M xenopi	

[a] Most common species.

Data from Patel R, Roberts GD, Keating MR, et al. Infections due to nontuberculous mycobacteria in kidney, heart, and liver transplant recipients. Clin Infect Dis 1994;19(2):263–73; and Doucette K, Fishman JA. Nontuberculous mycobacterial infection in hematopoietic stem cell and solid organ transplant recipients. Clin Infect Dis 2004;38(10):1428–39.

o higher risk include direct exposure of transplanted organ to the environment, the presence of structural abnormalities that can interfere with host defenses against infection and the immunologic deficiencies from intense immunosuppression.[11] Mortality was demonstrated higher in lung transplant recipients[24,28] and any SOT recipient with MOTT infection during the first year of transplant.[29] Most infections present at the late posttransplant period with a median time of 10 months for liver transplants, 13 months for lung transplants, 15 months for heart transplants, and 20 months for kidney transplants.[30]

DIAGNOSIS
Clinical Presentation

MOTT can cause various types of infections. In immunocompetent individuals, common pulmonary infections are due to *Mycobacterium avium* complex (MAC) and *Mycobacterium kansasii*, whereas *Mycobacterium marinum* causes skin infections. In immunocompromised individuals, the spectrum of the presentation (**Table 2**) can be broad including pulmonary, skin/soft tissue infection, intestinal infection, hepatic abscess, pericarditis, graft infection, endophthalmitis, and bone/joint infections.[22,30–35] Clinicians should have a high index of suspicion for MOTT infections in SOT, especially in those who have a poor response to treatment and/or lack of an identifiable pathogen with conventional cultures.

Clinical Diagnosis

Skin and soft tissue infection is the most common type of infection owing to MOTT in SOT recipients. Certain MOTT have characteristic clinical findings and associated exposure history that raises clinical suspicion. Infection owing to *M marinum* can present as painful papules that progress to ulceration and scar formation, and occasionally similar to sporotrichoid disease (multiple ascending lesions) often occurring after water exposure (fish tank granuloma). Rapidly growing Mycobacteria, *M abscessus*, *Mycobacterium fortuitum*, and *Mycobacterium chelonae* can often cause skin and soft tissue infection in the setting of trauma, surgical procedures, or cosmetic-related procedures. The skin lesions can present as one of the following: sporotrichoid, localized nonlymphocutaneous, folliculitis, and furuncles. Both rapidly growing and slow growing mycobacteria can cause tenosynovitis or osteomyelitis, often with a history of previous traumatic injury or surgical procedure. Radiographic imaging is warranted if bone involvement is suspected.

Table 2
Clinical presentation of *Mycobacterium* species other than tuberculosis in solid organ transplant recipients

Skin Soft Tissue[22,30–32]	Pulmonary[22,30–32]	Disseminated
M avium complex	M avium complex	M avium complex[33–35]
M marinum	M kansasii	M abscessus[25,36–38]
M haemophilium	M xenopi	M kansasii[39,40]
M szulgai	M malmoense	M haemophilium[41–45]
M abscessus	M szulgai	M chelonae[46–48]
M chelonae	M genavense	M immunogenum[49]
M fortuitum	M abscessus	M genavense[50–54]
	M chelonae	M lentifalvium[55]
	M fortuitum	M gordonae[56]
		M marinum[57]

Pulmonary disease is the second most common presentation of MOTT infection in SOT. Patients can present with chronic cough with or without sputum production and fatigue. Infrequently, dyspnea, fever, hemoptysis, and weight loss can be present. However, in SOT, symptoms may be blunted owing to the degree of net immunosuppression. Radiographic imaging may range from bronchiectasis, to reticulonodular disease, to cavitary lesions.[58]

Disseminated disease in SOT can be due to various MOTT species (see **Table 2**). It is the second most common presentation in renal transplant recipients after skin/soft tissue infection and the third most common presentation in heart and lung transplant recipients after skin/soft tissue and pulmonary disease.[31]

Laboratory Diagnosis

Appropriate specimen should be obtained based on clinical presentation. The biopsied tissue, aspirated fluid, or respiratory specimen (expectorated sputum, bronchoalveolar lavage) should be sent for acid-fast staining, mycobacterial cultures, and pathology review. Individuals with MOTT infections may have positive tuberculin skin testing owing to shared protein components between mycobacterial species.[59] In contrast, interferon-gamma release assays for *Mycobacterium tuberculosis* complex use antigens that are present in *M marinum, M kansasii,* and *Mycobacterium szulgai,* resulting in cross-reactivity.[60] Of note, not all MOTT have been studied for cross-reactivity with interferon-gamma release assays. For pulmonary disease, diagnosis is difficult because one has to distinguish colonization or laboratory contamination from true disease. Guidelines published by the American Thoracic Society and Infectious Diseases Society of America set the microbiologic criteria for lung disease due to MOTT (**Box 1**).[58]

In the setting of suspected disseminated disease, mycobacterial isolator blood cultures should be collected. Certain mycobacterial species may require specific handling or processing. *Mycobacterium haemophilium* and *Mycobacterium genavense* require special supplementation such as iron-containing compounds and mycobactin J, respectively, in culture media to grow. The traditional method of MOTT species

---

Box 1
Summary of 2007 American Thoracic Society/Infectious Diseases Society of America Diagnostic Criteria for MOTT Lung Disease

Should meet clinical, radiographic, and microbiological criteria, and exclude other diagnoses
  Clinical symptoms
    Based on the presence of pulmonary symptoms, which could be one of the following: chronic or recurring cough, sputum production, dyspnea, hemoptysis (less common), and chest pain
  Radiographic data
    Presence of nodules or cavities, multifocal bronchiectasis with multiple small nodules in radiographic imaging (chest radiograph, computed tomography scan)
  Microbiologic data
    At least 2 expectorated sputa or at least 1 bronchial lavage with positive culture for MOTT
    Or
    Transbronchial or lung biopsy showing the presence of granulomatous inflammation or acid-fast bacilli with 1 or more sputa or bronchial washings culture positive for MOTT

Abbreviation: MOTT, *Mycobacterium* species other than tuberculosis.
Adapted from Griffith DE, Aksamit T, Brown-Elliott BA, et al. An official ATS/IDSA statement: diagnosis, treatment, and prevention of nontuberculous mycobacterial diseases. Am J Respir Crit Care Med 2007;175(4):379; with permission.

identification depends on phenotypic characteristics determined by biochemical testing, pigment production, growth characteristics, and colony appearance.[61] However, this process is limited by subjectivity and low specificity. Newer techniques such as molecular probes, high-performance liquid chromatography, and 16S rDNA sequencing[61,62] are currently in use to provide rapid and accurate identification of MOTT. More recently, matrix-assisted laser desorption/ionization time-of-flight mass spectrometry is increasingly used to speciate mycobacteria.[63,64] Communication between the treating clinician and the microbiology laboratory is essential in determining the extent of identification analysis of a clinically relevant MOTT isolate.[58]

TREATMENT

Treatment of MOTT is species specific. Treatment of mycobacterial disease uses the fundamental principle of using more than 1 active agent for a prolonged duration to avoid the emergence of resistance. **Tables 3** and **4** summarize the standard therapy and dosing for MOTT based on the recommendations of the American Thoracic Society/Infectious Diseases Society of America.[58] Antimicrobial susceptibility testing can assist in therapeutic decision making for specific MOTT species. Guidelines recommended solely clarithromcyin susceptibility testing for either new, untreated MAC isolates or those who failed macrolided treatment or prevention. Newly diagnosed, untreated *M kansasii* should be tested in vitro to rifampin only. If it is rifampin resistant, other agents should be requested, which include rifabutin, ethambutol, isoniazid, clarithromycin, fluoroquinolones, amikacin, and sulfonamides. Only *M marinum* does not require routine testing given its consistent susceptibility to clarithromycin and ethambutol. Antimicrobial susceptibility testing may be warranted periodically in cases of persistent positive cultures after 6 months of treatment or in those with extended therapy.[65]

There are limited data in new treatment regimens for difficult-to-treat MOTT infections. Clofazimine as a salvage therapy has been used in 3 lung transplant, 1 kidney, and 1 liver transplant recipients after a standard course of MAC treatment was given.[66] Microbiological clearance and resolution of disease were documented in 2 of these 5 patients. Bedaquiline, an oral antimycobacterial drug belonging to the class diarylquinolines that have been approved for treatment of *M tuberculosis*, was used off-label for treatment failure of lung disease caused by MAC (n = 6), and *M abscessus* (n = 4).[67] Out of the 10 patients, 8 had macrolid-resistant isolates. All 10 patients received bedaquiline for 6 months, and 6 patients achieved the microbiologic response. This study suggests the potential of bedaquiline in those with advanced disease, but it remains to be validated in more extensive studies. Tedizolid, a new oxazolidinone, has better in vitro and intracellular activity against some MOTT species when compared with linezolid. Tedizolid was demonstrated to have equivalent or lower minimum inhibitory concentration (MIC)$_{50}$ and MIC$_{90}$ values than linezolid for rapidly growing mycobacteria, including *M abscessus* and *M fortuitum*, *M marinum*, MAC, and *Mycobacterium simiae*.[68] Future studies are needed to evaluate its role as a potential treatment for MOTT. The combination of tigecycline and clarithromycin has synergistic activity against rapidly growing mycobacteria; however, its use might be limited by gastrointestinal side effects.[69] Novel delivery of the already established antimycobacterial drug, such as amikacin, has been shown to reduce potential drug toxicities. The addition of inhaled amikacin to standard drug therapy of refractory *M abscessus* and MAC improved symptoms and decreased both smear quantity and mycobacterial culture growth.[70] Inhalational liposomal amikacin seems to be promising, as demonstrated by the efficacy data in a murine mouse model for *M avium* and *M abscessus*.[71] Studies are needed to confirm its clinical efficacy and safety in humans.

Table 3
Treatment recommendations for *Mycobacterium* other than tuberculosis

Mycobacterial Species	Preferred[a]	Susceptibility Testing
M avium complex	Nodular/bronchiectasis Clarithromycin + Ethambutol + Rifampin Cavitary Clarithromycin + Ethambutol + Rifampin ± Streptomycin or amikacin Advanced or previously treated disease Clarithromycin or Azithromycin + Ethambutol + Rifampin + Streptomycin or amikacin for the first 2-3 months of therapy Disseminated disease Clarithromycin or + Ethambutol + Rifampin	Recommended for macrolides

M kansasii	Pulmonary
	Rifampin
	+ Ethambutol
	+ Isoniazid
	+ Pyridoxine
	Rifampin-resistant:
	   Alternative options include clarithromycin/
	   azithromycin, moxifloxacin, ethambutol,
	   sulfamethoxazole, or streptomycin
		Recommended for rifampin

M xenopi	Isoniazid + Rifampin +Ethambutol + Clarithromycin ± Streptomycin	
M szulgai	Rifampin + Ethambutol + Clarithromycin or moxifloxacin	
M malmoense	Rifampin + Ethambutol + Isoniazid ± Clarithromycin or moxifloxacin	

M genavense	Optimal therapy not determined
	Multidrug therapy with clarithromycin has
	   been reported effective
	Other drugs to consider: amikacin, rifampin,
	   fluoroquinolones	

M marinum	Clarithromycin + Ethambutol Add rifampin for severe disease	Recommended only if failing treatment

(*continued on next page*)

Table 3 (continued)		
Mycobacterial Species	**Preferred[a]**	**Susceptibility Testing**
M haemophilum	Clarithromycin +Rifampin +Ciprofloxacin	No standardized method for susceptibility testing
M abscessus	Skin/soft tissue or bone infection Clarithromycin + One of the following: amikacin, cefoxitin, or imipenem Pulmonary Clarithromycin + Amikacin + Cefoxitin or imipenem Surgical debridement or resection of localized infection may offer best chance for cure	Recommended for amikacin, doxycycline, fluoroquinolones, sulfonamide or TMP-SMX, cefoxitin, clarithromycin, linezolid
M chelonae	Clarithromycin + One of the following: Amikacin/ tobramcycin, linezolid, tigecycline or imipenem	Recommended for amikacin, tobramycin, doxycycline, fluoroquinolones, sulfonamide or TMP-SMX, cefoxitin, clarithromycin, linezolid
M fortuitum	Minimum of 2 agents: Amikacin, fluoroquinolone, macrolide,[b] doxycycline, imipenem or sulfonamides Surgery is indicated for extensive disease, abscess	Recommended for amikacin, doxycycline, imipenem, fluoroquinolones, sulfonamide or TMP-SMX, cefoxitin, imipenem, clarithromycin, linezolid

Abbreviation: TMP-SMX, trimethoprim-sulfamethoxazole.
[a] Rifabutin and azithromycin can be substituted for rifampin and clarithromycin, respectively.
[b] Macrolide should be used with caution owing to inducible erythromycin methylase (erm) gene.
Data from Griffith DE, Aksamit T, Brown-Elliott BA, et al. An official ATS/IDSA statement: diagnosis, treatment, and prevention of nontuberculous mycobacterial diseases. Am J Respir Crit Care Med 2007;175(4):367–416.

The duration of therapy is defined by organ involvement, MOTT species, the severity of illness, and the overall net state of immunosuppression. Certain MOTT infections, which are considered limited in immunocompetent patients such as M marinum, may have an aggressive clinical course and may warrant a longer course of antibiotic treatment in immunocompromised hosts.[72] The duration of therapy in immunocompromised hosts is extrapolated from current guidelines.[58] Pulmonary disease, in general, should be treated until sputum cultures are negative over a 12-month period. Skin and soft tissue infections are treated for a minimum of 4 months, and bone infection requires at least 6 months of therapy. The recommended treatment duration of disseminated disease in patients infected with the human immunodeficiency virus is 6 to 12 months after immune reconstitution. In contrast, treatment duration in SOT

Table 4
Dosing of anti-mycobacterial drugs and interaction with immunosuppressive drugs

Antimicrobial	Dose	Drug–Drug Interaction	
		Calcineurin Inhibitor	mTOR Inhibitor
Macrolides			
Azithromycin	250–500 mg PO daily 500–600 mg PO 3 times a week (MAC nodular/bronchiectasis)	↑	↑
Clarithromycin	250–500 mg PO BID 1000 mg PO 3 times a week (MAC nodular/bronchiectatic disease)	↑↑↑	↑↑↑
Ethambutol	15 mg/kg/day 25 mg/kg/day 3 times a week (MAC nodular/bronchiectatic disease)	No	No
Rifamycins			
Rifabutin	150–300 mg/day PO	↓↓	↓↓
Rifampin	450–600 mg/day PO 600 mg PO 3 times a week (MAC nodular/bronchiectatic disease)	↓↓↓	↓↓↓
Fluoroquinolones			
Ciprofloxacin	500 mg PO BID or 400 mg IV BID	↑	No
Levofloxacin	500–750 mg PO/IV daily	↑ (Cyclosporine only)	No
Moxifloxacin	400 mg PO/IV daily	No	No
Aminoglycosides			
Amikacin	10–15 mg/kg IV or IM daily or 25 mg/kg 3 times a week	No	No
Streptomycin	500–1000 mg IV or IM daily or 3 times a week	No	No
Tobramycin	5 mg/kg IV or IM daily or 3 times a week	No	No
Tetracyclines			
Doxycycline	100 mg PO or IV BID	No	No
Minocycline	100 mg PO daily	No	No
Tigecycline	Loading dose 100 mg IV followed by 50 mg IV BID	↑	No
Beta-Lactams			
Cefoxitin	8–12 g/day IV in divided doses	No	No
Imipenem	500 mg IV every 6 h	No	No
Others			
Linezolid	600 mg PO or IV BID	No	No
Isoniazid	5 mg/kg/day up to 300 mg PO daily with pyridoxine 50 mg PO daily	No	No
Trimethoprim/ sulfamethoxazole	800–1600 mg (sulfa component) PO/IV BID	No	No

Abbreviations: BID, twice a day; IM, intramuscular; IV, intravenous; MAC, *Mycobacterium avium* complex; mTOR, mammalian target of rapamycin; PO, oral; ↑, slight potential for increased immunosuppressive drug level owing to CYP inhibition; ↑↑↑, severe interaction resulting in increased immunosuppressive drug level owing to CYP inhibition; ↓↓, moderately decreases immunosuppressive drug level owing to CYP induction; ↓↓↓, severe interaction resulting in decreased immunosuppressive drug level owing to CYP induction.
Data from Refs.[58,75,76]

recipients is not well-defined given their need for long-term immunosuppression to preserve the allograft. In the setting of severe disease, reduction of immunosuppression may be warranted. However, caution should be exercised as potential immune reconstitution inflammatory syndrome can occur.[73] Adjunct treatment such as surgical intervention may be necessary in certain instances to decrease the microbial burden in the setting of abscesses or bone and joint infections. Of note, treatment outcomes in SOT recipients have been variable. Cure rates of MOTT infections were estimated as 42% in lung, 47% in heart, 62% in kidney, and 64% in liver transplantation.[32] Secondary prophylaxis in SOT is not well-studied, and no expert consensus has been made to recommend this as the standard of care. However, experts have suggested suppression for those with severe disseminated or recurrent disease.[31]

Treatment of MOTT can be complicated owing to potential toxicities that warrant close monitoring of patients. Adverse effects may include but not limited to nephrotoxicity (aminoglycosides), ototoxicity or vestibular dysfunction (aminoglycosides), hepatotoxicity (isoniazid), peripheral neuropathy (linezolid, isoniazid), optic neuritis (ethambutol), myelosuppression (linezolid), tendonitis (fluoroquinolones), and gastrointestinal intolerance (macrolide, tetracycline). An additional complexity to the treatment of MOTT in SOT is the consideration of drug–drug interactions with immunosuppressive drugs, particularly the rifamycins and macrolides (see **Table 4**). Rifampin is a potent inducer of the CYP3A4 enzyme that can decrease the level of the calcineurin inhibitor and sirolimus and consequently cause rejection. An alternative drug for rifampin is rifabutin, which is a less potent inducer of the CYP3A4 enzyme and has less of an effect on the metabolism of the calcineurin inhibitors, tacrolimus and cyclosporine A, and sirolimus. Clarithromycin, in contrast, is a moderate to strong inhibitor of CYP3A4 and decreases metabolism of the calcineurin inhibitors and sirolimus. A high level of calcineurin inhibitors has consequential nephrotoxicity. Azithromycin is a less potent inhibitor and preferred over clarithromycin for treatment of MOTT. If either or both a macrolide and rifamycin will be used for MOTT treatment, drug level monitoring of immunosuppressive agents is warranted to avoid rejection or drug toxicity. Modification of immunosuppression may be required if drug–drug interactions cannot be avoided. The use of belatacept in kidney transplant recipients instead of calcineurin inhibitors may be an option to consider.[74]

SUMMARY

MOTT are important pathogens to consider in SOT recipients. A delay in recognition and treatment may incur significant morbidity and mortality. Management of MOTT infections requires knowledge of treatments specific for each species, interpretation of drug susceptibility testing, and drug–drug interactions between antimicrobial and immunosuppressive drugs. Therapy in SOT recipients can be prolonged and may require a reduction in immunosuppression to improve outcomes.

REFERENCES

1. Johnson MM, Odell JA. Nontuberculous mycobacterial pulmonary infections. J Thorac Dis 2014;6(3):210–20.
2. Brown-Eliott B, Wallace R. Infections caused by nontuberculous mycobacteria other than Mycobacterium avium complex. In: Mandell, Douglas and Bennett's principles and practice of infectious diseases, Vol. 2. Philadelphia: Elsevier Saunders; 2015. p. 2844–52.
3. Covert TC, Rodgers MR, Reyes AL, et al. Occurrence of nontuberculous mycobacteria in environmental samples. Appl Environ Microbiol 1999;65(6):2492–6.

4. Tichenor WS, Thurlow J, McNulty S, et al. Nontuberculous mycobacteria in household plumbing as possible cause of chronic rhinosinusitis. Emerg Infect Dis 2012; 18(10):1612–7.

5. Schulze-Robbecke R, Janning B, Fischeder R. Occurrence of mycobacteria in biofilm samples. Tuber Lung Dis 1992;73(3):141–4.

6. Jarlier V, Nikaido H. Mycobacterial cell wall: structure and role in natural resistance to antibiotics. FEMS Microbiol Lett 1994;123(1–2):11–8.

7. Baker AW, Lewis SS, Alexander BD, et al. Two-phase hospital-associated outbreak of Mycobacterium abscessus: investigation and mitigation. Clin Infect Dis 2017;64(7):902–11.

8. Aitken ML, Limaye A, Pottinger P, et al. Respiratory outbreak of Mycobacterium abscessus subspecies massiliense in a lung transplant and cystic fibrosis center. Am J Respir Crit Care Med 2012;185(2):231–2.

9. Ison MG, Nalesnik MA. An update on donor-derived disease transmission in organ transplantation. Am J Transplant 2011;11(6):1123–30.

10. Green M, Covington S, Taranto S, et al. Donor-derived transmission events in 2013: a report of the Organ Procurement Transplant Network Ad Hoc Disease Transmission Advisory Committee. Transplantation 2015;99(2):282–7.

11. Longworth SA, Vinnard C, Lee I, et al. Risk factors for nontuberculous mycobacterial infections in solid organ transplant recipients: a case-control study. Transpl Infect Dis 2014;16(1):76–83.

12. Costa JM, Meyers AM, Botha JR, et al. Mycobacterial infections in recipients of kidney allografts. A seventeen-year experience. Acta Med Port 1988;1(1):51–7.

13. Delaney V, Sumrani N, Hong JH, et al. Mycobacterial infections in renal allograft recipients. Transplant Proc 1993;25(3):2288–9.

14. Hall CM, Willcox PA, Swanepoel CR, et al. Mycobacterial infection in renal transplant recipients. Chest 1994;106(2):435–9.

15. Higgins RM, Cahn AP, Porter D, et al. Mycobacterial infections after renal transplantation. Q J Med 1991;78(286):145–53.

16. Lloveras J, Peterson PK, Simmons RL, et al. Mycobacterial infections in renal transplant recipients. Seven cases and a review of the literature. Arch Intern Med 1982;142(5):888–92.

17. Spence RK, Dafoe DC, Rabin G, et al. Mycobacterial infections in renal allograft recipients. Arch Surg 1983;118(3):356–9.

18. Vandermarliere A, Van Audenhove A, Peetermans WE, et al. Mycobacterial infection after renal transplantation in a Western population. Transpl Infect Dis 2003; 5(1):9–15.

19. Jie T, Matas AJ, Gillingham KJ, et al. Mycobacterial infections after kidney transplant. Transpl Proc 2005;37(2):937–9.

20. Queipo JA, Broseta E, Santos M, et al. Mycobacterial infection in a series of 1261 renal transplant recipients. Clin Microbiol Infect 2003;9(6):518–25.

21. Novick RJ, Moreno-Cabral CE, Stinson EB, et al. Nontuberculous mycobacterial infections in heart transplant recipients: a seventeen-year experience. J Heart Transplant 1990;9(4):357–63.

22. Patel R, Roberts GD, Keating MR, et al. Infections due to nontuberculous mycobacteria in kidney, heart, and liver transplant recipients. Clin Infect Dis 1994; 19(2):263–73.

23. Kesten S, Chaparro C. Mycobacterial infections in lung transplant recipients. Chest 1999;115(3):741–5.

24. Huang HC, Weigt SS, Derhovanessian A, et al. Non-tuberculous mycobacterium infection after lung transplantation is associated with increased mortality. J Heart Lung Transplant 2011;30(7):790–8.

25. Knoll BM, Kappagoda S, Gill RR, et al. Non-tuberculous mycobacterial infection among lung transplant recipients: a 15-year cohort study. Transpl Infect Dis 2012; 14(5):452–60.

26. Malouf MA, Glanville AR. The spectrum of mycobacterial infection after lung transplantation. Am J Respir Crit Care Med 1999;160(5 Pt 1):1611–6.

27. Henkle E, Winthrop KL. Nontuberculous mycobacteria infections in immunosuppressed hosts. Clin Chest Med 2015;36(1):91–9.

28. George IA, Santos CA, Olsen MA, et al. Epidemiology and outcomes of nontuberculous mycobacterial infections in solid organ transplant recipients at a midwestern center. Transplantation 2016;100(5):1073–8.

29. Longworth SA, Blumberg EA, Barton TD, et al. Non-tuberculous mycobacterial infections after solid organ transplantation: a survival analysis. Clin Microbiol Infect 2015;21(1):43–7.

30. Knoll BM. Update on nontuberculous mycobacterial infections in solid organ and hematopoietic stem cell transplant recipients. Curr Infect Dis Rep 2014; 16(9):421.

31. Doucette K, Fishman JA. Nontuberculous mycobacterial infection in hematopoietic stem cell and solid organ transplant recipients. Clin Infect Dis 2004;38(10): 1428–39.

32. Abad CL, Razonable RR. Non-tuberculous mycobacterial infections in solid organ transplant recipients: an update. J Clin Tuberc Other Mycobact Dis 2016; 4:1–8.

33. Todd JL, Lakey J, Howell D, et al. Portal hypertension and granulomatous liver disease in a lung transplant recipient due to disseminated atypical mycobacterial infection. Am J Transpl 2007;7(5):1300–3.

34. Verbeke F, Vogelaers D, Vanholder R, et al. Disseminated Mycobacterium avium complex infection in a renal transplant patient. Eur J Intern Med 2005;16(1):53–5.

35. Haas S, Scully B, Cohen D, et al. Mycobacterium avium complex infection in kidney transplant patients. Transpl Infect Dis 2005;7(2):75–9.

36. Taylor JL, Palmer SM. Mycobacterium abscessus chest wall and pulmonary infection in a cystic fibrosis lung transplant recipient. J Heart Lung Transpl 2006;25(8):985–8.

37. Garrison AP, Morris MI, Doblecki Lewis S, et al. Mycobacterium abscessus infection in solid organ transplant recipients: report of three cases and review of the literature. Transpl Infect Dis 2009;11(6):541–8.

38. Morales P, Ros JA, Blanes M, et al. Successful recovery after disseminated infection due to Mycobacterium abscessus in a lung transplant patient: subcutaneous nodule as first manifestation–a case report. Transpl Proc 2007;39(7):2413–5.

39. Kaur P, Fishman JA, Misdraji J, et al. Disseminated Mycobacterium kansasii infection with hepatic abscesses in a renal transplant recipient. Transpl Infect Dis 2011;13(5):531–5.

40. Fraser DW, Buxton AE, Naji A, et al. Disseminated Mycobacterium kansasii infection presenting as cellulitis in a recipient of a renal homograft. Am Rev Respir Dis 1975;112(1):125–9.

41. Lau SK, Curreem SO, Ngan AH, et al. First report of disseminated Mycobacterium skin infections in two liver transplant recipients and rapid diagnosis by hsp65 gene sequencing. J Clin Microbiol 2011;49(11):3733–8.

42. Brix SR, Iking-Konert C, Stahl RA, et al. Disseminated Mycobacterium haemophilum infection in a renal transplant recipient. BMJ Case Rep 2016;2016 [pii: bcr2016216042].
43. Munster S, Zustin J, Derlin T. Atypical mycobacteriosis caused by Mycobacterium haemophilum in an immunocompromised patient: diagnosis by (18)F-FDG PET/CT. Clin Nucl Med 2013;38(4):e194–5.
44. Fairhurst RM, Kubak BM, Pegues DA, et al. Mycobacterium haemophilum infections in heart transplant recipients: case report and review of the literature. Am J Transpl 2002;2(5):476–9.
45. Lin JH, Chen W, Lee JY, et al. Disseminated cutaneous Mycobacterium haemophilum infection with severe hypercalcaemia in a failed renal transplant recipient. Br J Dermatol 2003;149(1):200–2.
46. Chatzikokkinou P, Luzzati R, Sotiropoulos K, et al. Disseminated cutaneous infection with Mycobacterium chelonae in a renal transplant recipient. Cutis 2015; 96(5):E6–9.
47. Tebas P, Sultan F, Wallace RJ Jr, et al. Rapid development of resistance to clarithromycin following monotherapy for disseminated Mycobacterium chelonae infection in a heart transplant patient. Clin Infect Dis 1995;20(2):443–4.
48. Mehta R, Oliver LD, Melillo D, et al. Disseminated Mycobacterium chelonei infection following cadaveric renal transplantation: favorable response to cefoxitin. Am J Kidney Dis 1983;3(2):124–8.
49. Biggs HM, Chudgar SM, Pfeiffer CD, et al. Disseminated Mycobacterium immunogenum infection presenting with septic shock and skin lesions in a renal transplant recipient. Transpl Infect Dis 2012;14(4):415–21.
50. Doggett JS, Strasfeld L. Disseminated Mycobacterium genavense with pulmonary nodules in a kidney transplant recipient: case report and review of the literature. Transpl Infect Dis 2011;13(1):38–43.
51. Lhuillier E, Brugiere O, Veziris N, et al. Relapsing Mycobacterium genavense infection as a cause of late death in a lung transplant recipient: case report and review of the literature. Exp Clin Transplant 2012;10(6):618–20.
52. Hoefsloot W, van Ingen J, Peters EJ, et al. Mycobacterium genavense in the Netherlands: an opportunistic pathogen in HIV and non-HIV immunocompromised patients. An observational study in 14 cases. Clin Microbiol Infect 2013; 19(5):432–7.
53. Charles P, Lortholary O, Dechartres A, et al. Mycobacterium genavense infections: a retrospective multicenter study in France, 1996-2007. Medicine (Baltimore) 2011;90(4):223–30.
54. Ombelet S, Van Wijngaerden E, Lagrou K, et al. Mycobacterium genavense infection in a solid organ recipient: a diagnostic and therapeutic challenge. Transpl Infect Dis 2016;18(1):125–31.
55. Thomas G, Hraiech S, Dizier S, et al. Disseminated Mycobacterium lentiflavum responsible for hemophagocytic lymphohistocytosis in a man with a history of heart transplantation. J Clin Microbiol 2014;52(8):3121–3.
56. den Broeder AA, Vervoort G, van Assen S, et al. Disseminated Mycobacterium gordonae infection in a renal transplant recipient. Transpl Infect Dis 2003;5(3): 151–5.
57. Gombert ME, Goldstein EJ, Corrado ML, et al. Disseminated Mycobacterium marinum infection after renal transplantation. Ann Intern Med 1981;94(4 pt 1): 486–7.

58. Griffith DE, Aksamit T, Brown-Elliott BA, et al. An official ATS/IDSA statement: diagnosis, treatment, and prevention of nontuberculous mycobacterial diseases. Am J Respir Crit Care Med 2007;175(4):367–416.

59. Chaparas SD, Maloney CJ, Hedrick SR. Specificity of tuberculins and antigens from various species of mycobacteria. Am Rev Respir Dis 1970; 101(1):74–83.

60. Andersen P, Munk ME, Pollock JM, et al. Specific immune-based diagnosis of tuberculosis. Lancet 2000;356(9235):1099–104.

61. Cook VJ, Turenne CY, Wolfe J, et al. Conventional methods versus 16S ribosomal DNA sequencing for identification of nontuberculous mycobacteria: cost analysis. J Clin Microbiol 2003;41(3):1010–5.

62. Jagielski T, Minias A, van Ingen J, et al. Methodological and clinical aspects of the molecular epidemiology of Mycobacterium tuberculosis and other mycobacteria. Clin Microbiol Rev 2016;29(2):239–90.

63. Rodriguez-Sanchez B, Ruiz-Serrano MJ, Marin M, et al. Evaluation of matrix-assisted laser desorption ionization-time of flight mass spectrometry for identification of nontuberculous mycobacteria from clinical isolates. J Clin Microbiol 2015;53(8):2737–40.

64. Rodriguez-Temporal D, Perez-Risco D, Struzka EA, et al. Impact of updating the MALDI-TOF MS database on the identification of nontuberculous mycobacteria. J Mass Spectrom 2017;52(9):597–602.

65. Brown-Elliott BA, Nash KA, Wallace RJ Jr. Antimicrobial susceptibility testing, drug resistance mechanisms, and therapy of infections with nontuberculous mycobacteria. Clin Microbiol Rev 2012;25(3):545–82.

66. Cariello PF, Kwak EJ, Abdel-Massih RC, et al. Safety and tolerability of clofazimine as salvage therapy for atypical mycobacterial infection in solid organ transplant recipients. Transpl Infect Dis 2015;17(1):111–8.

67. Philley JV, Wallace RJ Jr, Benwill JL, et al. Preliminary results of bedaquiline as salvage therapy for patients with nontuberculous mycobacterial lung disease. Chest 2015;148(2):499–506.

68. Brown-Elliott BA, Wallace RJ Jr. In vitro susceptibility testing of tedizolid against nontuberculous mycobacteria. J Clin Microbiol 2017;55(6):1747–54.

69. Huang CW, Chen JH, Hu ST, et al. Synergistic activities of tigecycline with clarithromycin or amikacin against rapidly growing mycobacteria in Taiwan. Int J Antimicrob Agents 2013;41(3):218–23.

70. Olivier KN, Shaw PA, Glaser TS, et al. Inhaled amikacin for treatment of refractory pulmonary nontuberculous mycobacterial disease. Ann Am Thorac Soc 2014; 11(1):30–5.

71. Rose SJ, Neville ME, Gupta R, et al. Delivery of aerosolized liposomal amikacin as a novel approach for the treatment of nontuberculous mycobacteria in an experimental model of pulmonary infection. PLoS One 2014;9(9):e108703.

72. Pandian TK, Deziel PJ, Otley CC, et al. Mycobacterium marinum infections in transplant recipients: case report and review of the literature. Transpl Infect Dis 2008;10(5):358–63.

73. Lemoine M, Laurent C, Hanoy M, et al. Immune reconstitution inflammatory syndrome secondary to Mycobacterium kansasii infection in a kidney transplant recipient. Am J Transpl 2015;15(12):3255–8.

74. Vincenti F, Rostaing L, Grinyo J, et al. Belatacept and long-term outcomes in kidney transplantation. N Engl J Med 2016;374(4):333–43.

75. Keating MR, Daly JS, AST Infectious Diseases Community of Practice. Nontuberculous mycobacterial infections in solid organ transplantation. Am J Transpl 2013;13(Suppl 4):77–82.
76. Trofe-Clark J, Lemonovich TL, AST Infectious Diseases Community of Practice. Interactions between anti-infective agents and immunosuppressants in solid organ transplantation. Am J Transpl 2013;13(Suppl 4):318–26.

Prevention and Treatment of *Clostridium difficile*-Associated Diarrhea in Solid Organ Transplant Recipients

Stephanie M. Pouch, MD, MS*, Rachel J. Friedman-Moraco, MD

KEYWORDS

- *Clostridium difficile* infection • Solid organ transplant • Prevention • Infection control
- Antimicrobial stewardship • Treatment • Fecal microbiota transplant

KEY POINTS

- *Clostridium difficile* infection is a significant cause of morbidity and mortality in solid organ transplant recipients.
- Antimicrobial stewardship and infection control are the mainstays of *C difficile* infection prevention.
- Novel approaches to primary and secondary prevention of *C difficile* infection are on the horizon but require formal evaluation in the solid organ transplant population.
- Fecal microbiota transplantation is a promising treatment modality for *C difficile* infection in solid organ transplant recipients.

INTRODUCTION

Clostridium difficile is among the most frequently encountered nosocomial pathogens and is associated with significant morbidity, mortality, and excess health care expenditures.[1–4] Compared with other patient populations, solid organ transplant (SOT) recipients are disproportionately affected by this pathogen; reported rates of posttransplant *C difficile* infection (CDI), defined as diarrhea with evidence of *C difficile* toxin, toxigenic *C difficile*, or pseudomembranous colitis,[5] are as high as 30%.[6] The estimated incidence of CDI varies by organ transplanted, but ranges from 1.5% to 7.8% in kidney-pancreas recipients, 3% to 19% in liver recipients, 3.5% to 16.0%

Disclosure Statement: Neither Dr S.M. Pouch nor Dr R.J. Friedman has any relationship with a commercial company that has a direct financial interest in subject matter or materials discussed in the article or with a company making a competing product.
Division of Infectious Diseases, Emory University School of Medicine, 101 Woodruff Circle, WMB #2101, Atlanta, GA 30322, USA
* Corresponding author.
E-mail address: spouch@emory.edu

Infect Dis Clin N Am 32 (2018) 733–748
https://doi.org/10.1016/j.idc.2018.05.001
0891-5520/18/© 2018 Elsevier Inc. All rights reserved.

id.theclinics.com

in kidney recipients, 8% to 15% in heart recipients, 9% in intestinal recipients, and 7% to 31% in lung recipients.[6,7] SOT recipients may be at higher risk for adverse outcomes related to CDI, including fulminant colitis and death, than immunocompetent hosts[8,9] Further, CDI has also been associated with allograft loss in SOT recipients.[10]

The incidence of CDI after SOT is greatest within the first 3 months of transplantation, likely owing to frequent hospitalization, increased exposure to antimicrobials, and receipt of induction immunosuppression.[6,7,11] Although antimicrobial use is the most significant risk factor for CDI acquisition,[6] up to 25% of patients have no history of antibiotic exposure during the month preceding CDI.[12,13] This discordance may be explained by other characteristics that have been associated with disruption of the intestinal microbiome and are common in SOT recipients, such as advancing age, uremia, gastrointestinal surgery, severity of underlying disease, and the use of gastric acid-suppressing medications.[14] Additional potential risk factors for CDI unique to SOT recipients include hypogammaglobulinemia, retransplantation, use of antithymocyte globulin and prophylactic ganciclovir, and receipt of corticosteroids before transplantation.[6,7,11,13,15,16]

The incidence and potential for significant adverse outcomes among SOT recipients with CDI highlight the evolving need for strategic CDI risk factor modification and novel approaches to disease management in this patient population. This review focuses on current concepts related to the prevention and treatment of CDI in SOT recipients.

PREVENTION OF *CLOSTRIDIUM DIFFICILE* INFECTION IN SOLID ORGAN TRANSPLANT RECIPIENTS

The prevention of CDI among SOT recipients requires interdisciplinary engagement between transplant physicians, nurses, pharmacists, infection control, the microbiology laboratory, environmental services, information technology, and hospital administration.[14,17] To date, strategies for CDI prevention have largely focused on antimicrobial stewardship and reduction of horizontal *C difficile* transmission within the inpatient setting; however, immunization and therapeutics targeted toward the maintenance of a diverse intestinal microbiome are being studied as potential prophylactic approaches. As with other patient populations, the mitigation of other risk factors, including the use of gastric acid suppressants, is also essential.

Antimicrobial Stewardship

Because antibiotic exposure remains the most significant modifiable risk factor for CDI, antimicrobial stewardship programs (ASPs) are pivotal to CDI prevention and recommended in the most recent Infectious Diseases Society of America (IDSA) and Society for Healthcare Epidemiology of America (SHEA) CDI guidelines.[5] ASPs aim to coordinate "interventions designed to improve and measure the appropriate use of [antibiotic] agents by promoting the selection of the optimal [antibiotic] drug regimen including dosing, duration of therapy, and route of administration."[18] Interventions, including formulary restriction, prospective audit and feedback, use of antibiotic time-outs, and provider education, aim to improve patient outcomes and antibiotic susceptibility rates and optimize the use of resources.[18] Several recent studies have shown that implementation of ASPs, particularly those that limit the use of broad-spectrum or high-risk antibiotics such as fluoroquinolones, cephalosporins, and clindamycin, decrease the incidence of CDI by as much as 48%.[19–21]

Most academic medical centers performing SOT procedures within the United States have active institutional ASPs.[22] However, although SOT recipients likely benefit from facility-wide stewardship efforts, the efficacy of transplant-specific antimicrobial stewardship initiatives has not been evaluated systematically. Further, diagnostic and therapeutic uncertainty pose unique challenges to the implementation of dedicated transplant stewardship programs.[22,23] Nonetheless, recent literature suggests that the use of exceedingly broad-spectrum empiric antimicrobials, lack of deescalation, and prolonged duration of therapy provide opportunities for antimicrobial stewardship in this patient population.[23] The implementation of SOT-specific antibiograms may also assist in guiding empiric antimicrobial therapy.[24] Collectively, these stewardship interventions should minimize prolonged and excess exposure to antimicrobials and thereby help to reduce the risk of intestinal dysbiosis and CDI in SOT recipients.

Diagnostic stewardship is another critical component of initiatives targeting CDI reduction among SOT recipients. High rates of *C difficile* colonization may complicate the diagnosis of CDI in SOT recipients and lead to unintentional overtreatment.[25] In a population already prone to intestinal dysbiosis, this circumstance may further promote the downstream consequences of diminished colonization resistance and the increased risk of multidrug-resistant nosocomial pathogen acquisition.[26] Optimization of CDI diagnostic algorithms for SOT recipients is therefore warranted. In a recent study, CDI testing limited to patients who were not receiving laxatives and who met clinical criteria for diarrhea led to a significant decline in CDI rates and the use of oral vancomycin therapy; no adverse outcomes were noted.[27] Similar policies are gaining traction at centers caring for immunocompromised hosts,[25] but future studies addressing diagnostic stewardship specific to SOT are needed.

Therapeutics for Primary and Secondary Prevention of Clostridium difficile in Solid Organ Transplant Recipients

There is currently no well-established prophylaxis against *C difficile*. However, agents that preserve or promote diversity of the intestinal microbiome, as well as immunologic approaches to CDI prevention, are under investigation and are discussed herein.

Probiotics have been suggested as a mechanism for CDI prevention, particularly among patients receiving antibiotics, owing to the potential restoration of enteric flora, promotion of *C difficile* colonization resistance, and stimulation of the immune system.[28] Results of trials assessing the role of probiotics for primary and secondary CDI prophylaxis have been inconsistent.[5,28] However, a recent Cochrane review evaluating the effectiveness of probiotics in preventing CDI among individuals taking antibiotics showed that probiotics were effective in preventing CDI, particularly in patients with a baseline CDI risk of greater than 5%; further, there was no difference in adverse outcomes among patients receiving probiotics versus placebo.[29] Nonetheless, results of these studies should be interpreted with caution in the context of SOT, as probiotics have not been evaluated systematically in immunocompromised patients. Further, probiotic formulations are not standardized, and the administration of preparations containing *Saccharomyces boulardii* have been associated with fungemia in immunocompromised hosts.[30] Additional research is required to assess the safety and efficacy of probiotics as CDI prophylaxis in SOT recipients.

Although not endorsed in the national CDI guidelines,[5] small retrospective studies have suggested that oral vancomycin therapy may be effective for secondary prevention of CDI in nontransplanted patients receiving systemic antimicrobial therapy.[31,32] The use of oral vancomycin for secondary CDI prophylaxis in SOT recipients has not been well-established. However, a recent study suggested that oral vancomycin dosed 125 mg twice daily may decrease the risk of CDI recurrence in kidney transplant recipients receiving concomitant broad-spectrum antibiotics.[33] Further study of this strategy in SOT recipients is needed, both in terms of clinical efficacy and impact on the intestinal microbiome.

There are currently no data regarding the use of oral vancomycin as primary prophylaxis for CDI in SOT recipients. However, this strategy is being evaluated in other immunocompromised populations. In a study of 105 patients with hematologic malignancies undergoing allogeneic stem cell transplantation, the incidence of CDI was 0% (0 of 50) in those receiving oral vancomycin 125 mg twice daily compared with 20% (11 of 55) in patients who did not receive oral vancomycin prophylaxis; no cases of vancomycin-resistant enterococcal bloodstream infections were reported in the vancomycin prophylaxis arm.[34] Primary oral vancomycin prophylaxis in solid organ and stem cell transplant recipients may prove valuable in the peritransplant period owing to the receipt of immunosuppressant and chemotherapeutic agents that could alter the microbiome. However, the risks and benefits of this strategy warrant further systematic evaluation.

Over the past decade, there has been increasing interest in the development of novel β-lactamases targeting enteric degradation of antibiotics, thereby reducing intestinal antibiotic concentrations and preventing dysbiosis.[35,36] In a recent phase IIa clinical trial, SYN-004 (ribaxamase), an investigational β-lactamase orally administered with parenteral β-lactams, was shown to effectively degrade ceftriaxone excreted into the intestine.[37,38] In a subsequent trial, 412 patients receiving parenteral ceftriaxone for lower respiratory tract infections were randomly assigned to receive ribaxamase versus placebo. After 6 weeks, ribaxamase seemed to confer relative risk reductions in CDI and new colonization with vancomycin-resistant Enterococci of 71% and 44%, respectively. Although these agents are still in their infancy, they may have promise for CDI prevention in patients receiving β-lactam antibiotics. However, larger studies assessing safety, efficacy, and impact on immunosuppressive drug absorption will be needed before widespread use in SOT recipients.

Early studies of novel microbiome therapeutics, including spores from both nontoxigenic C difficile strains or multiple species of Firmicutes, have shown that microbial-based therapeutics may be efficacious in the secondary prevention of CDI.[39,40] Although these microbiome therapeutics have not been formally studied in SOT recipients, fecal microbiota transplantation (FMT) has been used for the treatment of recurrent or refractory CDI in SOT recipients and may also gain traction as a mechanism for CDI prevention. There are a growing number of studies on ClinicalTrials.gov assessing the use of FMT for prevention and treatment of intestinal dysbiosis in SOT recipients and primary CDI prophylaxis in patients undergoing hematopoietic stem cell transplantation. These studies may ultimately have a significant impact on CDI prevention in immunocompromised hosts, including SOT recipients.

Therapeutic strategies for secondary prevention of CDI also include the adjunctive use of monoclonal antibodies against C difficile toxin. An early study of patients with CDI receiving standard therapy showed that concomitant administration of actoxumab and bezlotoxumab, human monoclonal antibodies binding C difficile toxins A and B, respectively, decreased the rate of recurrent CDI.[41] Two subsequent phase III randomized clinical trials, MODIFY I and II, demonstrated that administration of antitoxin B antibody in conjunction with standard oral therapy reduced CDI recurrence by 38% through 12 weeks compared with standard oral therapy alone. In these studies, actoxumab was not efficacious when given alone with standard therapy, nor provided additional efficacy when coadministered with bezlotoxumab.[42] The MODIFY I and II trials included immunocompromised patients based on underlying disease or use of immunosuppressive agents, and the use of bezlotoxumab compared with placebo seems to be cost effective in this population.[42,43] However, the adjunctive use of bezlotoxumab for the secondary prevention of CDI in SOT recipients has not been evaluated formally. Further studies are also required to assess role of bezlotoxumab with respect to other mechanisms of secondary prevention, including FMT, among SOT recipients.

Infection Control

The prevention of nosocomial *C difficile* transmission relies on the implementation of contact precautions and strict adherence to hand hygiene. Upon the diagnosis of CDI, patients should be placed into contact precautions for the duration of diarrhea and ideally transferred to a private room.[5] Health care providers and visitors should also be educated about proper hand hygiene measures. Because alcohol-based hand rubs are not sporicidal and are less effective than soap and water at removing *C difficile* spores,[44] the use of soap and water is the preferred method of hand hygiene during outbreaks or in areas with high rates of CDI.[5,14]

Although preventing the transmission of *C difficile* from patients with active CDI has been a significant focus of infection control initiatives, emerging data suggest that more than 25% of hospital-onset CDI cases may result from transmission by asymptomatic carriers.[45–47] In a recent quasi-experimental study, patients admitted through the emergency department were screened for *C difficile* colonization by polymerase chain reaction; if colonized, patients were placed into modified contact precautions requiring the use of dedicated medical equipment and gloves only. Hospital-associated CDI decreased from 6.9 per 10,000 patient-days to 3.0 per 10,000 patient-days after this intervention ($P<.001$), suggesting that screening for *C difficile* colonization and isolation of asymptomatic carriers may be effective in decreasing CDI among hospitalized patients.[48] The screening and isolation of SOT recipients with asymptomatic *C difficile* carriage has not been evaluated, but may represent an adjunctive approach to minimize the incidence of CDI in transplant units. Further studies are also warranted to determine whether asymptomatic colonization with toxigenic versus nontoxigenic strains of *C difficile* pose different risks for transmission among hospitalized SOT recipients.

C difficile spores are resistant to standard disinfectants and may persist on environmental surfaces for weeks to years. Current guidelines suggest that environmental sources potentially harboring spores, particularly digital rectal thermometers, should be replaced with disposables whenever possible.[5] In addition, the use of sporicidal cleansers, including bleach- or chlorine-containing solutions, are recommended for daily and terminal room cleaning, and health care facilities should implement measures of cleaning effectiveness to ensure quality environmental disinfection.[5,14] Evidence supporting the use of ultraviolet rays for the disinfection of hospital surfaces is emerging.[49–52] The efficacy of ultraviolet rays is dose dependent,[49] and the impact of terminal cleaning with adjunctive use of ultraviolet on nosocomial CDI transmission remains unclear. Future studies addressing the optimization of *C difficile* disinfection methods for hospital rooms occupied by SOT recipients are needed.

TREATMENT OF *CLOSTRIDIUM DIFFICILE* INFECTION IN SOLID ORGAN TRANSPLANT RECIPIENTS

General Treatment Recommendations

Patients with suspected CDI should be placed in isolation with enteric contact precautions pending results of testing if testing results cannot be obtained the same day. If severe or complicated CDI is suspected, it is appropriate to initiate empiric treatment while awaiting test results, and any potentially inciting antimicrobials should be discontinued as soon as possible. Clinical data seem to demonstrate increased risk of CDI with use of proton pump inhibitors; however, there are multiple potential confounders in previous studies that make it difficult to estimate the true risk.[5,53–55] Although blanket discontinuation of proton pump inhibitors is not recommended in the current CDI treatment guidleines,[5] discontinuation of unnecessary acid-suppressing medications is advised. Supportive care should be administered with intravenous fluid resuscitation and electrolyte replacement, and antidiarrheals should be avoided.[5]

Therapy Based on Disease Severity

Consensus guidelines for the treatment CDI have been published by the IDSA and SHEA, as well as the European Society of Clinical Microbiology and Infectious Diseases (ESCMID).[5,56] Recommendations are divided by initial CDI episode versus recurrent CDI and further stratified based on CDI severity.

Mild or moderate CDI is defined by a white blood cell count of less than 15,000 cells/mm^3 and a serum creatinine level of less than 1.5 times the premorbid level.[5,56] Severe CDI is defined by a white blood cell count of 15,000 cells/mm^3 or greater and a serum creatinine level of greater than 1.5 times the premorbid level.[5,56] Severe, complicated, or fulminant CDI is defined by at least one of the following characteristics: admission to the intensive care unit, hypotension with or without shock, fever of 38.5°C or higher, ileus, toxic megacolon or acute abdomen, mental status changes, white blood cell count of 35,000 cells/mm^3 or greater or less than 2000 cells/mm^3, serum lactate greater than 2.2 mmol/L, or any evidence of end-organ failure.[5,56]

Initial episode of Clostridium difficile infection

Treatment of an initial CDI episode is the same for both SOT recipients and nontransplant patients.[15] The choice of antimicrobial therapy for an initial CDI episode depends disease severity (**Fig. 1**).

Initial Episode	First Recurrence	Multiple Recurrences
Mild to Moderate • Vancomycin 125 mg orally every 6 h for 10 d OR • Fidaxomicin 200 mg orally twice daily for 10 d • Metronidazole 500 mg orally three times daily for 10 d (only if vancomycin and fidaxomicin are unavailable)	• Vancomycin 125 mg orally every 6 h for 10 d followed by vancomycin taper and pulse OR • Fidaxomicin 200 mg orally twice daily for 10 d	• Vancomycin 125 mg orally every 6 h for 10 d followed by vancomycin taper and pulse OR • Vancomycin 125 mg orally every 6 h for 10 d followed by rifaximin 400 mg orally three times daily for 20 d
Severe • Vancomycin 125 mg orally every 6 h for 10 d OR • Fidaxomicin 200 mg orally twice daily for 10 d		OR • Fidaxomicin 200 mg orally twice daily for 10 d
Fulminant • Vancomycin 500 mg orally or by nasogastric tube every 6 h • Consider vancomycin retention enema and metronidazole 500 mg intravenously every 8 h if ileus is present		OR • FMT

Fig. 1. Approach to the management of *Clostridium difficile* infection (CDI) in solid organ transplant recipients. FMT, fecal microbiota transplantation.

For mild-to-moderate CDI, the most recent IDSA guidelines now recommend either oral vancomycin or fidaxomicin as first-line therapy over metronidazole.[5,56] The recommended dosage for vancomycin is 125 mg orally every 6 hours for 10 days, and the recommended dosage for fidaxomicin is 200 mg orally twice daily for 10 days.[5,57] Cost and access can be prohibitive factors in the use of fidaxomicin in particular as first-line therapy for an initial episode of CDI.[58] In resource-limited settings where both oral vancomycin and fidaxomicin are unavailable, metronidazole 500 mg orally every 8 hours for 10 days can used for an initial mild to moderate CDI episode.[5] Metronidazole is a weak CYP3A4 inhibitor, and there have been scattered case reports of supratherapeutic tacrolimus levels in the setting of concomitant metronidazole administration.[59] A retrospective review of 52 SOT recipients treated for CDI found no difference in tacrolimus adjustments in patients treated with metronidazole versus vancomycin.[60] Metronidazole is still recommended if vancomycin and fidaxomicin are not available, although tacrolimus serum levels should be monitored. Metronidazole is not recommended beyond the first episode of CDI or for long-term therapy owing to the potential risk of cumulative neurotoxicity.[5]

For severe CDI, vancomycin 125 mg orally every 6 hours or fidaxomicin 200 mg orally twice daily for 10 days are the recommended first-line therapies.[5,56] In cases of fulminant or complicated CDI (including ileus or toxic megacolon), vancomycin doses of up to 500 mg every 6 hours can be given via nasogastric tube.[5] In addition to oral therapy, vancomycin can also be administered via retention edema (500 mg in approximately 100 mL normal saline per rectum every 6 hours).[5] Intravenous metronidazole 500 mg every 8 hours should be co-administered with vancomycin in cases of fulminant CDI particularly if ileus is present.[5] Surgical management with total abdominal colectomy with ileostomy should be performed in cases of colonic perforation, toxic megacolon, or severe ileus that is not responding to antibiotic therapy.[5,56]

Of note, although 10 days is the recommended treatment duration for initial CDI episodes, treatment can be extended to 14 days if there is a delay in treatment response.[5,56]

Recurrent Clostridium difficile infection
Recurrence is defined as CDI that occurs within 8 weeks of a previous episode, and symptoms from the prior episode need to have resolved with the initial treatment regimen.[61]

Treatment for a first recurrence of CDI depends on which treatment regimen was used for the initial CDI episode, also accounting for disease severity[5] (see **Fig. 1**). If metronidazole was used for the initial episode, then vancomycin 125 mg orally every 6 hours is recommended for the first recurrence.[5] If vancomycin was used for the initial episode, strategies for treating the first recurrence include using prolonged, tapered, or pulsed vancomycin regimens or giving fidaxomicin 200 mg orally twice daily for 10 days.[5] Fidaxomicin may be particularly efficacious for those patients who are at risk of multiple recurrences.[15,56]

Fidaxomicin is a bactericidal, narrow spectrum macrocyclic antibiotic with less disruption of the bowel flora compared with oral vancomycin and metronidazole.[62,63] It has been found to have similar cure rates to vancomycin; however, significantly fewer patients treated with fidaxomicin compared with vancomycin experienced a recurrence.[64–66] This decrease in the recurrence rate was primarily seen in patients with the non-North American Pulsed Field type 1 (NAP1/BI/027) strain.[66] Cost-effectiveness studies have also shown that fidaxomicin is cost effective compared with vancomycin for the treatment of recurrent CDI.[67] Patients with inflammatory bowel disease were specifically excluded from the large phase III trials evaluating fidaxomicin versus vancomycin, but there was no specific mention of other immunocompromised groups.[64,66] Clutter and colleagues[68] evaluated fidaxomicin versus conventional therapy (vancomycin and metronidazole) in 59 SOT (liver and kidney) and hematopoietic stem cell transplant recipients. Fidaxomicin was well-tolerated and did not have an appreciable impact on serum tacrolimus levels. Cure rates were comparable with conventional therapy (67% vs 89%; $P = 0.06$). Of note, there was no new vancomycin-resistant *Enterococcus* colonization with fidaxomicin therapy compared with 36% of patients receiving conventional therapy. This study also showed no difference in *Candida* colonization.

Clostridium difficile infection with multiple recurrences

Per the ESCMID guidelines, risk factors for recurrent CDI include those greater than 65 years of age, continued use of non-CDI antibiotics after diagnosis of CDI and/or after CDI treatment, history of prior CDI, use of antacid medications, and initial disease severity.[56] SOT recipients also seem to be at greater risk for recurrent CDI. Studies in heart and lung transplant recipients demonstrated that 28.6% to 33.0% of patients had one or more recurrences, although these events were not distinguished from new CDI infections.[69]

Currently recommended treatment strategies for multiple CDI recurrences (defined as ≥ 2 recurrences) include (see **Fig. 1**)[5,14,56]:

- Fidaxomicin 200 mg orally twice daily for 10 days, or
- Vancomycin 125 mg orally 4 times a day for 10 days followed by either an oral vancomycin taper or pulse dosing, or
- Vancomycin 125 mg orally 4 times a day for 10 days followed by rifaximin 400 mg orally 3 times daily for 20 days, or
- FMT.

There is no standardized recommendation for vancomycin taper or pulse dosing. Per the IDSA guidelines, vancomycin can be given orally 125 mg 4 times daily for 10 to 14 days, followed by twice daily for one week, once daily for one week, and then every 2 to 3 days for 2 to 8 weeks.[5] Dubberke and colleagues[14] suggested the following taper and pulse regimens for SOT recipients: vancomycin tapering by decreasing the total dose by 125 mg per day each week and vancomycin pulsing by treating with vancomycin 3 times per week for 4 weeks.

Rifaximin

Small studies have also looked at the use of rifaximin as a chaser to vancomycin therapy for CDI with multiple recurrences.[70–72] In these studies, rifaximin was typically given 400 mg orally twice daily for 14 to 28 days after either a standard treatment regimen or a vancomycin taper. Cure rates have ranged from 53% to 100%.[70–72] Neff at al[73] published a case series of 3 liver transplant recipients with multiple CDI recurrences and persistent diarrhea despite standard of care therapy, including long-term vancomycin in 2 of the 3 recipients. These patients had a rapid and durable resolution of chronic diarrhea after treatment with rifaximin, although they were given a dose of 400 mg orally 3 times a day for 28 days.[73] Rifaximin was well-tolerated in these patients. Further randomized, controlled trials are needed to assess the use of rifaximin for recurrent CDI, particularly in SOT recipients, although it may be considered as adjunctive therapy for recurrent CDI after treatment with oral vancomycin.

Fecal microbiota transplantation

FMT has been shown to be effective for treating recurrent CDI, although trials have previously excluded SOT recipients.[74–78] Additionally, FMT was found to be the most cost-effective initial treatment for recurrent CDI compared with metronidazole, vancomycin, and fidaxomicin.[79] FMT is recommended for multiply recurrent CDI in the current ESCMID and IDSA/SHEA guidelines[5,56] There has been understandable concern about infection risk associated with FMT, particularly enteric translocation of bacterial infections in immunocompromised patients.[80] In 2014, the first case reports were published of a renal transplant and lung transplant recipient with multiply recurrent CDI who were successfully treated with FMT.[81] No infectious complications were noted; however, both patients required 2 FMT procedures before cure. It was hypothesized that SOT recipients may have more severe alterations in their intestinal microbiota and, thus, sequential FMT may be needed to correct dysbiosis. There have been a few additional case reports documenting the successful treatment of recurrent CDI in SOT recipients.[82,83]

Kelly and colleagues[69] conducted a retrospective review of 80 immunocompromised patients who underwent FMT for either recurrent or refractory CDI, including 19 SOT recipients. Patients were observed for a minimum of 12 weeks after FMT. Of the 80 patients, 62 (78%) were cured after a single FMT. Twelve patients underwent a second FMT, of whom 8 had CDI resolution, which gave an overall CDI cure rate of 89%. Serious adverse events were reported in 15% of patients; however, there were no infectious complications related to the FMT procedure. There were two deaths reported, both of which occurred in SOT recipients. One death was due to pneumonia. The other death was due to an aspiration event that occurred at the time of sedation for FMT. Woodworth and colleagues[84] published a summary of donor screening recommendations for fecal donors. This regimen did not include screening for cytomegalovirus, which is a significant problem in SOT recipients, and more robust fecal donor screening may be needed in this population. It is not fully known how changes in the microbiome after FMT may affect immunosuppressant metabolism, which may impact the risk of rejection. For example, Lee and colleagues[85] noted increased *Faecalibacterium prausnitzii* in patients who required increased tacrolimus doses. A small series did not note any changes in tacrolimus concentration to dose ratio after FMT, although data from greater numbers of patients are needed to fully assess the effects of FMT on immunosuppressant levels.[86]

There have also been concerns about the effects of FMT-induced alterations in the recipient microbiome and risk of obesity. Fischer and colleagues[87] analyzed data from both an observational cohort and randomized clinical trial and found no statistically significant differences in body mass index up to 48 weeks after a single FMT among recipients who received an FMT from normal weight, overweight, or obese donors.

Further studies are needed to fully evaluate the efficacy and safety of FMT for SOT recipients, as well as to evaluate the optimal number of FMT procedures needed to correct the dysbiosis of SOT recipients. Although there are no specific recommendations for FMT in SOT recipients at this time,[14,15] given the compelling efficacy data in other populations and current IDSA/SHEA treatment guidelines,[5] FMT should be strongly considered for recurrent CDI in this population.

Other Pharmacologic Therapies for Clostridium difficile Infection

Intravenous immunoglobulins

The use of pooled intravenous immunoglobulins (IVIG) has been proposed for treatment of severe or refractory CDI and CDI with multiple recurrences. IVIG neutralizes primarily toxin A through antitoxin A immunoglobulin (Ig)G antibodies.[88] There are clustered case reports and small retrospective studies showing successful use of concomitant IVIG for severe or multiply recurrent CDI, although there was variation in dose and duration of IVIG therapy.[88] Patients reported in these case reports and small studies also seem to have had low total serum IgG or antitoxin A IgG levels when tested.[88] Thus, the effect of concomitant IVIG therapy in patients with normal IgG levels is uncertain. IVIG can be considered as adjunctive therapy in cases of severe, refractory, or multiply recurrent CDI; however, further randomized, controlled trials evaluating the efficacy of IVIG are needed.

Cholestyramine and tolevamer

Cholestyramine is bile acid sequestrant that falls within the category of luminal toxin-binding agents, which have been shown to bind toxin A and toxin B within the intestinal lumen.[89,90] These luminal toxin-binding agents have minimal systemic absorption and thus a lesser risk of adverse side effects. There is also less risk of microbiota disruption with these agents. There are case reports of multiply relapsed CDI being cured with prolonged courses of cholestyramine.[91,92] Randomized, controlled trials evaluating the use of cholestyramine for CDI are currently lacking. There is also the concern that cholestyramine binds vancomycin, and it is recommended that vancomycin be administered either 1 hour before or 4 to 6 hours after cholestyramine.[89] This schedule can be a significant challenge because vancomycin is administered 4 times daily and cholestyramine 3 times daily. The bioavailability of metronidazole and of mycophenolic acid may also be reduced with cholestyramine, each posing different therapeutic issues.[89,93] There is insufficient evidence at this time to recommend cholestyramine for the treatment of CDI in SOT recipients.

Tolevamer is another luminal toxin-binding agent that is not currently available in the United States. It was found to be inferior to both metronidazole and vancomycin for the treatment of CDI in 2 large, randomized, controlled trials.[94]

Tigecycline

Tigecycline is a glycycline antibiotic that has activity against resistant gram-positive organisms, enteric gram-negative organisms, and anaerobes, including *C difficile*. There have been case reports and small retrospective series reporting successful use of tigecycline both alone, or in combination with vancomycin and/or metronidazole for patients with severe CDI.[95–97] There are few data on the use of tigecycline to treat CDI in immunosuppressed patients. A single-center retrospective review of 66 oncology patients treated for CDI found no significant benefit to tigecycline treatment compared with conventional treatment.[98] The majority of these patients were classified as having severe or fulminant CDI. Furthermore, they found an 18.1% incidence of non-CDI breakthrough infections in patients treated with tigecycline and had 4 cases of CDI develop in patients who were already receiving tigecycline therapy for an alternate infection.[98] Further prospective studies are needed to fully evaluate the efficacy of tigecycline therapy for CDI and to further analyze the risk of developing breakthrough multidrug-resistant infections while on tigecycline therapy. Tigecycline should not be used as first-line therapy for CDI, but can be considered as adjunctive salvage therapy in patients with fulminant or refractory CDI failing therapy with vancomycin and intravenous metronidazole.

SUMMARY

CDI disproportionately affects SOT recipients, and recurrences are common. To date, strategies for CDI prevention have largely focused on important factors such as infection control interventions to reduce rates of horizontal *C difficile* transmission and minimizing unnecessary antibiotic use through the development of ASPs. However, our understanding of intestinal dysbiosis and its impact on the pathogenesis of CDI is evolving. FMT seems to be safe and efficacious for the treatment of CDI in SOT recipients, and novel therapeutics aimed at maintaining a diverse intestinal microbiome may hold promise for the treatment and prevention of CDI in SOT recipients.

REFERENCES

1. Leffler DA, Lamont JT. Clostridium difficile infection. N Engl J Med 2015;373(3): 287–8.
2. Zilberberg MD, Shorr AF, Kollef MH. Increase in adult Clostridium difficile-related hospitalizations and case-fatality rate, United States, 2000-2005. Emerg Infect Dis 2008;14(6):929–31.
3. Dubberke ER, Olsen MA. Burden of Clostridium difficile on the healthcare system. Clin Infect Dis 2012;55(Suppl 2):S88–92.
4. Lofgren ET, Cole SR, Weber DJ, et al. Hospital-acquired Clostridium difficile infections: estimating all-cause mortality and length of stay. Epidemiology 2014; 25(4):570–5.
5. McDonald LC, Gerding DN, Johnson S, et al. Clinical practice guidelines for Clostridium difficile infection in adults and children: 2017 update by the Infectious Diseases Society of America (IDSA) and Society for Healthcare Epidemiology of America (SHEA). Clin Infect Dis 2018;66(7):987–94.
6. Riddle DJ, Dubberke ER. Clostridium difficile infection in solid organ transplant recipients. Curr Opin Organ Transplant 2008;13(6):592–600.
7. Boutros M, Al-Shaibi M, Chan G, et al. Clostridium difficile colitis: increasing incidence, risk factors, and outcomes in solid organ transplant recipients. Transplantation 2012;93(10):1051–7.
8. Dallal RM, Harbrecht BG, Boujoukas AJ, et al. Fulminant Clostridium difficile: an underappreciated and increasing cause of death and complications. Ann Surg 2002;235(3):363–72.
9. Lee JT, Kelly RF, Hertz MI, et al. Clostridium difficile infection increases mortality risk in lung transplant recipients. J Heart Lung Transplant 2013;32(10):1020–6.
10. Cusini A, Beguelin C, Stampf S, et al. Clostridium difficile infection is associated with graft loss in solid organ transplant recipients. Am J Transplant 2018. [Epub ahead of print].
11. Honda H, Dubberke ER. Clostridium difficile infection in solid organ transplant recipients. Curr Opin Infect Dis 2014;27(4):336–41.
12. Bignardi GE. Risk factors for Clostridium difficile infection. J Hosp Infect 1998; 40(1):1–15.
13. Len O, Rodriguez-Pardo D, Gavalda J, et al. Outcome of Clostridium difficile-associated disease in solid organ transplant recipients: a prospective and multicentre cohort study. Transpl Int 2012;25(12):1275–81.
14. Dubberke ER, Burdette SD, American Society of Transplantation Infectious Diseases Community of Practice. Clostridium difficile infections in solid organ transplantation. Am J Transplant 2013;13(Suppl 4):42–9.
15. Nanayakkara D, Nanda N. Clostridium difficile infection in solid organ transplant recipients. Curr Opin Organ Transplant 2017;22(4):314–9.
16. Bruminhent J, Cawcutt KA, Thongprayoon C, et al. Epidemiology, risk factors, and outcome of Clostridium difficile infection in heart and heart-lung transplant recipients. Clin Transplant 2017;31(6). https://doi.org/10.1111/ctr.12968.
17. Dubberke ER, Carling P, Carrico R, et al. Strategies to prevent Clostridium difficile infections in acute care hospitals: 2014 update. Infect Control Hosp Epidemiol 2014;35(6):628–45.

18. Barlam TF, Cosgrove SE, Abbo LM, et al. Implementing an antibiotic stewardship program: guidelines by the Infectious Diseases Society of America and the Society for Healthcare Epidemiology of America. Clin Infect Dis 2016;62(10):e51–77.
19. Feazel LM, Malhotra A, Perencevich EN, et al. Effect of antibiotic stewardship programmes on Clostridium difficile incidence: a systematic review and meta-analysis. J Antimicrob Chemother 2014;69(7):1748–54.
20. Baur D, Gladstone BP, Burkert F, et al. Effect of antibiotic stewardship on the incidence of infection and colonisation with antibiotic-resistant bacteria and Clostridium difficile infection: a systematic review and meta-analysis. Lancet Infect Dis 2017;17(9):990–1001.
21. Shea KM, Hobbs ALV, Jaso TC, et al. Effect of a health care system respiratory fluoroquinolone restriction program to alter utilization and impact rates of Clostridium difficile infection. Antimicrob Agents Chemother 2017;61(6). https://doi.org/10.1128/AAC.00125-17.
22. Seo SK, Lo K, Abbo LM. Current state of antimicrobial stewardship at solid organ and hematopoietic cell transplant centers in the United States. Infect Control Hosp Epidemiol 2016;37(10):1195–200.
23. So M, Yang DY, Bell C, et al. Solid organ transplant patients: are there opportunities for antimicrobial stewardship? Clin Transplant 2016;30(6):659–68.
24. Rosa R, Simkins J, Camargo JF, et al. Solid organ transplant antibiograms: an opportunity for antimicrobial stewardship. Diagn Microbiol Infect Dis 2016;86(4):460–3.
25. Robilotti E, Holubar M, Seo SK, et al. Feasibility and applicability of antimicrobial stewardship in immunocompromised patients. Curr Opin Infect Dis 2017;30(4):346–53.
26. Lewis BB, Buffie CG, Carter RA, et al. Loss of microbiota-mediated colonization resistance to Clostridium difficile infection with oral vancomycin compared with metronidazole. J Infect Dis 2015;212(10):1656–65.
27. Truong CY, Gombar S, Wilson R, et al. Real-time electronic tracking of diarrheal episodes and laxative therapy enables verification of Clostridium difficile clinical testing criteria and reduction of Clostridium difficile infection rates. J Clin Microbiol 2017;55(5):1276–84.
28. Parkes GC, Sanderson JD, Whelan K. The mechanisms and efficacy of probiotics in the prevention of Clostridium difficile-associated diarrhoea. Lancet Infect Dis 2009;9(4):237–44.
29. Goldenberg JZ, Yap C, Lytvyn L, et al. Probiotics for the prevention of Clostridium difficile-associated diarrhea in adults and children. Cochrane Database Syst Rev 2017;(12):CD006095.
30. Enache-Angoulvant A, Hennequin C. Invasive saccharomyces infection: a comprehensive review. Clin Infect Dis 2005;41(11):1559–68.
31. Van Hise NW, Bryant AM, Hennessey EK, et al. Efficacy of oral vancomycin in preventing recurrent Clostridium difficile infection in patients treated with systemic antimicrobial agents. Clin Infect Dis 2016;63(5):651–3.
32. Carignan A, Poulin S, Martin P, et al. Efficacy of secondary prophylaxis with vancomycin for preventing recurrent Clostridium difficile infections. Am J Gastroenterol 2016;111(12):1834–40.
33. Splinter LE, Kerstenetzky L, Jorgenson MR, et al. Vancomycin prophylaxis for prevention of Clostridium difficile infection recurrence in renal transplant patients. Ann Pharmacother 2018;52(2):113–9.
34. Ganetsky A, HJ, Hughes ME, et al. Oral vancomycin is highly effective in preventing Clostridium difficile infection in allogeneic hematopoietic stem cell transplant

recipients. Presented at the 58th ASH Annual Meeting and Exposition. [abstract: 2225]. San Diego, CA, December 3–6, 2016.

35. Pitout JD. IPSAT P1A, a class A beta-lactamase therapy for the prevention of penicillin-induced disruption to the intestinal microflora. Curr Opin Investig Drugs 2009;10(8):838–44.

36. Tarkkanen AM, Heinonen T, Jogi R, et al. P1A recombinant beta-lactamase prevents emergence of antimicrobial resistance in gut microflora of healthy subjects during intravenous administration of ampicillin. Antimicrob Agents Chemother 2009;53(6):2455–62.

37. Kokai-Kun JF, Roberts T, Coughlin O, et al. The oral beta-lactamase SYN-004 (ribaxamase) degrades ceftriaxone excreted into the intestine in phase 2a clinical studies. Antimicrob Agents Chemother 2017;61(3). https://doi.org/10.1128/AAC.02197-16.

38. Kokai-Kun J, Roberts T, Coughlin O, et al. SYN-004 (ribaxamase) prevents new onset Clostridium difficile infection by protecting the integrity of the gut microbiome in a phase 2b study. Oral abstract 136. IDWeek. San Diego, CA, October 4–8, 2017.

39. Gerding DN, Meyer T, Lee C, et al. Administration of spores of nontoxigenic Clostridium difficile strain M3 for prevention of recurrent C. difficile infection: a randomized clinical trial. JAMA 2015;313(17):1719–27.

40. Khanna S, Pardi DS, Kelly CR, et al. A novel microbiome therapeutic increases gut microbial diversity and prevents recurrent Clostridium difficile infection. J Infect Dis 2016;214(2):173–81.

41. Lowy I, Molrine DC, Leav BA, et al. Treatment with monoclonal antibodies against Clostridium difficile toxins. N Engl J Med 2010;362(3):197–205.

42. Wilcox MH, Gerding DN, Poxton IR, et al. Bezlotoxumab for prevention of recurrent Clostridium difficile infection. N Engl J Med 2017;376(4):305–17.

43. Prabhu VS, Dubberke ER, Dorr MB, et al. Cost-effectiveness of bezlotoxumab compared with placebo for the prevention of recurrent Clostridium difficile infection. Clin Infect Dis 2018;66(3):355–62.

44. Oughton MT, Loo VG, Dendukuri N, et al. Hand hygiene with soap and water is superior to alcohol rub and antiseptic wipes for removal of Clostridium difficile. Infect Control Hosp Epidemiol 2009;30(10):939–44.

45. Curry SR, Muto CA, Schlackman JL, et al. Use of multilocus variable number of tandem repeats analysis genotyping to determine the role of asymptomatic carriers in Clostridium difficile transmission. Clin Infect Dis 2013;57(8):1094–102.

46. Lanzas C, Dubberke ER, Lu Z, et al. Epidemiological model for Clostridium difficile transmission in healthcare settings. Infect Control Hosp Epidemiol 2011;32(6):553–61.

47. Lanzas C, Dubberke ER. Effectiveness of screening hospital admissions to detect asymptomatic carriers of Clostridium difficile: a modeling evaluation. Infect Control Hosp Epidemiol 2014;35(8):1043–50.

48. Longtin Y, Paquet-Bolduc B, Gilca R, et al. Effect of detecting and isolating Clostridium difficile carriers at hospital admission on the incidence of C difficile infections: a quasi-experimental controlled study. JAMA Intern Med 2016;176(6):796–804.

49. Boyce JM, Farrel PA, Towle D, et al. Impact of room location on UV-C irradiance and UV-C dosage and antimicrobial effect delivered by a mobile UV-C light device. Infect Control Hosp Epidemiol 2016;37(6):667–72.

50. Pegues DA, Han J, Gilmar C, et al. Impact of ultraviolet germicidal irradiation for no-touch terminal room disinfection on Clostridium difficile infection incidence

among hematology-oncology patients. Infect Control Hosp Epidemiol 2017;38(1): 39–44.

51. Anderson DJ, Chen LF, Weber DJ, et al. Enhanced terminal room disinfection and acquisition and infection caused by multidrug-resistant organisms and Clostridium difficile (the Benefits of Enhanced Terminal Room Disinfection study): a cluster-randomised, multicentre, crossover study. Lancet 2017;389(10071): 805–14.

52. Liscynesky C, Hines LP, Smyer J, et al. The effect of ultraviolet light on Clostridium difficile spore recovery versus bleach alone. Infect Control Hosp Epidemiol 2017; 38(9):1116–7.

53. Chitnis AS, Holzbauer SM, Belflower RM, et al. Epidemiology of community-associated Clostridium difficile infection, 2009 through 2011. JAMA Intern Med 2013;173(14):1359–67.

54. Kwok CS, Arthur AK, Anibueze CI, et al. Risk of Clostridium difficile infection with acid suppressing drugs and antibiotics: meta-analysis. Am J Gastroenterol 2012; 107(7):1011–9.

55. Janarthanan S, Ditah I, Adler DG, et al. Clostridium difficile-associated diarrhea and proton pump inhibitor therapy: a meta-analysis. Am J Gastroenterol 2012; 107(7):1001–10.

56. Debast SB, Bauer MP, Kuijper EJ, European Society of Clinical Microbiology and Infectious Diseases. European Society of Clinical Microbiology and Infectious Diseases: update of the treatment guidance document for Clostridium difficile infection. Clin Microbiol Infect 2014;20(Suppl 2):1–26.

57. Crobach MJ, Planche T, Eckert C, et al. European Society of Clinical Microbiology and Infectious Diseases: update of the diagnostic guidance document for Clostridium difficile infection. Clin Microbiol Infect 2016;22(Suppl 4):S63–81.

58. Bartsch SM, Umscheid CA, Fishman N, et al. Is fidaxomicin worth the cost? An economic analysis. Clin Infect Dis 2013;57(4):555–61.

59. Page RL 2nd, Klem PM, Rogers C. Potential elevation of tacrolimus trough concentrations with concomitant metronidazole therapy. Ann Pharmacother 2005; 39(6):1109–13.

60. Early CR, Park JM, Dorsch MP, et al. Effect of metronidazole use on tacrolimus concentrations in transplant patients treated for Clostridium difficile. Transpl Infect Dis 2016;18(5):714–20.

61. Surawicz CM, Brandt LJ, Binion DG, et al. Guidelines for diagnosis, treatment, and prevention of Clostridium difficile infections. Am J Gastroenterol 2013; 108(4):478–98 [quiz: 499].

62. Venugopal AA, Johnson S. Fidaxomicin: a novel macrocyclic antibiotic approved for treatment of Clostridium difficile infection. Clin Infect Dis 2012;54(4):568–74.

63. Johnson AP. Drug evaluation: OPT-80, a narrow-spectrum macrocyclic antibiotic. Curr Opin Investig Drugs 2007;8(2):168–73.

64. Cornely OA, Crook DW, Esposito R, et al. Fidaxomicin versus vancomycin for infection with Clostridium difficile in Europe, Canada, and the USA: a double-blind, non-inferiority, randomised controlled trial. Lancet Infect Dis 2012;12(4): 281–9.

65. Crook DW, Walker AS, Kean Y, et al. Fidaxomicin versus vancomycin for Clostridium difficile infection: meta-analysis of pivotal randomized controlled trials. Clin Infect Dis 2012;55(Suppl 2):S93–103.

66. Louie TJ, Miller MA, Mullane KM, et al. Fidaxomicin versus vancomycin for Clostridium difficile infection. N Engl J Med 2011;364(5):422–31.

67. Nathwani D, Cornely OA, Van Engen AK, et al. Cost-effectiveness analysis of fidaxomicin versus vancomycin in Clostridium difficile infection. J Antimicrob Chemother 2014;69(11):2901–12.

68. Clutter DS, Dubrovskaya Y, Merl MY, et al. Fidaxomicin versus conventional antimicrobial therapy in 59 recipients of solid organ and hematopoietic stem cell transplantation with Clostridium difficile-associated diarrhea. Antimicrob Agents Chemother 2013;57(9):4501–5.

69. Kelly CR, Ihunnah C, Fischer M, et al. Fecal microbiota transplant for treatment of Clostridium difficile infection in immunocompromised patients. Am J Gastroenterol 2014;109(7):1065–71.

70. Johnson S, Schriever C, Galang M, et al. Interruption of recurrent Clostridium difficile-associated diarrhea episodes by serial therapy with vancomycin and rifaximin. Clin Infect Dis 2007;44(6):846–8.

71. Johnson S, Schriever C, Patel U, et al. Rifaximin redux: treatment of recurrent Clostridium difficile infections with rifaximin immediately post-vancomycin treatment. Anaerobe 2009;15(6):290–1.

72. Mattila E, Arkkila P, Mattila PS, et al. Rifaximin in the treatment of recurrent Clostridium difficile infection. Aliment Pharmacol Ther 2013;37(1):122–8.

73. Neff G, Zacharias V, Kaiser TE, et al. Rifaximin for the treatment of recurrent Clostridium difficile infection after liver transplantation: a case series. Liver Transpl 2010;16(8):960–3.

74. Bakken JS, Borody T, Brandt LJ, et al. Treating Clostridium difficile infection with fecal microbiota transplantation. Clin Gastroenterol Hepatol 2011;9(12):1044–9.

75. Kassam Z, Lee CH, Yuan Y, et al. Fecal microbiota transplantation for Clostridium difficile infection: systematic review and meta-analysis. Am J Gastroenterol 2013;108(4):500–8.

76. van Nood E, Vrieze A, Nieuwdorp M, et al. Duodenal infusion of donor feces for recurrent Clostridium difficile. N Engl J Med 2013;368(5):407–15.

77. Kelly CR, Khoruts A, Staley C, et al. Effect of fecal microbiota transplantation on recurrence in multiply recurrent Clostridium difficile infection: a randomized trial. Ann Intern Med 2016;165(9):609–16.

78. Cammarota G, Masucci L, Ianiro G, et al. Randomised clinical trial: faecal microbiota transplantation by colonoscopy vs. vancomycin for the treatment of recurrent Clostridium difficile infection. Aliment Pharmacol Ther 2015;41(9):835–43.

79. Konijeti GG, Sauk J, Shrime MG, et al. Cost-effectiveness of competing strategies for management of recurrent Clostridium difficile infection: a decision analysis. Clin Infect Dis 2014;58(11):1507–14.

80. Di Bella S, Gouliouris T, Petrosillo N. Fecal microbiota transplantation (FMT) for Clostridium difficile infection: focus on immunocompromised patients. J Infect Chemother 2015;21(4):230–7.

81. Friedman-Moraco RJ, Mehta AK, Lyon GM, et al. Fecal microbiota transplantation for refractory Clostridium difficile colitis in solid organ transplant recipients. Am J Transplant 2014;14(2):477–80.

82. Bilal M, Khehra R, Strahotin C, et al. Long-term follow-up of fecal microbiota transplantation for treatment of recurrent Clostridium difficile infection in a dual solid organ transplant recipient. Case Rep Gastroenterol 2015;9(2):156–9.

83. Ehlermann P, Dosch AO, Katus HA. Donor fecal transfer for recurrent Clostridium difficile-associated diarrhea in heart transplantation. J Heart Lung Transplant 2014;33(5):551–3.

84. Woodworth MH, Carpentieri C, Sitchenko KL, et al. Challenges in fecal donor selection and screening for fecal microbiota transplantation: a review. Gut Microbes 2017;8(3):225–37.
85. Lee JR, Muthukumar T, Dadhania D, et al. Gut microbiota and tacrolimus dosing in kidney transplantation. PLoS One 2015;10(3):e0122399.
86. Woodworth MH, Kraft CS, Meredith EJ, et al. Tacrolimus concentration to dose ratio in solid organ transplant patients treated with fecal microbiota transplantation for recurrent Clostridium difficile infection. Transpl Infect Dis 2018;20(2):e12857.
87. Fischer M, Kao D, Kassam Z, et al. Stool donor body mass index does not affect recipient weight after a single fecal microbiota transplantation for Clostridium difficile infection. Clin Gastroenterol Hepatol 2017 [pii:S1542-3565(17)31448-9].
88. Abougergi MS, Kwon JH. Intravenous immunoglobulin for the treatment of Clostridium difficile infection: a review. Dig Dis Sci 2011;56(1):19–26.
89. McCoy RM, Klick A, Hill S, et al. Luminal toxin-binding agents for Clostridium difficile infection. J Pharm Pract 2016;29(4):361–7.
90. Weiss K. Toxin-binding treatment for Clostridium difficile: a review including reports of studies with tolevamer. Int J Antimicrob Agents 2009;33(1):4–7.
91. Moncino MD, Falletta JM. Multiple relapses of Clostridium difficile-associated diarrhea in a cancer patient. Successful control with long-term cholestyramine therapy. Am J Pediatr Hematol Oncol 1992;14(4):361–4.
92. Kunimoto D, Thomson AB. Recurrent Clostridium difficile-associated colitis responding to cholestyramine. Digestion 1986;33(4):225–8.
93. Mignat C. Clinically significant drug interactions with new immunosuppressive agents. Drug Saf 1997;16(4):267–78.
94. Johnson S, Louie TJ, Gerding DN, et al. Vancomycin, metronidazole, or tolevamer for Clostridium difficile infection: results from two multinational, randomized, controlled trials. Clin Infect Dis 2014;59(3):345–54.
95. Navalkele BD, Lerner SA. Intravenous tigecycline facilitates cure of severe Clostridium difficile infection (CDI) after failure of standard therapy: a case report and literature review of tigecycline use in CDI. Open Forum Infect Dis 2016;3(2):ofw094.
96. Britt NS, Steed ME, Potter EM, et al. Tigecycline for the treatment of severe and severe complicated Clostridium difficile infection. Infect Dis Ther 2014;3(2):321–31.
97. Bishop EJ, Tiruvoipati R, Metcalfe J, et al. The outcome of patients with severe and severe-complicated Clostridium difficile infection treated with tigecycline combination therapy: a retrospective observational study. Intern Med J 2018. [Epub ahead of print].
98. Brinda BJ, Pasikhova Y, Quilitz RE, et al. Use of tigecycline for the management of Clostridium difficile colitis in oncology patients and case series of breakthrough infections. J Hosp Infect 2017;95(4):426–32.

Management of *Strongyloides* in Solid Organ Transplant Recipients

Justin Hayes, MD, Anoma Nellore, MD*

KEYWORDS

- Strongyloides • Transplant • Hyperinfection syndrome • Corticosteroids
- Autoinfection • Th2 immune response • Antihelminthic therapy

KEY POINTS

- Solid organ transplant recipients are vulnerable to the most severe manifestations of strongyloidiasis.
- Travel to or residence in an endemic region is a risk factor for disease among donors and recipients.
- Limited diagnostic strategies and lack of alternative agents to oral ivermectin make the diagnosis and management of strongyloidiasis challenging.
- Targeted screening for *Strongyloides stercoralis* infection in the solid organ transplant population is recommended, but universal screening may be beneficial depending on transplant center geography.
- Ivermectin is the treatment of choice for *Strongyloides stercoralis* and should be initiated before organ transplantation if possible.

INTRODUCTION

First reported in 1876 among French soldiers in Vietnam with initial fatal case reports after immunocompromise were described in 1966,[1] *Strongyloides stercoralis* is a threadworm parasite that has a complex life cycle with both free-living and parasitic phases (**Fig. 1**). Its free-living cycle starts after rhabditiform larvae pass from stool to soil, molt, and emerge as adult free-living worms.[2] Adult free-living worms undergo sexual reproduction and generate further rhabditiform larvae, which molt into filariform larvae. Filariform larvae are able to infect humans or develop into adult worms to continue the free-living life cycle. The parasitic life cycle involves infection of humans with filariform larvae via penetration through skin with subsequent invasion of the

Disclosure Statement: Neither author has any disclosures.
University of Alabama at Birmingham, THT229, 1720 2nd Avenue South, Birmingham, AL 35294-0006, USA
* Corresponding author.
E-mail address: anellore@uabmc.edu

Infect Dis Clin N Am 32 (2018) 749–763
https://doi.org/10.1016/j.idc.2018.04.012   id.theclinics.com
0891-5520/18/Published by Elsevier Inc.

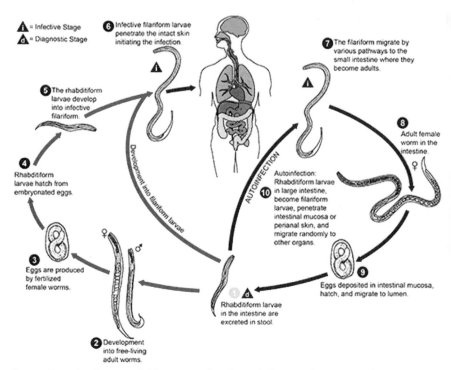

Fig. 1. Life cycle of *Strongyloides stercoralis*. The cycle begins after rhabditiform larvae pass from the stool to the soil, molt, and emerge as adult worms. Female adult worms then lay eggs producing rhabditiform larvae, which develop into filariform larvae. Filariform larvae can then infect humans via penetration of the skin with eventual migration to the small intestine to become adult worms. The female adult worms then lay eggs that are excreted in stool as rhabditiform larvae. However, in a process unique to *S stercoralis* called autoinfection, some rhabditiform larvae are not excreted in stool but instead become filariform larvae. These infective filariform larvae invade the intestinal wall or perianal skin, leading to a hyperinfection syndrome or disseminated infection in the immunosuppressed transplant patient. (*From* https://www.cdc.gov/dpdx/strongyloidiasis/index.html.)

systemic circulation after passage through subcutaneous lymphatics. Ultimately, the filiariform larvae reach the pulmonary circulation, invade the alveolus, ascend the tracheobronchial ,tree and are aspirated into the gastrointestinal tract, where they molt into adult females. These females lay eggs that are excreted into stool as rhabditiform larvae. Unlike other helminths, *S stercoralis* is able to complete an entire life cycle in the human host in a unique process termed autoinfection. In autoinfection, rhabditiform larvae are not excreted in human stool, but instead invade the intestinal wall or perianal skin leading to hyperinfection syndrome or disseminate through the venous circulation. Mortality rates for immunocompromised patients with *S stercoralis* infection have been reported to be as high as 60% to 85%.[1] This article reviews the epidemiology, clinical manifestations, host immune responses, diagnostics, and modalities for treatment of *S stercoralis* in the context of solid organ transplantation.

EPIDEMIOLOGY AND RISK FACTORS

Strongyloides is present in temperate, tropical, and subtropical environments[3] and is believed to infect as many as 30 to 100 million individuals globally.[1] In North America,

Strongyloides is endemic to the southeast, particularly Appalachia,[4] and to the Caribbean. Although the published studies confirming the presence of *S stercoralis* in the soil of Appalachia were performed in the 1980s,[4] as recently as 2013, surveillance of 102 residents in rural Kentucky showed evidence of *S stercoralis* asymptomatic infection.[5] Poor hygiene, drinking water, or general sanitary conditions permit spread of this organism. Nosocomial spread has also been documented among institutionalized individuals.[6] In the United States, low socioeconomic status, occupational exposure to soil contaminated with waste (eg, coal miners and farmers), alcoholism, Caucasian race, and male gender have been associated with *Strongyloides* infection.[2] Rates of *Strongyloides* infection in North America have also been associated with immigrants or returning travelers from endemic countries. Underscoring this epidemiologic association, there is a documented 23.0% prevalence from Sudanese refugees in the United States,[7] a 4.0% prevalence in migrant farm workers in Maryland,[8] and a 2.5% prevalence among Asian refugees in Seattle.[9]

The actual incidence of *Strongyloides* infection after solid organ transplantation is not defined. Although cases of infection have been documented in liver, heart, lung, heart–kidney, intestine, and pancreas transplant recipients,[3] cases have been more frequently reported after kidney transplantation. This may be due to the fact that kidney transplantation is a frequent transplant modality, that *S stercoralis* organisms have been found in the urine, or that intraperitoneal placement of the transplanted kidney renders the organ peculiarly susceptible to extraintestinal *Strongyloides* invasion.[2]

CLINICAL MANIFESTATIONS

Strongyloides infection after solid organ transplantation may occur by (1) de novo acquisition via travel or residence in endemic areas after transplantation,[10] (2) reactivation of disease in the recipient, or (3) donor-derived transmission. Reactivation of prior disease in the recipient is most common. Donor-derived strongyloidiasis typically presents early after transplantation, although there are some reports of diagnosis as late as 9 months after transplantation.[11] Reactivation disease generally presents within 6 months of transplantation, although diagnosis can be delayed owing to nonspecific symptoms.[11] Herein we review the common clinical manifestations of acute, chronic, and disseminated *Strongyloides* infection.

Acute Infection

At the site of larval entry, a local serpiginous, urticarial rash occurs initially that may persist for weeks.[12] Cough from tracheal irritation occurs days after invasion and within 2 weeks nonspecific abdominal cramping, diarrhea, and bloating develop. Larvae appear in the stool as early as 4 weeks after acute infection. Because the symptoms of acute infection are nonspecific, diagnosis of *Strongyloides* infection at this stage is challenging.

Chronic Infection

Chronic infection may be asymptomatic or may be characterized by end-organ dysfunction at usual sites of infection. In the gastrointestinal tract, recurring gastrointestinal complaints such as diarrhea are common. Intestinal obstruction, ileus, and gastrointestinal bleeding have also been associated with chronic infection. Skin manifestations like repeated pruritus ani, urticarial rashes, and larva currens rashes have been reported. Persistent asthma develops with repeated pulmonary insults from *Strongyloides*.[13–16]

Hyperinfection Syndrome and Disseminated Disease

Hyperinfection has not been defined clearly, but is generally associated with immuno-suppression and increased *Strongyloides* larval migration at sites associated with the pulmonary autoinfective life cycle, for example, the pulmonary and gastrointestinal tracts.[2] Diagnostic criteria include exacerbation of gastrointestinal or pulmonary symptoms and increased larvae in the stool or sputum. Usual gastrointestinal symptoms associated with hyperinfection syndrome include diarrhea, pain, bloating, anorexia, weight loss, and bleeding as well as parenchymal obstruction and ileus.[17] A protein-losing enteropathy[17] or nephrotic syndrome[18] with associated hypoalbuminemia may also result. Pathologic examination of intestinal tissue after hyperinfection has demonstrated pseudomembranous colitis, proctitis, mucosal ulceration particularly at the small intestine, crypt distortion, inflammation, and necrosis.[19] Pulmonary manifestations and downstream cardiac complications after hyperinfection include chronic cough or wheeze, pleuritic chest pain, palpitations, atrial fibrillation, and respiratory alkalosis. Sputum may demonstrate larvae, both filariform and rhabditiform, as well as eggs.[20] Adult parasites have been identified in sputum samples, suggesting that the lung may provide a local replicative environment for the parasite independent of migration from the gastrointestinal tract.[21] On pathology, lung tissues may demonstrate alveolar hemorrhage or hemorrhage of the tracheobronchial mucosa. Chronic skin manifestations of hyperinfection syndrome include vasculitis, and petechial and purpuric rashes.[22,23]

In contrast with hyperinfection, disseminated disease refers to the migration of *Strongyloides* larvae outside the pulmonary autoinfective cycle via the venous system. This spread may include central nervous system disease. Larvae have been identified in cerebrospinal fluid, meningeal vessels, and dura, as well as epidural, subdural and subarachnoid spaces. Meningitis from primary *S stercoralis* infection is associated with aseptic cerebrospinal fluid studies without eosinophilia.[24] Importantly, hyperinfection and disseminated disease have been linked to the development of polymicrobial and enteric gram-negative rod bacteremia and meningitis. These organisms are believed to access the systemic circulation or the brain space via the extraintestinal migration of the larvae themselves or via translocation through the gastrointestinal mucosal ulcerations generated by the hyperinfection syndrome. In the context of solid organ transplantation, both hyperinfection and disseminated disease have been reported to be up to 50% fatal, underscoring the clinical gravity of this level of parasitic burden.[25]

HOST RESPONSE TO *STRONGYLOIDES*

Limited animal models have compromised our ability to understand the *Strongyloides* host–pathogen interaction. In rodents, *S stercoralis* penetrate skin, migrate to the lungs, and move to skeletal muscle.[26] Other species of *Strongyloides*—*Strongyloides ratti* and *Strongyloides venezuelensis*—also infect rodents, but lack an autoinfective cycle.[26] Thus, rodent models neither reproduce the intestinal phase of *S stercoralis* infection nor the autoinfective cycle seen in humans. Only severe combined immunodeficiency (SCID) mice, deficient in T and B cells, develop an intestinal phase of infection with *S stercoralis*.[26] Most recently, a NOD SCID gamma mouse model with reduced innate and adaptive immunity has been shown to develop *S stercoralis* human hyperinfection upon steroid receipt.[27] However, the high cost to maintain and breed these mice may make it difficult to apply these models widely for understanding *S stercoralis* pathogenesis. Similarly expensive animal models, dogs, primates, and more recently gerbils have been shown to be susceptible to *S stercoralis* infection.[28]

Gerbils, like the NOD SCID gamma mice, develop hyperinfection syndrome only when administered steroids, thus closely phenocopying human disease in the context of immunosuppression.[29]

Another technical challenge associated with the study of *S stercoralis* in animal models is the difficulty of quantifying parasite burden given rapid parasite migration. Diffusion chambers inoculated with parasite and transcutaneously placed in animal models are used to understand parasite survival in the context of host immune responses.[26] Despite the limited ability to assess host–pathogen response in vivo, certain immunologic insights into *S stercoralis* have been elucidated and are reviewed elsewhere in this article.

Innate Immune Responses to Strongyloides

The innate response represents the arm of the immune system that responds rapidly and in a nonspecific manner to a pathogenic insult. In the context of *S stercoralis* infection, the innate immune response is mediated by neutrophils, eosinophils, and macrophages that accumulate at sites of infection. Isolated, purified neutrophils kill larvae in vitro via elaboration of the neutrophil-specific granular protein myeloperoxidase.[30] Defective neutrophil recruitment to infection in CXCR2 knockout mice is associated with a higher burden of disease.[31] In fact, injection of *S stercoralis*–soluble extract into mice cause neutrophils to release macrophage inflammatory protein-2 and keratinocyte-derived chemokine to recruit further neutrophils, suggesting that autocrine amplification of the neutrophil host response to *Strongyloides* infection is key to pathogen clearance.[26]

Parasite extract recruits eosinophils by direct eosinophil receptor stimulation.[32] Once activated, eosinophils have cytolytic activity against *S stercoralis* larvae, eggs, and worms.[33] Coating of the parasite with complement component C3 and immunoglobulin (Ig)E has been shown to be critical to eosinophilic cytotoxic activity against the parasite. *S stercoralis* larvae activate both the classical and alternative pathways of the complement cascade.[30,34–36]

In tandem with neutrophils, eosinophils play a role in the early host response to *Strongyloides*. Blockade of interleukin (IL)-5, key to the survival, differentiation, and maturation of eosinophils, compromises the ability to clear *S ratti* in murine primary infection.[37] Similarly, blockade of eosinophils via anti-chemokine receptor 3 monoclonal antibody also compromises protective immunity to infection.[31] PHIL mice that are constitutively deficient in eosinophils develop protective immunity to *Strongyloides* infection via the action of neutrophils, suggesting that eosinophils and neutrophils act in concert to effect the innate immune response to *Strongyloides*.[30] Underscoring the importance of eosinophils in pathogen clearance, eosinophil counts were lower in severe versus asymptomatic individuals with *Strongyloides* infection.[38]

Adaptive Immune Responses to Strongyloides

The adaptive immune response requires a parasite to be dissociated with immunogenic peptides presented by antigen-presenting cells to T cells. To study the adaptive immune response in isolation from the innate immune response, a model wherein mice immunized with *Strongyloides* extract and then given challenge infection has been used. After prior immunization, *Strongyloides* antigen pulsed eosinophils expand and upregulate T-cell costimulatory molecules and major histocompatibility class II antigens, serving as antigen-presenting cells to activate a cell-mediated immune response, termed the Th2 response.[39] The Th2 response, unlike its Th1 counterpart, elaborates cytokines like IL-4 and IL-5 and also promotes the production of the immunoglobulin IgE. Dynamic cytokine changes and multifunctional Th2 responses have been documented in human immunologic studies of *Strongyloides* infected individuals.[40,41]

The importance of the Th2 response to parasite clearance is underscored by the association between *S stercoralis* and human T-lymphotropic virus type 1 (HTLV-1). HTLV-1 is an RNA retrovirus that is endemic in Asia, the Caribbean, South America, and Africa, and is the etiologic agent of T-cell hematologic malignancies. HTLV-1 is known to skew an infected individuals response toward a Th1 type of response with increased interferon-γ levels and decreased IL-4, IL-5, and IgE production. This skewing may predispose HTLV-1–infected patients to contract *Strongyloides* infection.[26,38]

Protective cell-mediated immunity to *Strongyloides* requires CD4 T cells but not CD8 T cells,[42] which raises the question of which immune cell performs effector cytolytic function in the adaptive immune response to *Strongyloides*. Adequate protective adaptive immune responses develop after specific depletion of eosinophils either via monoclonal antibodies or use of PHIL mice.[30] This finding implies that degranulation of eosinophils is not an essential component of the adaptive immune response. Neutrophil deficient CXCR2$^{-/-}$ mice also develop adequate protective adaptive immunity to *Strongyloides*, similarly suggesting that neutrophils may not be necessary for the effector functions of the adaptive immune response to *Strongyloides*.[30,43] Although activation of host pattern recognition receptors, such as Toll-like receptors (TLR), typically initiate an innate immune response, TLR signaling may be more critical to the adaptive immune response in the context of *Strongyloides* challenge infection. Mice deficient in TLR4 signaling do not mount an adaptive immune response to *Strongyloides* owing to defective neutrophil cytotoxic response.[35] Thus, the combination of TLR4 signaling and neutrophil activation may play a role in the effector function of the adaptive immune response to *S stercoralis*.

The association between exogenous and endogenous steroid receipt and *Strongyloides* highlights the complexity of the immune response to *Strongyloides*. Steroids highjack this response by depressing innate immune eosinophilic function and by downregulating the adaptive Th2 immune response.[33,44] It has even been suggested that the organism itself has a membrane steroid receptor, thereby allowing glucocorticoids to act directly on the organism to augment pathogenesis.[45]

Finally, the humoral immune response is also an important arm of the adaptive immune response to *Strongyloides*. Hypogammaglobulinemia is associated with the development of hyperinfection.[46,47] μMT mice that lack B cells do not mount a protective serologic response after *Strongyloides* infection.[48] Serum IgG from individuals infected with *Strongyloides* provides passive immune protection to mice exposed to the parasite.[49] Mice immunized with *Strongyloides* larvae have increased titers of IgA, IgG1, and IgM in serum.[50] However, in this experimental model system, IgM exclusively conferred passive protective immunity, whereas IgG provided protection via antibody-dependent cellular cytotoxicity and required complement and neutrophils to effectively kill the worms. This effect may be due to antigenic differences between the isotypes. Collectively, these studies of humoral immune protection after in vivo *Strongyloides* infection raise hopes for an eventual effective vaccine against *Strongyloides*.[51,52] A more precise understanding of the host immune response to *Strongyloides* will allow for insights into such future therapeutic and preventative developments.

DIAGNOSIS

At present, noninvasive diagnostic modalities include parasitologic and serologic tests for the diagnosis of *S stercoralis*. Unfortunately, the performance of existing noninvasive tests is not optimal. In addition, there are no pathognomonic radiologic findings to assist in diagnosis of *S stercoralis*.[2] The current reference standard, fecal microscopy, has limited sensitivity because there is only intermittent shedding of rhabditiform larvae into stool during the acute, chronic, or autoinfective cycles of infection. A single specimen has a sensitivity of only 15% to 30%, but with serial stool examination in an expert laboratory, sensitivity increases to 100%.[53] Attempts at fecal concentration have been used to increase sensitivity of fecal examination for parasites, including the Harada-Mori technique, which uses the water tropism of larvae to concentrate them and the agar plate culture method, which microscopically counts tracks made by larvae on agar for diagnosis. However, despite fecal concentration, consecutive fecal samples must still be examined to increase diagnostic yield.[54]

Current categories of serologic testing include (1) in-house immunofluorescence antibody testing, which uses antibodies against intact *S stercoralis* filiariform larvae, (2) NIE assays, which use a 31-kD recombinant *S stercoralis* antigen (termed NIE) and use a detection system with either luciferase immunoprecipitation assay (NIE-LIPS) or enzyme-linked immunosorbent assay (NIE ELISA), and (3) commercial ELISAs (eg, assays from Bordier Affinity Products, which uses antigens from *S ratti* and IVD Research, which uses antigens from *S stercoralis*). A head-to-head comparison of these tests with the use of fecal microscopy as a reference standard as well as a composite serologic reference standard determined NIE-LIPS to be the most sensitive and specific.[55,56] All commercial ELISA assays were found to have excellent negative predictive value. Large-scale incorporation of NIE-LIPS assays to understand diagnostic accuracy of *S stercoralis* in the solid organ transplant population has yet to be performed. However, the sensitivity of serologic studies for *S stercoralis* is decreased in immunocompromised hosts and agar plate culture may be the more sensitive diagnostic modality in this population.[57]

Invasive diagnostic modalities have been used and include endoscopic sampling of the duodenal fluid, the string test, or actual duodenal biopsy. Endoscopic appearance after *S stercoralis* infection includes ulceration, spasm, bleeding, thickening of mucosal folds, or pustular lesions from larval burrowing.[58] The string test allows duodenal sampling and entails swallowing a gelatin capsule with a coiled string. Retrieval of the capsule by pulling back on the string and examination of associated gastric contents for *S stercoralis* may have better sensitivity than direct fecal examination.[59] Histologic examination of gastrointestinal tract biopsy has shown eosinophilic infiltration of the lamina propria and actual larval or worm forms in gastrointestinal tissue.[58] Procedures performed at sites outside the gastrointestinal tract, like skin biopsy of the larvae currens rash, ascites tap, or bronchoalveolar lavage for larvae, egg, and worm examination, may all assist in diagnosis.

Polymerase chain reaction (PCR)-based testing of stool represents an emerging noninvasive diagnostic modality.[54,60] Real-time PCR screens have been developed against the 18s rRNA, the cytochrome c oxidase subunit I gene or the 28S RNA gene of the organism.[54] The hypervariable regions of the 18s rRNA permit species-specific diagnostics.[61] PCR-based diagnostics of the stool have been used successfully to diagnose *S stercoralis* after transplantation and to document donor-to-recipient transmission. The sensitivity and specificity of PCR-based diagnostics is unclear, with 1 study showing a sensitivity and specificity of 100% in a limited number of subjects[62] and another study showing inferior sensitivity and specificity compared with direct fecal examination.[63] In the latter study, the amount of stool used for PCR diagnostics was far less than that used for direct fecal examination, and this may have influenced comparative diagnostic performance. In general, low or intermittent larval output in stool as well as variability in stool DNA extraction methods may compromise molecular diagnostic yields. However, decreased time to detection, opportunities for universal standardization, and application of assay to other body fluid types render molecular diagnostics attractive as a future testing modality for the solid organ transplantation population.[64]

SCREENING STRATEGIES

Screening strategies for *Strongyloides* infection in the context of solid organ transplantation fall into 2 categories: (1) screening of the donor and (2) screening of the recipient. Screening is generally performed via commercial serology. Screening of donors and at-risk recipients is critical to the prevention of hyperinfection or dissemination syndromes after immunosuppression as well as to the rapid evaluation and initiation of appropriate therapy should *S stercoralis* infection disseminate after transplantation.

Donor Screening

Although donor transmission of *S stercoralis* is rare, deceased donors experience a physiologic cortisol surge associated with the stress response from severe illness and also often receive a preconditioning steroid regimen, both of which may permit dissemination of donor *S stercoralis* larvae near the time of organ transfer and put potential recipients at risk.[65] The Organ Procurement and Transplantation Network has recently mandated infectious diseases screening of living donors for infectious diseases, in addition to already established screening of deceased donors. Screening is to include testing for endemic diseases that are pertinent to center specific geography.[66,67] Although these guidelines are in place, there is a paucity of evidence based data to help guide appropriate screening practices for donors with respect to *S stercoralis*. Expert opinion suggests screening for *S stercoralis* if there are epidemiologic risk factors (eg, veterans of wars in the South Pacific or southeast Asia), unexplained peripheral eosinophilia, or a known history of *S stercoralis* in the donor.[67] The New York Organ Donor Network implemented a screening strategy wherein deceased donors' next of kin were interviewed with a comprehensive questionnaire that elicited travel history with *S stercoralis* serologic testing performed if travel to endemic areas was reported. Of the 1103 potential donors screened by questionnaire, 21% (n = 233) met questionnaire criteria that prompted *S stercoralis* testing, with 4.3% of donors (n = 10) ultimately testing positive for *S stercoralis* antibody. The majority of recipients from these *S stercoralis*–exposed donors were treated for *S stercoralis* and no recipient developed disease.[65] The New York Organ Donor Network experience offers a template protocol to facilitate donor screening in other organ procurement centers.

Recipient Screening

The Infectious Diseases Society of America, the American Society of Transplantation, and the Centers for Disease Control and Prevention all recommend targeted serologic testing of potential solid organ recipients with peripheral eosinophilia or with travel or residence in an endemic region.[3,66,68] Treatment of seropositive recipients (see Treatment section) is recommended before organ transplantation if possible. If serologic testing is not possible, stool testing is recommended; if serologic testing is negative but clinical suspicion for disease is high, stool testing is warranted. It is important to note that, although eosinophilia is part of the accepted criteria to initiate *S stercoralis* screening, if screening is performed after organ transplantation or on candidates with underlying baseline immune suppression requiring steroid receipt (eg, autoimmune diseases), there may be no peripheral eosinophilia present despite disease. In addition, given the poor diagnostic performance of several serologic test modalities for *S stercoralis* especially after organ transplantation (reviewed elsewhere in this article), careful history taking and physical examination are key to identifying solid organ transplant recipients exposed to *S stercoralis*. Transplant providers may require specific education to assist in screening efforts as a recent study of health care professionals found that only 9% of US-trained professionals could accurately identify patients in need of *S stercoralis* screening.[69]

In contrast with prevailing expert recommendation, the University of South Florida recently reported the adoption of universal screening for *S stercoralis* among transplant recipients after an unscreened lung transplant recipient passed away from *S stercoralis* infection.[70] Over the course of 2 years of universal screening (2014–2016), 2351 solid organ transplant candidates were screened with 116 (4.9%) testing positive. Importantly, more than one-half of the solid organ transplant candidates who tested positive had no laboratory abnormality, epidemiologic risk factor or other flag to initiate targeted *S stercoralis* screening. Thirty-eight of the 116 solid organ transplant candidates went on to transplant with the majority receiving *S stercoralis* treatment and no known disease has been reported. Thus, in areas with relatively greater proportion of solid organ transplant candidates from endemic areas, a universal screening strategy for potential solid organ transplant recipients may be more appropriate.[70,71] Currently, there are no comparative cost-effective analyses to evaluate targeted versus universal screening strategies according to transplant center geography.[3,65]

TREATMENT AND PREVENTION
Antimicrobial Chemotherapy

Available agents with targeted antihelminth properties to treat strongyloidiasis are the azole drugs—namely, thiabendazole, mebendazole, and albendazole—as well as ivermectin. The calcineurin inhibitor, cyclosporine, may actually have intrinsic antihelminth activity.[2] Importantly, antihelminth agents have largely been studied only in the context of chronic *Strongyloides* infection and there are limited evidence based-data to guide agent selection or duration for treatment of hyperinfection syndrome or disseminated disease more commonly seen in immunocompromised states.[2] Thiabendazole has been available since 1963 and at a dose of 25 mg/kg twice daily for 3 days clears stool of *S stercoralis* larvae. Unfortunately, side effects occur in almost all patients who take thiabendazole, with nausea, malaise, dizziness, and neuropsychiatric effects frequently reported.[72] Mebendazole is poorly absorbed and may not reliably clear larvae.[2] Albendazole dosed at 400 mg twice daily for 3 days has a minimal side effect profile and has been shown to normalize serologies in 75% of chronically infected subjects with few reportable side effects.[73] Ivermectin, a semisynthetic macrocyclic lactone, causes paralysis of the parasite by acting on ion channels in the parasite cell membrane.[33] Although both ivermectin and albendazole have been reported to be effective in chronic as well as hyperinfection syndromes, clinical trials comparing ivermectin with albendazole in the treatment of chronic strongyloidiasis show that ivermectin has superior antihelminth activity and side effect profile.[74] Currently, ivermectin is the drug of choice for treatment of *S stercoralis* in solid organ transplant recipients.[28]

The ivermectin treatment schedule varies by clinical syndrome. Ideally, patients are diagnosed while being evaluated for solid organ transplant candidacy (see Screening strategies). If *S stercoralis* is diagnosed as a chronic asymptomatic infection with no history of hyperinfection syndrome, treatment to prevent hyperinfection is warranted.

In this clinical context, a course of ivermectin 200 μg/kg/d for 2 days with repeat dosing 2 weeks later, timed to the autoinfective larval cycle, is administered.[2] There are no formal recommendations regarding screening or administration of prophylactic ivermectin after such a treatment schedule, but a low threshold to reexamine stool for larval forms or blood for increase in serologic titer, particularly in the context of clinical symptomatology, is warranted.

Solid organ transplant recipients with hyperinfection syndrome carry a grave prognosis with mortality reported to be as high as 50% in a series of infected renal transplant recipients.[25] Initiation of daily ivermectin therapy for an extended period of time is critical to the management of hyperinfection, as is the tapering of immune suppression, particularly exogenous corticosteroids. Therapy should be continued as long as clinical samples remain positive for the parasite. Commonly sampled sites include stool, but urine and sputum samples may also need to be examined for clearance. Attention should be paid to surgical blind loops, because parasite concentration in these loops has been reported.[75] Concomitant empirical antibacterial or antifungal therapy may be appropriate given the increased incidence of these infections with disseminated and hyperinfection syndromes. Importantly, contact precautions in the hospital and among close contacts should be initiated to prevent spread of disease or reinfection of the recipient.

Although ivermectin has intravenous, subcutaneous, and oral formulations, it is approved by the US Food and Drug Administration for treatment in its oral form only. This modality presents a therapeutic challenge for the critically ill patient who is unable to tolerate oral medications or has paralytic ileus from hyperinfection syndrome with poor oral absorption. Intravenous ivermectin has been administered to 1 patient who ultimately did not survive.[76] In contrast, subcutaneous ivermectin has been successful in parasite eradication and patient survival in immunocompetent patients and transplant recipients. In these cases, doses of subcutaneous ivermectin have ranged from 75 to 200 μg/kg daily for a 3-day period.[76,77] After subcutaneous delivery, peak and trough serum ivermectin concentrations are similar to those achieved after oral ivermectin delivery. At this time, subcutaneous ivermectin can be obtained via an emergency use investigational drug application.[3] Treatment recommendations are summarized in **Box 1**.

After successful treatment of hyperinfection syndrome, organ transplant recipients may continue to shed larvae. Practice patterns for secondary prevention after hyperinfection are variable, with some providers prescribing ivermectin for extended periods. Continued periodic screening for S stercoralis in stool should be pursued after hyperinfection has resolved.[2]

Box 1
Treatment of the solid organ transplant population

Acute and chronic strongyloidiasis
  First line: ivermectin (oral) 200 μg/kg/d for 2 days with repeat dosing 2 weeks later
  Alternative: albendazole 400 mg twice daily for 7 days

Hyperinfection syndrome and disseminated strongyloidiasis
  First line: ivermectin (oral) 200 μg/kg/d until clinical samples are negative
  Alternative: intravenous and subcutaneous formulations of ivermectin (note approved by the US Food and Drug Administration) are potential treatment options for patients that are critically ill and/or experiencing malabsorption

[a] Immunosuppression should be reduced or stopped if possible.

SUMMARY

Infection with *S stercoralis* after organ transplantation carries a high mortality. A high index of suspicion is necessary to identify and treat patients with chronic infection owing to *S stercoralis* before the start of immunosuppression. Delayed diagnosis owing to imperfect diagnostics and limited alternative therapies to oral ivermectin render management of strongyloidiasis challenging. Recent advances in molecular diagnostics, newly identified preclinical therapeutic compounds with antihelminth activity,[28] as well as antigenic targets for rational therapeutic and preventative vaccine design hold promise for improved future outcomes in the transplant population after *Strongyloides* infection.

REFERENCES

1. Siddiqui AA, Berk SL. Diagnosis of Strongyloides stercoralis infection. Clin Infect Dis 2001;33(7):1040–7.
2. Keiser PB, Nutman TB. Strongyloides stercoralis in the immunocompromised population. Clin Microbiol Rev 2004;17(1):208–17.
3. Roxby AC, Gottlieb GS, Limaye AP. Strongyloidiasis in transplant patients. Clin Infect Dis 2009;49(9):1411–23.
4. Berk SL, Verghese A, Alvarez S, et al. Clinical and epidemiologic features of strongyloidiasis. A prospective study in rural Tennessee. Arch Intern Med 1987; 147(7):1257–61.
5. Centers for Disease Control and Prevention. Notes from the field: strongyloidiasis in a rural setting–Southeastern Kentucky, 2013. MMWR Morb Mortal Wkly Rep 2013;62(42):843.
6. Braun TI, Fekete T, Lynch A. Strongyloidiasis in an institution for mentally retarded adults. Arch Intern Med 1988;148(3):634–6.
7. Posey DL, Blackburn BG, Weinberg M, et al. High prevalence and presumptive treatment of schistosomiasis and strongyloidiasis among African refugees. Clin Infect Dis 2007;45(10):1310–5.
8. Ungar BL, Iscoe E, Cutler J, et al. Intestinal parasites in a migrant farmworker population. Arch Intern Med 1986;146(3):513–5.
9. Buchwald D, Lam M, Hooton TM. Prevalence of intestinal parasites and association with symptoms in Southeast Asian refugees. J Clin Pharm Ther 1995;20(5): 271–5.
10. Kotton CN. Travel and transplantation: travel-related diseases in transplant recipients. Curr Opin Organ Transplant 2012;17(6):594–600.
11. Le M, Ravin K, Hasan A, et al. Single donor-derived strongyloidiasis in three solid organ transplant recipients: case series and review of the literature. Am J Transplant 2014;14(5):1199–206.
12. Freedman DO. Experimental infection of human subject with Strongyloides species. Rev Infect Dis 1991;13(6):1221–6.
13. Pelletier LL Jr, Gabre-Kidan T. Chronic strongyloidiasis in Vietnam veterans. Am J Med 1985;78(1):139–40.
14. Friedenberg F, Wongpraparut N, Fischer RA, et al. Duodenal obstruction caused by Strongyloides stercoralis enteritis in an HTLV-1-infected host. Dig Dis Sci 1999; 44(6):1184–8.
15. Nonaka D, Takaki K, Tanaka M, et al. Paralytic ileus due to strongyloidiasis: case report and review of the literature. Am J Trop Med Hyg 1998;59(4):535–8.
16. Smith B, Verghese A, Guiterrez C, et al. Pulmonary strongyloidiasis. Diagnosis by sputum gram stain. Am J Med 1985;79(5):663–6.

17. Liepman M. Disseminated Strongyloides stercoralis. A complication of immunosuppression. JAMA 1975;231(4):387–8.
18. Wong TY, Szeto CC, Lai FF, et al. Nephrotic syndrome in strongyloidiasis: remission after eradication with anthelmintic agents. Nephron 1998;79(3):333–6.
19. Wurtz R, Mirot M, Fronda G, et al. Short report: gastric infection by Strongyloides stercoralis. Am J Trop Med Hyg 1994;51(3):339–40.
20. Kramer MR, Gregg PA, Goldstein M, et al. Disseminated strongyloidiasis in AIDS and non-AIDS immunocompromised hosts: diagnosis by sputum and bronchoalveolar lavage. South Med J 1990;83(10):1226–9.
21. Cirioni O, Giacometti A, Burzacchini F, et al. Strongyloides stercoralis first-stage larvae in the lungs of a patient with AIDS: primary localization or a noninvasive form of dissemination? Clin Infect Dis 1996;22(4):737.
22. Weiser JA, Scully BE, Bulman WA, et al. Periumbilical parasitic thumbprint purpura: strongyloides hyperinfection syndrome acquired from a cadaveric renal transplant. Transpl Infect Dis 2011;13(1):58–62.
23. Martin SJ, Cohen PR, MacFarlane DF, et al. Cutaneous manifestations of Strongyloides stercoralis hyperinfection in an HIV-seropositive patient. Skinmed 2011; 9(3):199–202.
24. Nutman TB. Human infection with Strongyloides stercoralis and other related Strongyloides species. Parasitology 2017;144(3):263–73.
25. DeVault GA Jr, King JW, Rohr MS, et al. Opportunistic infections with Strongyloides stercoralis in renal transplantation. Rev Infect Dis 1990;12(4):653–71.
26. Bonne-Annee S, Hess JA, Abraham D. Innate and adaptive immunity to the nematode Strongyloides stercoralis in a mouse model. Immunol Res 2011;51(2–3): 205–14.
27. Patton JB, Bonne-Annee S, Deckman J, et al. Methylprednisolone acetate induces, and Δ7-dafachronic acid suppresses, Strongyloides stercoralis hyperinfection in NSG mice. Proc Natl Acad Sci U S A 2018;115(1):204–9.
28. Mendes T, Minori K, Ueta M, et al. Strongyloidiasis current status with emphasis in diagnosis and drug research. J Parasitol Res 2017;2017:5056314.
29. Nolan TJ, Megyeri Z, Bhopale VM, et al. Strongyloides stercoralis: the first rodent model for uncomplicated and hyperinfective strongyloidiasis, the Mongolian gerbil (Meriones unguiculatus). J Infect Dis 1993;168(6):1479–84.
30. O'Connell AE, Hess JA, Santiago GA, et al. Major basic protein from eosinophils and myeloperoxidase from neutrophils are required for protective immunity to Strongyloides stercoralis in mice. Infect Immun 2011;79(7):2770–8.
31. Galioto AM, Hess JA, Nolan TJ, et al. Role of eosinophils and neutrophils in innate and adaptive protective immunity to larval Strongyloides stercoralis in mice. Infect Immun 2006;74(10):5730–8.
32. Stein LH, Redding KM, Lee JJ, et al. Eosinophils utilize multiple chemokine receptors for chemotaxis to the parasitic nematode Strongyloides stercoralis. J Innate Immun 2009;1(6):618–30.
33. Mobley CM, Dhala A, Ghobrial RM. Strongyloides stercoralis in solid organ transplantation: early diagnosis gets the worm. Curr Opin Organ Transplant 2017; 22(4):336–44.
34. Brigandi RA, Rotman HL, Yutanawiboonchai W, et al. Strongyloides stercoralis: role of antibody and complement in immunity to the third stage of larvae in BALB/cByJ mice. Exp Parasitol 1996;82(3):279–89.
35. Kerepesi LA, Hess JA, Leon O, et al. Toll-like receptor 4 (TLR4) is required for protective immunity to larval Strongyloides stercoralis in mice. Microbes Infect 2007; 9(1):28–34.

36. Kerepesi LA, Hess JA, Nolan TJ, et al. Complement component C3 is required for protective innate and adaptive immunity to larval Strongyloides stercoralis in mice. J Immunol 2006;176(7):4315–22.

37. Herbert DR, Lee JJ, Lee NA, et al. Role of IL-5 in innate and adaptive immunity to larval Strongyloides stercoralis in mice. J Immunol 2000;165(8):4544–51.

38. Iriemenam NC, Sanyaolu AO, Oyibo WA, et al. Strongyloides stercoralis and the immune response. Parasitol Int 2010;59(1):9–14.

39. Padigel UM, Hess JA, Lee JJ, et al. Eosinophils act as antigen-presenting cells to induce immunity to Strongyloides stercoralis in mice. J Infect Dis 2007;196(12): 1844–51.

40. Anuradha R, Munisankar S, Dolla C, et al. Parasite antigen-specific regulation of Th1, Th2, and Th17 responses in Strongyloides stercoralis Infection. J Immunol 2015;195(5):2241–50.

41. Anuradha R, Munisankar S, Bhootra Y, et al. Systemic cytokine profiles in Strongyloides stercoralis infection and alterations following treatment. Infect Immun 2015;84(2):425–31.

42. Rotman HL, Schnyder-Candrian S, Scott P, et al. IL-12 eliminates the Th-2 dependent protective immune response of mice to larval Strongyloides stercoralis. Parasite Immunol 1997;19(1):29–39.

43. O'Connell AE, Redding KM, Hess JA, et al. Soluble extract from the nematode Strongyloides stercoralis induces CXCR2 dependent/IL-17 independent neutrophil recruitment. Microbes Infect 2011;13(6):536–44.

44. Vadlamudi RS, Chi DS, Krishnaswamy G. Intestinal strongyloidiasis and hyperinfection syndrome. Clin Mol Allergy 2006;4:8.

45. Siddiqui AA, Stanley CS, Skelly PJ, et al. A cDNA encoding a nuclear hormone receptor of the steroid/thyroid hormone-receptor superfamily from the human parasitic nematode Strongyloides stercoralis. Parasitol Res 2000;86(1):24–9.

46. Najmuddin A, Hadique S, Parker J. Strongyloides hyperinfection syndrome complications: a case report and review of the literature. W V Med J 2012;108(1): 32–8.

47. Brandt de Oliveira R, Voltarelli JC, Meneghelli UG. Severe strongyloidiasis associated with hypogammaglobulinaemia. Parasite Immunol 1981;3(2):165–9.

48. Herbert DR, Nolan TJ, Schad GA, et al. The role of B cells in immunity against larval Strongyloides stercoralis in mice. Parasite Immunol 2002;24(2):95–101.

49. Kerepesi LA, Nolan TJ, Schad GA, et al. Human immunoglobulin G mediates protective immunity and identifies protective antigens against larval Strongyloides stercoralis in mice. J Infect Dis 2004;189(7):1282–90.

50. Ligas JA, Kerepesi LA, Galioto AM, et al. Specificity and mechanism of immunoglobulin M (IgM)- and IgG-dependent protective immunity to larval Strongyloides stercoralis in mice. Infect Immun 2003;71(12):6835–43.

51. Abraham D, Hess JA, Mejia R, et al. Immunization with the recombinant antigen Ss-IR induces protective immunity to infection with Strongyloides stercoralis in mice. Vaccine 2011;29(45):8134–40.

52. Kerepesi LA, Keiser PB, Nolan TJ, et al. DNA immunization with Na+-K+ ATPase (Sseat-6) induces protective immunity to larval Strongyloides stercoralis in mice. Infect Immun 2005;73(4):2298–305.

53. Sato Y, Kobayashi J, Toma H, et al. Efficacy of stool examination for detection of Strongyloides infection. Am J Trop Med Hyg 1995;53(3):248–50.

54. Requena-Mendez A, Chiodini P, Bisoffi Z, et al. The laboratory diagnosis and follow up of strongyloidiasis: a systematic review. PLoS Negl Trop Dis 2013; 7(1):e2002.

55. Bisoffi Z, Buonfrate D, Sequi M, et al. Diagnostic accuracy of five serologic tests for Strongyloides stercoralis infection. PLoS Negl Trop Dis 2014;8(1):e2640.

56. Anderson NW, Klein DM, Dornink SM, et al. Comparison of three immunoassays for detection of antibodies to Strongyloides stercoralis. Clin Vaccin Immunol 2014;21(5):732–6.

57. Luvira V, Trakulhun K, Mungthin M, et al. Comparative diagnosis of strongyloidiasis in immunocompromised patients. Am J Trop Med Hyg 2016;95(2):401–4.

58. Choudhry U, Choudhry R, Romeo DP, et al. Strongyloidiasis: new endoscopic findings. Gastrointest Endosc 1995;42(2):170–3.

59. Goka AK, Rolston DD, Mathan VI, et al. Diagnosis of Strongyloides and hookworm infections: comparison of faecal and duodenal fluid microscopy. Trans R Soc Trop Med Hyg 1990;84(6):829–31.

60. Gomez-Junyent J, Paredes-Zapata D, de las Parras ER, et al. Real-time polymerase chain reaction in stool detects transmission of Strongyloides stercoralis from an infected donor to solid organ transplant recipients. Am J Trop Med Hyg 2016; 94(4):897–9.

61. Hasegawa H, Hayashida S, Ikeda Y, et al. Hyper-variable regions in 18S rDNA of Strongyloides spp. as markers for species-specific diagnosis. Parasitol Res 2009;104(4):869–74.

62. Moghaddassani H, Mirhendi H, Hosseini M, et al. Molecular Diagnosis of Strongyloides stercoralis Infection by PCR Detection of Specific DNA in Human Stool Samples. Iran J Parasitol 2011;6(2):23–30.

63. Verweij JJ, Canales M, Polman K, et al. Molecular diagnosis of Strongyloides stercoralis in faecal samples using real-time PCR. Trans R Soc Trop Med Hyg 2009; 103(4):342–6.

64. O'Connell EM, Nutman TB. Molecular diagnostics for soil-transmitted helminths. Am J Trop Med Hyg 2016;95(3):508–13.

65. Abanyie FA, Gray EB, Delli Carpini KW, et al. Donor-derived Strongyloides stercoralis infection in solid organ transplant recipients in the United States, 2009-2013. Am J Transplant 2015;15(5):1369–75.

66. Levi ME, Kumar D, Green M, et al. Considerations for screening live kidney donors for endemic infections: a viewpoint on the UNOS policy. Am J Transplant 2014;14(5):1003–11.

67. Rosen A, Ison MG. Screening of living organ donors for endemic infections: understanding the challenges and benefits of enhanced screening. Transpl Infect Dis 2016. [Epub ahead of print].

68. Schwartz BS, Mawhorter SD, Practice AST Infectious Diseases Community of Practice. Parasitic infections in solid organ transplantation. Am J Transplant 2013;13(Suppl 4):280–303.

69. Boulware DR, Stauffer WM, Hendel-Paterson BR, et al. Maltreatment of Strongyloides infection: case series and worldwide physicians-in-training survey. Am J Med 2007;120(6):545.e1-8.

70. Castro R, Aslam S, Albers C, et al. Strongyloides stercoralis infection incidence, risk factors and outcomes among solid organ transplant candidates and recipients; a Florida Center experience. Open Forum Infect Dis 2017;4(Suppl 1):S10–1.

71. Fitzpatrick MA, Caicedo JC, Stosor V, et al. Expanded infectious diseases screening program for Hispanic transplant candidates. Transpl Infect Dis 2010; 12(4):336–41.

72. Grove DI. Treatment of strongyloidiasis with thiabendazole: an analysis of toxicity and effectiveness. Trans R Soc Trop Med Hyg 1982;76(1):114–8.

73. Archibald LK, Beeching NJ, Gill GV, et al. Albendazole is effective treatment for chronic strongyloidiasis. Q J Med 1993;86(3):191–5.
74. Datry A, Hilmarsdottir I, Mayorga-Sagastume R, et al. Treatment of Strongyloides stercoralis infection with ivermectin compared with albendazole: results of an open study of 60 cases. Trans R Soc Trop Med Hyg 1994;88(3):344–5.
75. Scowden EB, Schaffner W, Stone WJ. Overwhelming strongyloidiasis: an unappreciated opportunistic infection. Medicine (Baltimore) 1978;57(6):527–44.
76. Donadello K, Cristallini S, Taccone FS, et al. Strongyloides disseminated infection successfully treated with parenteral ivermectin: case report with drug concentration measurements and review of the literature. Int J Antimicrob Agents 2013; 42(6):580–3.
77. Barrett J, Broderick C, Soulsby H, et al. Subcutaneous ivermectin use in the treatment of severe Strongyloides stercoralis infection: two case reports and a discussion of the literature. J Antimicrob Chemother 2016;71(1):220–5.

Printed and bound by CPI Group (UK) Ltd, Croydon, CR0 4YY

08/05/2025

01864734-0001

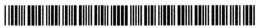